T0257990

Key Concepts of Ophthalmology

Key Concepts of Ophthalmology

Edited by **Ray George**

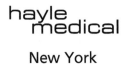

New York

Published by Hayle Medical,
30 West, 37th Street, Suite 612,
New York, NY 10018, USA
www.haylemedical.com

Key Concepts of Ophthalmology
Edited by Ray George

© 2015 Hayle Medical

International Standard Book Number: 978-1-63241-273-7 (Hardback)

This book contains information obtained from authentic and highly regarded sources. Copyright for all individual chapters remain with the respective authors as indicated. A wide variety of references are listed. Permission and sources are indicated; for detailed attributions, please refer to the permissions page. Reasonable efforts have been made to publish reliable data and information, but the authors, editors and publisher cannot assume any responsibility for the validity of all materials or the consequences of their use.

The publisher's policy is to use permanent paper from mills that operate a sustainable forestry policy. Furthermore, the publisher ensures that the text paper and cover boards used have met acceptable environmental accreditation standards.

Trademark Notice: Registered trademark of products or corporate names are used only for explanation and identification without intent to infringe.

Printed in the United States of America.

Contents

Preface   VII

Part 1   Retina and Vitreous   1

Chapter 1   Retinal Detachment –
An Update of the Disease and Its Epidemiology –
A Discussion Based on Research and Clinical Experience
at the Prince Charles Eye Unit, Windsor, England   3
Irina Gout, Faye Mellington, Vikas Tah, Mahmoud Sarhan,
Sofia Rokerya, Michael Goldacre and Ahmed El-Amir

Chapter 2   Induction of Branch Retinal
Vein Occlusion by Photodynamic
Therapy with Rose Bengal in a Rabbit Model   19
Xiao-Xu Zhou, Yan-Ping Song, Yu-Xing Zhao and Jian-Guo Wu

Chapter 3   Retinal Vascular Occlusions   29
Mario Bradvica, Tvrtka Benašić and Maja Vinković

Chapter 4   Retinitis Pigmentosa
in Northern Sweden – From Gene to Treatment   71
Irina Golovleva and Marie Burstedt

Chapter 5   A Novel Artificial Vitreous
Substitute – Foldable Capsular Vitreous Body   93
Qianying Gao

Chapter 6   Endophthalmitis   105
Phillip S. Coburn and Michelle C. Callegan

Chapter 7   Regulation of Angiogenesis in Choroidal
Neovascularization of Age Related Macular
Degeneration by Endogenous Angioinhibitors   127
Venugopal Gunda and Yakkanti A. Sudhakar

Chapter 8   **NRF2 and Age-Dependent RPE Degeneration**   **145**
Yan Chen, Zhenyang Zhao, Paul Sternberg and Jiyang Cai

Chapter 9   **Mechanisms of RDH12-Induced Leber**
Congenital Amaurosis and Therapeutic Approaches   **169**
Anne Kasus-Jacobi, Lea D. Marchette, Catherine Xu,
Feng Li, Huaiwen Wang and Mark Babizhayev

Part 2   **Eye Plastics and Orbital Disorders**   **193**

Chapter 10   **Eyelid and Orbital Infections**   **195**
Ayub Hakim

Chapter 11   **Extended Applications of Endoscopic**
Sinus Surgery to the Orbit and Pituitary Fossa   **217**
Balwant Singh Gendeh

Permissions

List of Contributors

Preface

Eye diseases are very common. This book deals with diverse features of ophthalmology - the medical discipline of analysis and management of eye diseases. It is separated into a variety of clinical sub-areas of expertise, such as cornea, cataract, glaucoma, uveitis, retina, neuro-opthalmology, pediatric ophthalmology, oncology, pathology, and oculoplastics. This book presents innovative improvements and forthcoming viewpoints in ophthalmology. This book includes an analysis of various issues related to retina, vitreous, eye plastics and orbital disorders. It intends to provide some fruitful information for experts and students involved in this field.

This book is a comprehensive compilation of works of different researchers from varied parts of the world. It includes valuable experiences of the researchers with the sole objective of providing the readers (learners) with a proper knowledge of the concerned field. This book will be beneficial in evoking inspiration and enhancing the knowledge of the interested readers.

In the end, I would like to extend my heartiest thanks to the authors who worked with great determination on their chapters. I also appreciate the publisher's support in the course of the book. I would also like to deeply acknowledge my family who stood by me as a source of inspiration during the project.

Editor

Part 1

Retina and Vitreous

Retinal Detachment – An Update of the Disease and Its Epidemiology – A Discussion Based on Research and Clinical Experience at the Prince Charles Eye Unit, Windsor, England

Irina Gout, Faye Mellington, Vikas Tah,
Mahmoud Sarhan, Sofia Rokerya, Michael Goldacre and Ahmed El-Amir
Oxford University
England

1. Introduction

Retinal detachment is a potentially blinding condition. It is caused by separation of neurosensory retina from the underlying retinal pigment epithelium. Despite treatment advances, functional results remain poor (with only 42% achieving 6/12 vision and only 28% if the macula is involved). There are three distinct types of retinal detachment: rhegmatogenous (RRD), tractional and exudative. For the purpose of this chapter we will focus on RRD.

RRD demonstrates wide geographical variation with incidence reported between 6.3 and 17.9 per 100, 000[1] with 7300 new cases estimated annually in the UK[29]. Risk factors include myopia, increasing age and certain vitreoretinal conditions. Horseshoe tears, giant tears and round holes have been shown the most common along with lattice degeneration[7].

Vitreoretinal traction is responsible for most RRD. As the vitreous becomes syneretic (liquefied) with age, a posterior vitreous detachment (PVD) occurs. In most cases, the vitreous separates from the retina without any sequelae. However, in certain eyes, strong vitreoretinal adhesions are present and the occurrence of a PVD can lead to a retinal tear; then, fluid from the liquefied vitreous can enter the sub-retinal space through the tear, leading to a retinal detachment.

Several studies have investigated the epidemiology and risk factors associated with RRD. These differ in their methodology making comparison of data difficult [1,2,4,6,11,29]. RRD incidence varies with ethnicity and is strongly associated with increasing age, myopia and certain vitreoretinal degenerations including lattice degeneration and round holes. Abnormal vitreoretinal adhesions, which may be visible or invisible, are present in many eyes. Among the visible ones are lattice degeneration and cystic retinal tufts. When a PVD occurs and encounters such an area, a retinal tear may form. Due to changes in cataract surgery trends, the proportion of pseudophakic retinal detachment presenting to specialised

centres appears to be increasing. The incidence is lower in phacoemulsification than extra
and intracapsular cataract extraction.

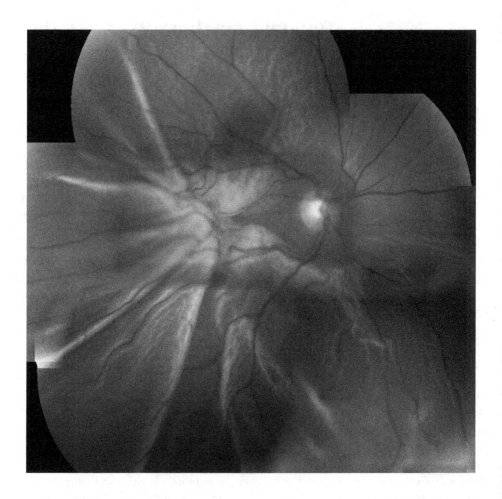

Fig. 1. Retinal detachment

Obtaining an accurate estimate of rhegmatogenous retinal detachment incidence in
England and associated risk factors is essential in understanding the healthcare burden
related to this disorder. We investigated the epidemiology of rhegmatogenous retinal
detachment and associated clinical features by analysing routinely collected hospital
statistics for England, using the Hospital In-patient Enquiry (HIPE) and Hospital Episode
Statistics (HES) from 1968 to 2004, and for the Oxford National Health Service Region
using the Oxford Record Linkage Study (ORLS) from 1963 to 2004. A literature review is
also presented.

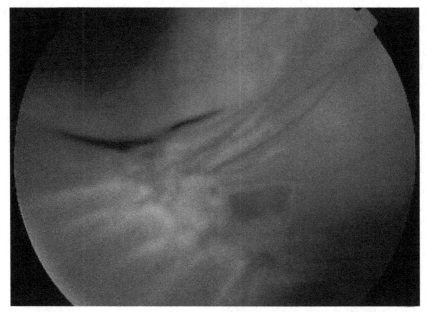

Fig. 2. Retinal break

2. Methods

At the start date for our national analysis, 1968, national hospital statistics for England were collected as the HIPE. This system ceased in 1985 and was replaced, though not until 1989 by HES. Both HIPE and HES are statistical databases of demographic, medical and administrative information about each episode of hospital care. HES include data on all "day cases" or office procedures, as well as patients admitted for overnight stay, whereas the HIPE did not include day cases.. The Oxford Record Linkage Study (ORLS) was also used for all patients treated in the Oxford Regional Health Authority area.

The International Classification for Disease (ICD) by the World Health Organisation was used to identify rhegmatogenous retinal detachment. The codes included ICD-7 (1955) code 386, ICD-8 (1965) code 376, ICD-9 (1977) codes 361.0, 361.1, 361.8 and 361.9, ICD-10 (1992) codes H33.0, H33.2, H33.4 and H33.5.

National HES for England were analysed to produce a geographical profile of hospital admission for retinal detachment by the Local Authority (LA) between 1998 and 2005. The data were used to construct a map showing the person-based admission rate per 100 000 resident population for each LA, expressed as an average annual rate. The LAs were arranged into quintiles: the fifth of LAs with the lowest rates are shown with the lightest colour, and the fifth of LAs with the highest rates are shown with the darkest colour.

The association with affluence was studied using the Index of Multiple Deprivation score for 1998-2005 (n= 57,949) as a measure of deprivation levels. The study population was split into quintiles from least deprived to the most deprived. Standardised admission ratios and 95% confidence intervals were calculated to evaluate statistical significance. Seasonal variation by monthly analysis was studied for detachment surgery from 1989-2006 (n=169,417).

The datasets were anonymised; approval to analyse them in a programme of research undertaken by the Unit and affiliated University, was obtained through the NHS Central Office for Research Ethics Committees (reference 04/Q2006/176).

3. Incidence

The English National and ORLS admission rates for retinal detachment surgery were just over 10 episodes per 100 000 population in the late 1960s. They rose nationally steadily, but gradually, to around 22 episodes per 100 000 population by 2004.

The ORLS data show rates based on the number of people admitted to hospital for retinal detachment surgery as well as the number of episodes of care for surgery (episodes of separate admission or transfers within an admission, or both). The scale of multiple admissions per person was small, although an increase in multiple recording is evident in recent years as seen in the recent divergence between the rates for episodes and people (figure 3). The figure confirms that the increase in hospital episodes in the 1990s represents an increase in the number of people treated (all RRD admissions were operated). It also shows more accurately than the English figures (which omit data for 1986–8) that the start of rapid increase in surgery was about 1989–90.

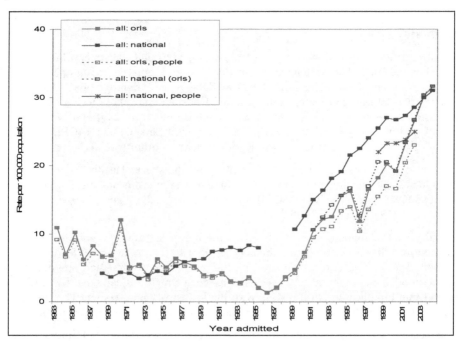

Fig. 3. Hospital admission rates 1963-2004 for Retinal surgery for ORLS and National data measured as episodes and people per year, male and female, all ages, all sources of admission, any mention

The reported annual incidence of rhegamatogenous retinal detachment in other studies around
the world varies from 4-17.9 per 100 000 population [1,2,4,8,10,12,13,32,38]. Studies with small sample size,
potential for sampling error and varied methodologies underlie these different results.

4. Geographic variation

The people rate for the national data is at its peak at 16 per 100,000 in 2004. There is a
suggestion that the rate has reached its peak as the rate fluctuated between15-16 per 100,000
from 1998 to 2004. The people rate for the Oxford data continues to show a rise to 20 per
100,000 in 2004. This can be explained by the fact that Oxford remains a tertiary referral
centre for retinal detachment and serves patients from outside the region and so the service
throughput may not represent the local population. Bilaterality was not investigated but
most series support a bilateral rate of retinal detachment of between 5-15%.

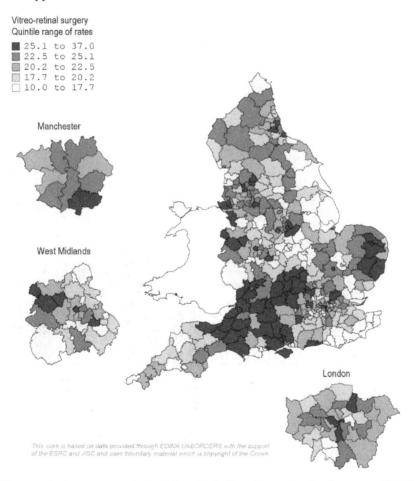

Fig. 4. Vitreo-retinal surgery: males and females indirectly standardised rate per 100 000:
each local authority in England any mention of operation: 1998/99 to 2004/05

Figure 4 shows a geographical profile of the annual rate of retinal detachment surgery by LA. LAs showed a wide variation in rates of retinal detachment surgery, ranging from 7 to 23 people per 100 000 population. This reflects the relative infancy of retinal surgery service provision in comparison to cataract surgery for example and highlights the need for more service provision for patients in England.

5. Age distribution

The prevalence of PVD increases with age; occurring in 11% of 60-69 year olds, 46% of 80-89 year olds and occurring earlier in myopes. The highest incidence rate of detachment was found in the 70-74 age group with rates of 60 per 100,000. The incidence rate in under 20 year old females was the lowest noted; <3 per 100,000. The bimodal distribution with a secondary peak in younger ages (24-30 years) reflects the highly myopic group.

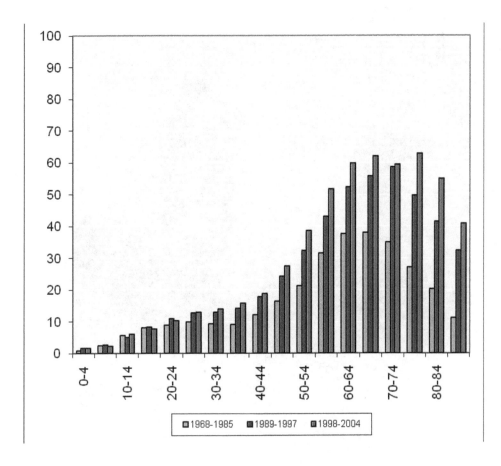

Fig. 5. Admission rates for retinal detachment per 100,000 population: all sources, males, National data

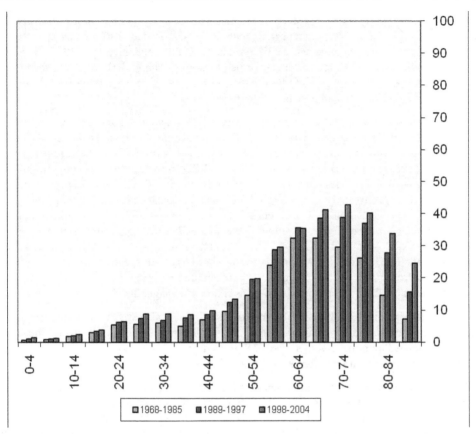

Fig. 6. Admission rates for retinal detachment per 100,000 population: all sources, females,
National data

6. Gender

Figures 5 and 6 presents national and ORLS admission rates for retinal detachment surgery
analysed by age and sex, and over three time periods (1968–1985, 1989–1997 and 1998–2004)
for men and women separately. Three contrasting time periods were selected: one relatively
long historical period, when rises in rates were fairly modest, and two more recent periods,
when rises were more evident. Over these time periods, the rate of retinal detachment
surgery shows a bi-modal distribution with peaks at the 24-30 and 70-74 age groups for both
men and women. There was a 6 times higher risk in the 70-74 age group for both males and
females. The rate of retinal detachment surgery for all age groups shows a 1.5 times male
preponderance.

While some reports indicate a sex distribution corresponding with that of the general
population, most indicate a male preponderance[2-6]. This may be related to an inherent
gender risk, though an increased rate of ocular trauma may be contributory. Furthermore,
the higher proportion of myopia in young males may partly explain this.

In a prospective study which involved 1130 cases of RRD in Scotland over a 2-year period from 2007-2009, Mitry *et al.*, reported that PVD -associated RRD showed a male preponderance of 61.7% male vs. 38.2% female (P<0.001). Notably, 1 in 10 cases were associated with a recent history of ocular or head trauma.[7] The underlying sex distribution could not account for this gender discrepancy but higher rates of traumatic RRD or an inherent increased risk in men may be influential.[8]

Exclusion of traumatic retinal detachments from analysis may negate or even reverse gender differences in RRD incidence. The Beijing Rhegmatogenous Retinal Detachment Study Group prospectively reviewed 528 patients diagnosed with RRD from October 1999-September 2000. It reported a greater incidence of RRD in males (8.98/100000 population; 95% CI 8.07 – 10.13 in males, and 6.78/100000 population; 95% CI 5.97 – 7.76 in females). However, on subgroup analysis, although there was a greater incidence of traumatic RRD in males, there was no significant difference between males and females in nontraumatic, phakic, aphakic and pseudophakic retinal detachments.[11] A Swedish retrospective study of 590 cases of RRD over a 10-year period from 1971 to 1981 reported a higher incidence of non-traumatic RRD in females.[12] However in another large retrospective case-control study (1032 cases from 1995 to 2001), the male predominance persisted even after excluding trauma-related RRD, with a reported 2.15 odds ratio for male gender.[13]

The sex difference, that is a higher incidence of RRD in men, also appears to apply to retinal detachment incidence after cataract surgery. A small retrospective study from Olmstead County, Minnesota, found that men were 2.9 times more likely to have a retinal detachment after cataract surgery than women (P<0.001; 95%CI 1,8-4.4).[14]

Other possible explanations include increased myopia and axial length in men, as well as gender differences in the anatomy of the vitreoretinal base. [15, 16] Myopia is a well-known risk factor for retinal detachment and an increase in axial length is significantly associated with an increased risk of RRD.[17-19] Axial length is related to height and men tend to be taller than women.[20] Anatomical differences in the vitreoretinal base (with males having larger eyes hence longer vitreous chambers as described in 1912 by Salzmann's Anatomy and Histology of the Human Eyeball) can be in the form of greater migration of the posterior vitreous base towards the retina in males as reported by Wang et al, in their study of donor eyes.[21] This may predispose males to retinal breaks after PVD, either from greater dynamic vitreoretinal traction and/or an increase in vitreoretinal irregularities of the posterior border.

7. Cataract extraction and other ophthalmic operations

Cataract operation is the most common ophthalmic surgical procedure worldwide. Even with the best technique and in healthy eyes this procedure is associated with an increased risk of retinal detachment. There is a higher rate of PVD after cataract extraction and a lower hyaluronic acid concentration causing vitreous collapse 5. Increased rates of cataract surgery (phacoemulsification, internal and external capsular cataract extraction) and higher life expectancy may also contribute to retinal detachment. The cumulated six year risk of detachment after cataract surgery is increased by a factor of 6 to 8, increasing linearly for 20 years[22].

The risk is increased if there are complications during cataract surgery. There is a
statistically significant higher incidence of RRD after posterior capsule rupture and
anterior vitrectomy than after uncomplicated phacoemulsification, 16% versus 0.75%
according to one study[23].The estimated risk of retinal detachment after cataract surgery is
5 to 16 per 1000 uncomplicated cataract operations[24].The risk may be much higher in
those who are highly myopic, with a frequency of 7% reported in one study[25].Young age
at cataract removal further increased risk in this study. A vitreo-retinal centre in London
analysed cases of rhegmatogenous retinal detachment in 1980 and again in 1999 finding
that pseudophakia rose from 0.8% to 24%. This may explain the steady rise in retinal
detachment we found as shown in figure 7 in England over the last 4 decades. Most series
report that about 50% of RRD occur during the first year following cataract surgery. Long
term risk of retinal detachment after extracapsular and phacoemulsification cataract
surgery at 2, 5, and 10 years was estimated in one study to be 0.36%, 0.77%, and 1.29%,
respectively[26].

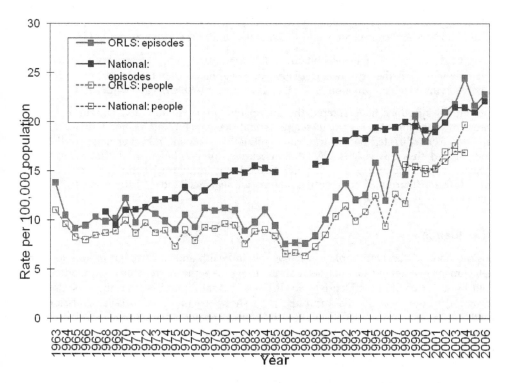

Fig. 7. Hospital admission rates (per 100,000 population) for retinal detachment: National &
ORLS data 1963-2004(06) measured as episodes and people per year, all ages, males and
females, all sources, any mention

The exact mechanism contributing to retinal detachment related to cataract surgery is not
fully known, however several hypothesis have been postulated. It is well known that

cataract extraction alters the physiology of the eye. Removal of a larger cataractous lens in aphakia or its replacement with a smaller lens implant in pseudophakia is responsible for the anterior shift of the iris lens diaphragm resulting in a relative increase in volume of the vitreous cavity. The removal of the lens and its anterior capsule also disturbs the diffusion barriers and results in a more liquefied vitreous with a reduced hyaluronic acid content . This is associated with a higher rate of PVD. Direct evidence between cataract surgery and PVD comes from a recently published study from New Zealand [33]. The study showed that among 149 patients aged 50 to 60 years who underwent unilateral cataract surgery, the incidence of PVD after five years was 51 per cent in the treated eyes, compared to only 21 per cent in their unoperated fellow eyes. Other possible mechanisms leading to a retinal detachment have been implicated to be the inflammatory vitreoretinal adhesions and retinal breaks caused by surgical trauma.

ND:Yag capsulotomy following cataract operation carries a potential to induce PVD, and thereby cause a retinal detachment [23]. The risk factors include myopia, lattice degeneration and retinal detachment in the fellow eye. No relationship has been established between energy application and incidence of retinal detachment. According to one study the incidence of RD following Nd:YAG laser capsulotomy was 0.82% , with a mean time of 32 months between cataract surgery and capsulotomy and 13.5 months between capsulotomy and RD.[23]

The incidence of retinal detachment following penetrating keratoplasty is variable, dependent on whether the eye is phakic or pseuphakic or whether the procedure has involved vitreous manipulation. Several series report 2.4-6.8% of cases with RRD[28]

Intravitreal injections have entered the therapeutic arena recently and remain a potential threat to causation of a rhegmatogenous retinal detachment. Iaterogenic retinal tears and rips due to misdirected needles can cause retinal detachment, however most studies have documented that this risk is low. A consecutive, interventional, multicenter case series measured the incidence of RD in patients receiving intravitreal anti-vascular endothelial growth factor. During 36 consecutive months the incidence rate of RRD was 0.013% (5/35 942) (1 per 7188 injections)[29] .

8. Affluence

Socio-economic deprivation plays a major role in health and disease, but its role in retinal detachment in England has not been studied. Figure 8 shows the study population being split by Index of Multiple Deprivation (IMD) scores into quintiles from the least deprived (group 1) to the most deprived (group 5). As shown by the standardised admission ratio (with lower and upper 95% CIs) there is a gradient with deprivation score showing a significant relationship, though not strong, between affluence (least deprived) and retinal detachment surgery. There's about a 10% difference between the least deprived quintile and the most deprived (n= 57,949).

The Scottish Retinal Detachment Study Group, based on 12 months prospective research between 1 November 2007 and 31 October 2008, assessed 572 patients diagnosed with primary retinal detachment[29]. They came to the conclusion that retinal detachment is twice as common among the more affluent than those living in areas of deprivation. This might be as those in poorer areas may present later if at all to medical services and the more affluent tend to have greater myopic prevalence.

IMD Group	Index of Multiple Deprivation Score	No. of LA's	Observed	Expected	o/e	SAR	Confidence Interval (Lower)	Confidence Interval (Upper)
1 Least Deprived	8,36	71	9924	9150,1	1,08	108,5	106,3	110,6
2	12,68	70	9807	9615,1	1,02	102,0	100,0	104,0
3	17,13	70	9585	9793,4	0,98	97,9	95,9	99,9
4	22,92	70	11701	11903,7	0,98	98,3	96,5	100,1
5 Most Deprived	33,35	71	16932	17486,6	0,97	96,8	95,4	98,3
Total			57949	57949,0		100,0		

Fig. 8.

High myopia is one of the risk factors in patients with retinal detachment. It was documented that there is an association of short sightedness with intelligence quotient (IQ) and thus higher income and socio-economic status[31,32]. Saw et al. report the association between retinal detachment and educational achievement in a study of 1204 school children aged 10 to 12 in Singapore. Using the nonverbal Raven Standard Progressive Matrix test Intelligence Quotient they concluded that non-verbal IQ is a strong risk factor for myopia[32]. Higher prevalence of myopia in the most affluent quartile could explain the increased incidence in this group.

However, we cannot exclude the possibility that affluence is associated with some other, hitherto undefined, risk factor such as genetic factors. The latest evaluation by the Scottish Retinal Detachment Study Group investigated the influence of genetic predilection on primary RRD in 2011. They show a doubled risk of the condition in those having an affected sibling[33]. Whilst ethnicity could not be studied we know that the incidence of retinal detachment is lower in Asians and in Blacks[34].

As the risk of retinal detachment has direct connection with the most affluent group of population, there are implications for service planning, as there is likely to be a greater need for vitreoretinal services in wealthier areas.

9. Seasonality

Seasonal variation in RRD incidence has been widely reported. Most studies describe a summer peak and winter trough; others vice versa and some no seasonal variation at all[35-39]. This is likely attributed to increased sun exposure and outdoor activities in summer[36].

Figure 9 shows that the rate of retinal detachment surgery is higher in summer peaking in July with the lowest rates being in January-February. This pattern is most striking in males under

40 in whom there is relatively lower presentation in winter (lower incidence in December-February). The association with season was statistically significant at the level of p=0.01.

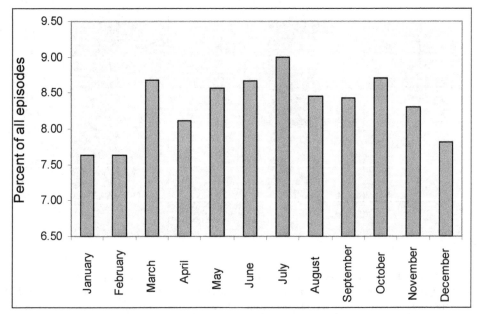

Fig. 9. Retinal detachment: monthly percentages of all FCEs, National data, male and females, any mention 1989-2006

We found a statistically significant summer peak and winter trough at the level of p=0.01 (n=115,450). The effect of light and temperature on the vitreous has been implicated. This study showed that the seasonal variation was most striking in younger males suggesting another association other than the season itself. Could this subgroup of patient be more active during the summer months and be more likely to experience trauma and PVD formation?

In a large retrospective review of 2314 patients with primary RRD in Germany, Thelen *et al.* (1997) reported a significant mid-summer peak incidence (n in July = 228) and winter trough (mean n December to January = 161) with a difference of 36% between the two periods. They noted a close correlation between seasonal incidence of RRD and seasonal incidence of light hours per day and considered a potential role of light-induced changes on vitreoretinal adhesion.[35]

Mansour *et al.* (2009) retrospectively reviewed the charts of 211 patients undergoing idiopathic RRD repair in one referral centre in Lebanon over a 13-year period. They reported a significant (P<0.05) increase in RRD in spring and summer compared to autumn and winter (56% vs. 44%). Interestingly, there was a significantly younger age of onset of RRD in the warmer months (47 vs. 54, P= 0.007).[36]

In contrast, a retrospective evaluation of RRD in Kuwait from 1981 to 1987 reported a peak incidence in winter (with the highest level in November) and a trough in the summer months.[38] These findings have not been replicated elsewhere.

Studies reporting no apparent seasonal variation in RRD incidence include the large prospective population-based study by the Beijing Rhegmatogenous Retinal Detachment Study Group. There were no seasonal differences in incidence even after further classification of retinal detachments into blunt traumatic, aphakic and pseudophakic and non-traumatic phakic.[39]

Possible explanations for seasonal variation in RRD incidence include: variations in light and temperature affecting vitreous structure, and increased outdoor activity and consequent trauma during periods of longer daylight hours and warmer weather [35].

Posterior vitreous detachment (PVD) is widely accepted as a contributory factor in RRD. Mitry et al. (2011) found that more than 85% of RRDs are associated with PVD and associated tractional retinal tears.[40] The influence of climatic variables namely seasonality, air temperature, solar radiation and humidity on PVD rates was elegantly evaluated by Rahman et al. (2002).[41] They retrospectively reviewed 567 patient records diagnostically coded as PVD in the Oxford Eye Casualty over a 2-year period. They excluded cases with a precipitating cause for PVD such as blunt trauma, retinal vascular disease and diabetes, and looked for a correlation between ambient temperatures, humidity and solar radiance and PVD incidence. Interestingly, they found no statistically significant difference in the total numbers of new patients attending the Eye casualty over the summer months compared to winter (912 from April to September vs. 839 October to March). They did however note a strong association (P= 0.035) between weekly average air temperatures and PVD incidence. Air temperatures of the previous week also correlated positively with PVD incidence (P = 0.028). The higher the average air temperature the higher the weekly rate of PVD. As such, increased physical activity and dehydration associated with higher ambient temperatures may alter vitreous structure and thereby increase the incidence of PVD and, in turn, RRD. Further investigation into the role of increased temperature on the biochemical structure of the vitreous and retinal detachment rates is needed.

10. Conclusion

The data on overall incidence of RRD worldwide has been inconsistent. The incidence varies with the population studied and is limited by study design and inclusion criteria. Few recent estimates of incidence have used large samples sizes. These studies show national data and provides longitudinal information, a more inclusive estimate of incidence and its' variation over time.

The highest annual incidence of RRD in England is in the 70-74 year age group with a secondary peak in young myopes and a higher overall incidence in males. Retinal detachment is correlated with affluence and season in England and there is geographic variation. This data sheds light into understanding the epidemiology of RRD in England. This would be particularly useful in designing and developing vitreo-retinal services to meet local needs.

11. Clinical features and management summary

Patients perceive flashing lights and floaters acutely. It probably arises from the mechanical stimulation of vitreoretinal traction on the retina. Floaters are opacities in the vitreous cavity that cast a shadow in the patient's visual field. Cobwebs are caused by condensation of the collagen fibers. Floaters can also indicate fresh blood due to the rupture of a retinal vessel during an acute PVD. Patients often describe a black curtain (visual field defect) once the subretinal fluid accumalates. When the macula becomes detached (ie, extension of subretinal fluid into the macula), the patient experiences a drop in central vision.

Cell and flare may be seen in the anterior chamber and the intraocular pressure is usually lower in the affected eye. Pigment in the anterior vitreous ('tobacco dusting' or a Shaffer sign) is usually present and this represents release of retinal pigment epithelium through the retinal break. Once the retina becomes detached, it assumes a slightly opaque color secondary to intraretinal edema. It has a corrugated appearance and undulates freely with eye movements unless severe proliferative vitreoretinopathy is present.

Patients with a RRD should be referred to a vitreoretinal specialist immediately. Regardless of the surgical technique chosen, the surgical goals are to identify and close all the breaks with minimum iatrogenic damage. Closure of the breaks occurs when the edges of the retinal break are brought into contact with the underlying RPE. This is accomplished either by bringing the eye wall closer to the detached retina (using a scleral buckle) or by pushing the detached retina toward the eye wall (intraocular tamponade with a gas bubble or silicone oil). Sealing of the breaks is accomplished by creating a strong chorioretinal adhesion around the breaks; this may be completed with cryotherapy or laser photocoagulation.

Scleral buckles usually are made of solid silicone and silicone sponges. Indirect ophthalmoscopy is used to localize all the breaks. Once the breaks are localized, they are usually treated with cryotherapy. A buckling element is chosen and sutured over the breaks. The drainage of the subretinal fluid is a controversial topic among vitreoretinal specialists. The retina can be reattached by either technique and the technical details are outside the remit of this chapter.

Currently, many surgeons use pars plana vitrectomy surgery (PPV) to treat primary uncomplicated retinal detachments. A central core vitrectomy and removal of the vitreous from the margins of the breaks is the next step. Drainage of subretinal fluid through a break internally is then performed. Intraocular tamponade with either gas or silicone oil is chosen according to the surgeon's preference. The advantages of gas are that it has a higher surface tension than silicone oil and it dissipates on its own. The disadvantage is that it expands with changing atmospheric pressure. Patients with an intraocular gas bubble should not fly. Transconjunctival and suture-less small-gauge vitrectomy has gained popularity in the past few years. 23 and 25 gauge systems have several potential advantages over traditional 20-gauge vitrectomy including improved patient comfort, faster wound healing, decreased inflammation, less conjunctival scarring, and a decrease in surgical time in opening and closing.

More than 90% of RRD cases can expect anatomical success with reattachment following one operation. Further surgery is required in the failed cases.

12. References

[1] Mitry D, Charteris DG, Fleck BW, Campbell H, Singh J. 1The epidemiology of rhegmatogenous retinal detachment: geographical variation and clinical associations. . Br J Ophthalmol. 2010 Jun;94(6):678-84. Epub 2009 Jun 9.
[2] Pollinghorne PJ, Craig JP. Northern New Zealand Rhegmatogenous Retinal Detachment Study: epidemiology and risk factors. *Clin Experiment Ophthalmol.* 2004;32:159-63.

[3] Mowatt L, Shun-Shin G, Price N. Ethnic differences in the demand incidence of retinal detachments in two districts in the West Midlands. *Eye*. 2003;17:63-70.

[4] Limeira-Soares PH, Lira RP, Arieta CE, *et al*. Demand incidence of retinal detachment in Brazil. *Eye*. 2007;21:348-52.

[5] Ivanisevic M, Bojic I, Eterovic D. Epidemiological study of nontraumatic phakic rhegmatogenous retinal detachment. *Ophthalmic Res*. 2000;32:237-9.

[6] Rosman M, Wong TY, Ong SG *et al*. Retinal detachment in Chinese, Malay and Indian residents in Singapore: a comparative study on risk factors, clinical presentation and surgical outcomes. *Int Ophthalmol*. 2001;24:101-6.

[7] Mitry D, Singh J, Yorston D, Siddiqui MA, Wright A, Fleck BW, Campbell H, Charteris DG. The Predisposing Pathology and Clinical Characteristics in the Scottish Retinal Detachment Study. *Ophthalmology*. 2011 May 9. [Epub ahead of print].

[8] Mitry D, Chalmers J, Anderson K, Williams L, Fleck BW, Wright A, Campbell H. Temporal trends in retinal detachment incidence in Scotland between 1987 and 2006. *Br J Ophthalmol*. 2011;95:365-369

[9] Wong TY, Tielsch JM. A population-based study on the incidence of severe ocular trauma in Singapore. *Am J Ophthalmol*. 1999;128(3):345-51.

[10] Wong TY, Tielsch JM, Schein OD. Racial difference in the incidence of retinal detachment in Singapore. *Arch Ophthalmol*. 1999;117(3):379-83.

[11] Li X; Beijing Rhegmatogenous Retinal Detachment Study Group. Incidence and epidemiological characteristics of rhegmatogenous retinal detachment in Beijing, China. *Ophthalmology*. 2003;110(12):2413-7.

[12] Tornquist R, Stenkula S, Tornquist P. retinal detachment. A study of a population-based patient material in Sweden 1971-1981. I. Epidemiology. *Acta Ophthalmol (Copenh)*. 1987;65(2):213-22.

[13] Chou SC, Yang CH, Lee CH, Yang CM, Ho TC, Huang JS, Lin CP, Chen MS, Shih YF. Characteristics of primary rhegmatogenous retinal detachment in Taiwan. *Eye*. 2007;21:1056-1061.

[14] Rowe JA, Erie JC, Baratz KH, Hodge DO, Gray DT, Butterfield L, Robertson D. Retinal Detachment in Olmstead County, Minnesota, 1976 Through 1995. *Ophthalmology*. 1999;106(1):154-9.

[15] Bourne RR, Dineen BP. Ali SM, Noorul Huq DM, Johnson GJ. Prevalence of refractive error in Bangladeshi adults: results of the National Blindness and Low Vision Survey of Bangladesh. *Ophthalmology*. 2004;111(8):1150-60.

[16] Dandona R, Dandona L, Srinivas M, Giridhar P, McCarty CA, Rao GN. Population-based assessment of refractive error in India: the Andhra Pradesh eye disease study. *Clin Experiment Ophthalmol*. 2002; 30(2):84-93.

[17] Schepens CLDM. Data on the natural history of retinal detachment. *Arch Ophthalmol*. 1961;66:47-58.

[18] Cambiaggi A. Myopia and Retinal Detachment: statistical study of their relationships. *Am J Ophthalmol*. 1964;58:642-50.

[19] Sheu SJ, Ger LP, Chen JF. Male sex as a risk factor for pseudophakic retinal detachment after cataract extraction in Taiwanese adults. *Ophthalmology*. 114(10):1898-903.

[20] Tan CS, Chan YH, Wong TY, Gazzard G, Niti M, Ng TP, Saw SM. Prevalence and risk factors for refractive errors and ocular biometry parameters in an elderly Asian population: the Singapore Longitudinal Aging Study (SLAS). *Eye*. 2011 July 1 [Epub ahead of print].

[21] Wang J, McLeod D, Henson DB, Bishop PN. Age-dependent changes in the basal retinovitreous adhesion. *Invest Ophthalmol Vis Sci*. 2003;44(5):1793-800.

[22] Lois N, Wong D. Pseudophakic retinal detachment. *Surv Ophthalmol.* Sep-Oct 2003;48(5):467-87.

[23] Powell SK, Olson RJ. Incidence of retinal detachment after cataract surgery and neodymium: YAG laser capsulotomy. *J Cataract Refract Surg.* 1995 Mar;21(2):132-5.

[24] Ramos M, Kruger EF, Lashkari K (2002). "Biostatistical analysis of pseudophakic and aphakic retinal detachments". *Seminars in ophthalmology* 17 (3–4): 206–13.

[25] Hyams SW, Bialik M, Neumann E (1975). "Myopia-aphakia. I. Prevalence of retinal detachment". *The* British journal of *ophthalmology* 59 (9): 480–2.

[26] J.A. Rowe, J.C. Erie, K.H. Baratz et al. (1999). "Retinal detachment in Olmsted County, Minnesota, 1976 through 1995". Ophthalmology 106 (1): 154–159.

[27] Hilford D, Hilford M, Mathew A, Polkinghorne PJ. Posterior vitreous detachment following cataract surgery. *Eye 2009; 23:1388-1392.*

[28] Forstot SL, Binder PS, Fitzgerald C, Kaufman HE. The incidence of retinal detachment after penetrating keratoplasty. *Am J Ophthalmol.* Jul 1975;80(1):102-5.

[29] Meyer CH, Michels S, Rodrigues EB, Hager A, Mennel S, Schmidt JC, Helb HM, Farah ME. Incidence of rhegmatogenous retinal detachments after intravitreal antivascular endothelial factor injections. Acta Ophthalmol. 2011 Feb;89(1):70-5. doi: 10.1111/j.1755-3768.2010.02064.x. Epub 2010 Dec 22.

[30] Mitry D, Charteris DG, Yorston D, Siddiqui MA, Campbell H, Murphy AL, Fleck BW, Wright AF, Singh J; Scottish RD Study Group. The epidemiology and socioeconomic associations of retinal detachment in Scotland: a two-year prospective population-based study. Invest Ophthalmol Vis Sci. 2010 Oct;51(10):4963-8.

[31] Williams C, Miller LL, Gazzard G, Saw SM. A comparison of measures of reading and intelligence as risk factors for the development of myopia in a UK cohort of children. Br J Ophthalmol. 2008 Aug;92(8):1117-21.

[32] Saw SM, Tan SB, Fung D et al. IQ and the association with myopia in children. *Invest Ophthalmol Vis Sci.* 2004;45(9):2943–2948.

[33]Polkinghorne PJ, Craig JP. Northern New Zealand Rhegmatogenous Retinal Detachment Study: epidemiology and risk factors.Clin Experiment Ophthalmol. 2004 Apr;32(2):159-63.

[34] Mitry D, Williams L, Charteris DG, Fleck BW, Wright AF, Campbell H. Population-based estimate of the sibling recurrence risk ratio for rhegmatogenousretinal detachment. Invest Ophthalmol Vis Sci. 2011 Apr 20;52(5):2551-5.

[35] Thelen U, Gerding H, Clemens S. Rhegmatogenous retinal detachments. Seasonal variation and incidence. *Ophthalmologe.* 1997;94(9):638-41.

[36] Mansour AM, Hamam RN, Sibai TA, Farah TI, Mehio-Sibai A, Kanaan M. Seasonal variation of retinal detachment in Lebanon. *Ophthalmic Res.* 2009;41(3):170-4.

[37] Paavola M, Chehova S, Forsius H. Seasonal variations in retinal detachment in Northern Finland and Novosibirsk. *Acta Ophthalmol (Copenh).* 1983;61(5):806-12.

[38] Al Samarrai AR. Seasonal variations of retinal detachment among Arabs in Kuwait. *Ophthalmic Res.* 1990;22(4):220-3.

[39] Li X; Beijing Rhegmatogenous Retinal Detachment Study Group. Incidence and epidemiological characteristics of rhegmatogenous retinal detachment in Beijing, China. *Ophthalmology.* 2003;110(12):2413-7.

[40] Mitry D, Singh J, Yorston D, Siddiqui MA, Wright A, Fleck BW, Campbell H, Charteris DG. The Predisposing Pathology and Clinical Characteristics in the Scottish Retinal Detachment Study. *Ophthalmology.* 2011 May 9. [Epub ahead of print].#

[41] Rahman R, Ikram K, Rosen PH, Cortina-Borja M, Taylor ME. Do climatic variables influence the development of posterior vitreous detachment? *Br J Ophthalmol.* 2002;86(7):829.

Induction of Branch Retinal Vein Occlusion by Photodynamic Therapy with Rose Bengal in a Rabbit Model

Xiao-Xu Zhou[1], Yan-Ping Song[2], Yu-Xing Zhao[2] and Jian-Guo Wu[1,2]

[1]Tianjin Medical University Eye Center, Tianjin,
[2]Department of Ophthalmology of PLA Wuhan General Hospital, Wuhan,
People's Republic of China

1. Introduction

Branch retinal vein occlusion (BRVO) is a common vascular disorder that is frequently associated with severe vision loss due to its complications. There are two forms of BRVO, the ischaemic and the non-ischemic, both leading to loss of visual acuity. About 20-30% of the BRVOS are ischemic and the majority of them develop secondary glaucoma and rubeosis. [1] Although this disorder was first reported by J. von Michel in 1878, its pathogenesis has still not been fully understood, and no effective therapy has been developed for this disorder [1-3]. Comparative research on this disorder is based on clinical models of BRVO.

The pathological features of BRVO can be more accurately reproduced by a photodynamic method to induce thrombosis in retinal vessels[4-14] than by using other methods such as laser coagulation[15-17], electrocoagulation of the retinal vein via the vitreous body[18], intravenous thrombin instillation[19-21] and endothelin-I injection into the posterior vitreous body[22, 23]. In the photodynamic method, a photosensitizing agent, namely, rose Bengal, is injected intravenously. This dye absorbs light maximally at a specific wavelength of 550 nm. Dye activation in the presence of molecular oxygen leads to the generation of singlet oxygen, which in turn acts locally to injure or destroy the vascular endothelium. The altered endothelium provides a surface for platelet aggregation and subsequent thrombosis. By using this method, thrombi can be produced in vessels. Because relatively low light intensities are required to initiate this process, the thermal effects on the surrounding tissues are minimized.

In this investigation, we used a Xenon arc lamp as the light source, and visible light was transmitted through an intraocular fiber to induce BRVO in pigmented rabbits. The characteristics of BRVO were evaluated quantitatively, and histological studies were performed to support the clinical findings. The results provided a framework for future applications of this technique.

2. Materials and methods

2.1 Animals and husbandry

Thirty-two male Standard Chinchilla rabbits were purchased from the Experimental Animal Center of Tianjin Medical University (Tianjin, China) and allowed to acclimate upon arrival for 10 d before the initiation of the experiment. At the beginning of the study, the animals were aged 3–4 months and weighed 2.5–3.5 kg. All experimental animals were housed in individual cages under stable environmental conditions: diet, commercial pellet diet (Lushifu, Beijing, China) and tap water ad libitum; relative humidity, 45–55%; temperature, 18°C; and light-dark cycle, 12/12 h (intensity, 300 lux).

The study was approved by the Ethics Committee of Tianjin medical university. All animal experiments were performed in accordance with the conventions of the Association for Research in Vision and Ophthalmology (ARVO) for ethics in animal experimentation.

2.2 Experimental design

The 32 rabbits (32 eyes, 32 vessels) were randomly divided into 15 treatment groups (n = 2) and 1 control group (n = 2). The treatment groups were administered 5 different rose Bengal doses (3, 6, 9, 12 and 15 mg/kg) and exposed to light of 3 different intensities (600, 1000 and 1400 lux) 1 min later. In the control group rabbits, the vessels were exposed to a light intensity of 1400 lux for 20 min without injection of the rose Bengal dye.

2.3 Experimental procedure

In preparation for the treatment and follow-up examinations, the rabbits were fully anesthetized with an intramuscular injection of 60 mg/kg ketamine (Beijing Shuanghe Pharmaceuticals, Beijing, China) and 8 mg/kg xylazine (Beijing Shuanghe Pharmaceuticals, Beijing, China). The pupils were dilated using 0.5% tropicamide eye drops (Beijing Shuanghe Pharmaceuticals, Beijing, China).

Rose Bengal (tetrachloro-tetraiodo-fluorescein sodium; certified purity, 90%; Sigma, St. Louis, MO) was dissolved in normal saline (30 mg/ml), sterilized by passage through a 0.22-μm filter and injected intravenously in doses of 3, 6, 9, 12 or 15 mg/kg before the light treatment. A Xenon arc lamp (Anshijia Instrument Co. Ltd., Beijing, China) was used as a light source, and light was transmitted by using a 0.2-mm intraocular illumination fiber (Alcon (China) Ophthalmic Product Co. Ltd., Shanghai, China). Light intensity was measured using a digital lux meter (LX-9621; Landtek Instrument Co. Ltd., Guangzhou, China). Average values of 600, 1000 and 1400 lux, for the low, medium and high settings, respectively, were obtained with less than 3% variation in repeated measurements throughout the study.

According to the treatment protocol, the rabbits were placed on a stage under a surgical microscope (OPTON Universal S3; Germany). 2% methylcellulose solution (Zhengda Co. Ltd., Shandong, China) is dropped on the cornea to couple the input light into the 30-degree prism lens (Anshijia Instrument Co. Ltd., Beijing, China). The operations were observed by using a contact lens and a surgical microscope. A 25-gauge trocar (Alcon (China) Ophthalmic Product Co. Ltd., Shanghai, China) was used to make an incisions in the conjunctiva and sclera at the projection holes located supratemporally 3 mm from the corneal limbus, then the needle was removed and the intraocular fiber was inserted through the incision and its direction was toward optic disc, the depth was 10 mm. Rose Bengal was injected intravenously through the marginal ear vein. After 1 min, the trunk vessels adjacent to the optic disc of 1~ 3 mm were exposed to a beam of white light. The duration of continuous exposure to light did not exceed 20 min, and the exposure time was recorded if complete vascular occlusion was observed. The fiber finally was then taken out and the sclera was finally sutured.

Fundus fluorescein angiography (FFA) was performed using a fundus camera (Zeiss FF450IR; Carl Zeiss Far East Co. Ltd., Beijing, China) before the treatment and everyday after the treatment until the occluded vein reopened. The 5 mg aqueous fluorescein sodium (100 mg/ml, Baiyunshan Pharmaceuticals Co. Ltd., Guangzhou, China) was injected into ear veins immediately prior to FFA under anesthesia and pupil dilation those were as same as the prior.

2.4 Experimental observation

The rate and duration of vessel occlusion are confirmed with an ophthalmoscope and by FFA. The blood flow was confirmed by a scleral depressor transiently applied pressure on the equator of the eyeball, thereby the higher intraocular pressure (IOP) reduced the flow rate until freely moving red blood cells were seen. Once the scleral depressor was removed, a rapid uninterrupted column of blood flow passed through without the presence of stagnant red blood cells. [9] These dynamic phenomenons were monitored by an ophthalmoscope and it was the character of reperfused vessels.

When reperfusion was noted on post-treatment day 1, the number of days of occlusion was defined as 0. When the vessel was observed to be occluded on day 1 but not on day 2, the number of days of occlusion was defined as 1 and so on.

Two rabbits in the control group and 1 rabbit in the treatment groups in whom BRVO was confirmed by FFA were euthanized using intravenous overdose of pentobarbital sodium (Beijing Shuanghe Pharmaceuticals, Beijing, China). Their eyes were enucleated and prepared for light microscopic examination by using standard techniques. Sections (5-μm-thick) were stained with haematoxylin/eosin. The remaining rabbits were euthanized by administering an overdose of pentobarbital sodium at the end of the experiment.

2.5 Statistical analysis

A partial correlation coefficient was used to analyze the relationship between the time of thrombosis, the drug dose, and light intensity. A P value of 0.05 or less was considered statistically significant. All data were analysed with the SPSS 11.5 software.

3. Results

3.1 Evaluation of BRVO animal model

BRVO models were developed in 22 of the 30 rabbits in the treatment group. The fundus could be observed in detail by using a surgical microscope (please see supplemental video 1). In the site exposed to light, photodynamic injury resulted in white debris (plaque-like thrombi) and the stagnation of blood flow. FFA showed the engorged distal ends of the venules proximal to the occlusion site and peripheral retinal oedema in the BRVO area (Figure 1).

Histological sections were studied to confirm the presence and extent of the photodynamic lesions. Retinal vein damage was confined to the area of direct light exposure in the treatment groups. Histological examination revealed thrombi consisting of platelet aggregates, stagnant red blood cells and a few white blood cells. Occluded retinal vein histological section indicated that compact thrombus filled the entire vein cavity and occlusion is evident. (Figure 2).

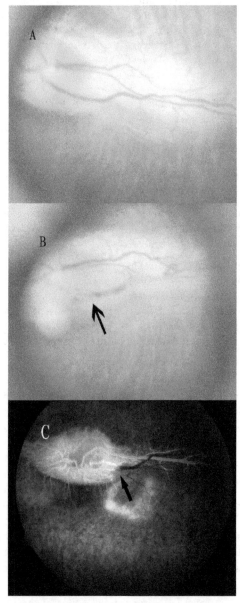

Fig. 1. **Photodynamic thrombosis of a branch retinal vein in a pigmented rabbit eye.** Initial formation of a thrombosis in the target vein (A) and complete obliteration of the vessel lumen (B). FFA showed a delay in the time required for angiosclerosis in the distal end of the vein and discontinuous intravenous blood flow in the vicinity of the optic disc (C). Arrows indicate the occlusion site and peripheral retinal oedema.

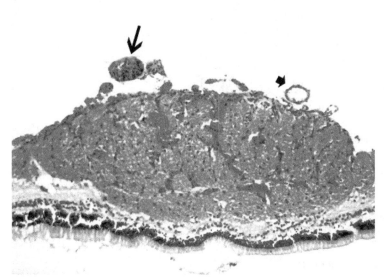

Fig. 2. **Histological findings.** Two hours after thrombosis, the thrombus filled the entire vein cavity (long arrow), and the artery was normal (short arrow). The thrombus consisted of platelet aggregates, stagnant red blood cells and a few white blood cells. Magnification, 200×.

The control vessels and the blood flow through them were as same as those in healthy animals. The histological sections from the rabbits that were not injected with rose Bengal showed no evidence of photochemical or thermal retinal damage in the site that was exposed to a light intensity of 1400 lux (maximum light intensity) for 20 min.

3.2 Dose- and light-response studies

Vein occlusion in the pigmented rabbits was considered as the end point for determining dose- and light-response relationships. In 22 successful BRVO models, the time required to produce an occlusion decreased with an increase in the dose of rose Bengal administered and the light intensity. Rose Bengal at doses of more than 9 mg/kg was effective in producing BRVO; a dose of 6 mg/kg was ineffective in producing BRVO at a light intensity of 600 lux. At a dose of 3 mg/kg, small plaques also developed in the target vessel; however, they did not progress to vascular occlusions in 20 min even if the light intensity was as high as 1400 lux. The total light energy required to produce an occlusion increased from an average of 600 lux with 9 mg/kg of rose Bengal to 1000 lux with 6 mg/kg of rose Bengal. The time of occurrence of thrombosis showed a negative correlation with the drug dose and light intensity. A decrease in the time required for the development of BRVO corresponded to a higher drug dose (partial $r = -0.7895$; $P < 0.001$) and a higher light intensity (partial $r = -0.9060$; $P < 0.001$) (Figure 3).

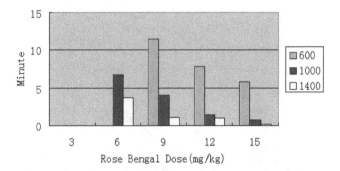

Fig. 3. **The relationship between the time required for thrombosis and the dose of rose Bengal and the light intensity.** The mean value of the time required for thrombosis was determined (n = 2). Complete BRVO formation did not occur when a dose of 3 mg/kg rose Bengal was used, and a dose of 6 mg/kg rose Bengal was ineffective in producing BRVO at a light intensity of 600 lux.

3.3 Duration of occlusion

In the early period of BRVO in the animal models, FFA and fundus photography documented the blood along the circuitous expanded vein, and retinal oedema that was similar to the lesion in humans. The area of the white thrombus gradually decreased with time, and the angiostenosis in the distal end of the retinal vein also gradually decreased. In 21 cases, the minimum duration record for the reopening of an occlusion was 3 d and the maximum, 10 d (Figure 4).

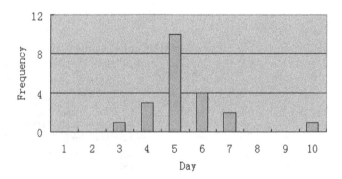

Fig. 4. **The frequency of the duration of vessel occlusion.** The duration of BRVO varied from 3 to 10 d. The data correspond to a Gaussian distribution (P < 0.01); the 95% confidence bound was 4.73–6.03 d, and the mean duration of vessel occlusion was 5.38 ± 1.43 d (n = 21).

4. Discussion

While developing an animal model, the following factors should be considered: the animal species used, the ease of development and reproducibility of the model and the degree of similarity of the model with the human disease. In this study, we focus on optimizing the method used to induce experimental thrombosis.

The animal species that are usually selected for the development of BRVO animal models are mouse, rat, rabbit, cat, pig, dog and monkey. Mice[14] and rats[5-7, 9] are suitable for the development of large numbers of RVO models for research because of their low price, easy availability and breeding management. Further, these models enable easy identification of the retinal artery and vein. However, the eye of mice or rats is too small to permit investigative surgical procedures. The structure of the retina in pigs[12, 15], cats[8] or dogs[4] is similar to that in humans except that it does not have a macular region. The retinal blood supply in rhesus monkeys[16, 17] is similar to that in human; however, the sources of these animals are limited, and they are difficult to breed and manage. Compared with the eyeballs of other animal species, the rabbit eyeball is sufficiently large to operate[19-23]. Further, rabbits are inexpensive, can be easily bred and the FFA of the rabbit eye is stable. Therefore, we selected pigmented rabbits for our study.

The combination of intraocular fibre illumination with the administration of rose Bengal should be classified as a photodynamic method of inducing BRVO because the wavelength of visible light include 550 nm. These findings correspond to Virchow's hypothesis of thrombosis in humans. Compared with the photodynamic method, laser coagulation[15-17] requires higher energy and a longer exposure time, which would inevitably result in heat injury and disruption of the vessel wall, and subsequently, frequent bleeding. Electrocoagulation of the retinal vein via the vitreous body[18] utilizes electrothermal energy to destroy the vascular endothelium and block the vessels, which is different from the process of thrombosis. In intravitreous thrombin instillation method[19-21], the location of the retinal thrombus could not be determined; thus, the thrombus may occlude other regions but not the target vessels. The injection of endothelin-I into the posterior vitreous body[22, 23] caused complete occlusion of the temporal retinal vessels, but this vasospastic mechanism is also unsuitable for application in the experimental induction of thrombosis because actual clinical BRVO was occluded at one or some spots in vein.

Presently, an argon (Ar) laser is often used as the excitation light source in the photodynamic method because its wavelength of 514 nm is similar to the light absorption peak of rose Bengal. However, heat injury from laser-coagulation to the retinal tissue and its vessels is observed. Moreover, due to the pulsed excitation of the laser, continuous exposure of the vessel to the laser beam is impossible. Consequently, it is difficult to adjust the level of energy used in this procedure: if the energy level is too low, no thrombus formation occurs and if it is too high, vessel hemorrhage occurs[8]. Some researchers utilize common light sources such as slit lamps and Xenon lamps to develop BRVO animal models. However, the use of these light sources resulted in an extensive arteriovenous obstruction caused due to the exposure of a large area to the light source, therefore, these light sources are not suitable for studying a typical BRVO[9, 10, 13]. In a previous study, we use a microsurgical illumination system, which comprised a 0.9-mm intraocular fibre that served as an endoilluminator to produce RVO in pigs[11]; the intraocular fibre illuminated the nearby retinal vascular target and by localizing energy, it is able to produce a thrombus as effectively as laser irradiation. However, the diameter of the retinal trunk vein in rabbits was only 150–200 μm, and the microsurgical system was too wide to the rabbit. Therefore, in this study, we used a Xenon arc lamp as a light source and designed a 0.2 mm fiber for illumination to ensure that the light beam irradiate the trunk vein and not the accompanying artery. We find that this is a simple and reliable system for developing BRVO models in rabbits.

The process of formation of BRVO in our rabbit model can be visualized and photographed using a surgical microscope. At the site exposed to light, the following course of thrombogenesis is recognized: photodynamic injury resulted in a decrease in the rate of venous blood flow; this is followed by the appearance of stagnant red blood cells in the vessel, the gradual accumulation of white debris (plaque-like thrombi) and the development of a vascular occlusion. The distal ends of the venules are engorged proximal to the occlusion site. The morphological and histopathological changes are similar to Kohner's results[24]. No changes were observe in the light microscopic images of the control vessels; this confirmes that illumination do not produce heat injury in the retinal vessels and tissue.

The dose- and light-response studies show that the time of occurrence of thrombosis correlate negatively with the drug dose and light intensity; further, the basic set of parameters require to produce an occlusion is an average light intensity of 600 lux, a rose Bengal dose of 9 mg/kg and an exposure time of 11.5 min or an average light intensity of 1000 lux, a rose Bengal dose of 6 mg/kg and an exposure time of 6.75 min. Thus, we suggest that the optimum parameters should be 1000 lux, 9 mg/kg of rose Bengal and an exposure time of 3–5 min. This suggestion is based on the following considerations: the experimental dose of rose Bengal in this model is maintained as low as possible to prevent the leakage of rose Bengal into the vitreous humour and the anterior chamber[12]; the energy level of the light used to induce thrombosis is higher than that in the breeding conditions (300 lux); this ensures that thrombosis occur only in the area exposed to the light and not in other vessels. On the other hand, the exposure time of 3–5 min was suitable for operation. The optimization of this method may aid investigators in controlling thrombus formation more precisely.

Clinical BRVO is a disease of long duration and various types [1-3]; however, the experimental occlusion is maintained for 3 to 10 d (average, 5.38 d) in our model. This may be attributed to the use of young and healthy experimental animals, the sudden generation of an obstruction in the normal vascular bed and the activation of an autochthonous repair mechanism; all these factors result in rapid thrombolysis. Therefore, this BRVO model is very suitable for observation of immediate therapy experiment, for example, surgery; and not suitable for long-term drug treatment studies.

5. References

[1] Hayreh SS, Podhajsky PA, Zimmerman MB. Branch retinal artery occlusion: natural history of visual outcome. Ophthalmology. 116:1188-94. e1-4(2009).

[2] Hayreh SS, Zimmerman B, McCarthy MJ, et al. Systemic diseases associated with various types of retinal vein occlusion. Am J Ophthalmol.131:61-77(2001).

[3] Shahid H, Hossain P, Amoaku WM. The management of retinal vein occlusion: is interventional ophthalmology the way forward?. Br J Ophthalmol. 90:627- 39(2006).

[4] Tameesh MK, Lakhanpal RR, Fujii GY, et al. Retinal vein cannulation with prolonged infusion of tissue plasminogen activator (t-PA) for the treatment of experimental retinal vein occlusion in dogs. Am J Ophthalmol. 138:829-39(2004)

[5] Kang SG, Chung H, Hyon JY. Experimental preretinal neovascularization by laser-induced thrombosis in albino rats. Korean J Ophthalmol. 13(2):65-70(1999)

[6] Ham DI, Chang K, Chung H. Preretinal neovascularization induced by experimental retinal vein occlusion in albino rats. Korean J Ophthalmol.11:60-64(1997)

[7] Shen W, He S, Han S, et al. Preretinal neovascularisation induced by photodynamic venous thrombosis in pigmented rat. Aust N Z J Ophthalmol. 24:50-52(1996)

[8] Si BX, Zhang MN, Huang HB, et al. [Experimental retinal vein occlusion in cats]. Chin Inter J Ophthalmol.7:987-989(2007)

[9] Wilson CA, Hatchell DL. Photodynamic retinal vascular thrombosis. Rate and duration of vascular occlusion. Invest Ophthalmol Vis Sci. 32:2357-2365(1991)

[10] Nanda SK, Hatchell DL, Tiedeman JS, et al. A new method for vascular occlusion. Photochemical initiation of thrombosis. Arch Ophthalmol. 105:1121-1124(1987)

[11] Zhang XL, Ma ZZ, Hu YT, et al. Direct tissue plasminogen activator administration through a microinjection device in a pig model of retinal vein thrombosis. Curr Eye Res. 24:263-267(2002)

[12] Zhang XL, Hu YT, Ma ZZ, et al. [Experimental retinal vein occlusion induced by photodynamic approach]. Chin J Ophthalmol. 39:220-223(2003)

[13] Royster AJ, Nanda SK, Hatchell DL, et al. Photochemical initiation of thrombosis. Fluorescein angiographic, histologic, and ultrastructural alterations in the choroid, retinal pigment epithelium, and retina. Arch Ophthalmol. 106:1608-1614(1988)

[14] Zhang H, Sonoda KH, Qiao H, et al. Development of a new mouse model of branch retinal vein occlusion and retinal neovascularization. Jpn J Ophthalmol. 51:251-257(2007)

[15] Pournaras CJ, Tsacopoulos M, Strommer K, et al. Experimental retinal branch vein occlusion in miniature pigs induces local tissue hypoxia and vasoproliferative microangiopathy. Ophthalmol. 97:1321-1328(1990)

[16] Hamilton AM, Kohner EM, Rosen D, et al. Experimental retinal branch vein occlusion in rhesus monkeys. I. Clinical appearances. Br J Ophthalmol. 63:377-387(1979)

[17] Minamikawa M, Yamamoto K, Okuma H, et al. [Experimental retinal branch vein occlusion]. Nippon Ganka Gakkai Zasshi. 93:691-697(1989)

[18] Chan CC, Green WR, Rice TA. Experimental occlusion of the retinal vein. Graefes Arch Clin Exp Ophthalmol. 224:507-512(1986)

[19] Matsumoto M. [Experimental study on earlier thrombogenic process in thrombin induced retinal venous obstruction in rabbit eye]. Nippon Ganka Gakkai Zasshi. 96:1132-1141(1992)

[20] Tamura M. Neovascularization in experimental retinal venous obstruction in rabbits. Jpn J Ophthalmol. 45:144-150(2001)

[21] Sakuraba T. [Experimental retinal vein obstruction induced by transadventitial administration of thrombin in the rabbit]. Nippon Ganka Gakkai Zasshi. 93:978-985(1989)

[22] Takei K, Sato T, Nonoyama T, et al. A new model of transient complete obstruction of retinal vessels induced by endothelin-1 injection into the posterior vitreous body in rabbits. Graefes Arch Clin Exp Ophthalmol. 231:476-481(1993)

[23] Sato T, Takei K, Nonoyama T, et al. [Endothelin-1-induced vasoconstriction in retinal blood vessels in the rabbit]. Nippon Ganka Gakkai Zasshi. 97:683-689(1993)

[24] Kohner EM, Dollery CT, Shakib M. Experimental retinal branch vein occlusion. Am J Ophthalmol. 69:7782−8251(1970)

3

Retinal Vascular Occlusions

Mario Bradvica, Tvrtka Benašić and Maja Vinković
University of Josip Juraj Strossmayer, Medical School Osijek, University Hospital Osijek
Croatia

1. Introduction

Retinal vascular occlusions are serious diseases and significant causes of blindness that include arterial and venous obstructions. The causes, pathogenesis, clinical characteristics, prognosis, and response to therapy are influenced by the location of the occlusion in the retinal vasculature and by the extent of retinal nonperfusion.

The hallmark of clinical presentation in the retinal occlusive disease is painless loss of vision, which can be asymptomatic, gradual with only mildly reduced visual acuity, or sudden and reduced to counting fingers depending on the extent of the irrigation area of the affected vessel. The clinical presentation aids in distinguishing the type of the occlusion, which may be classified according to the anatomical site of the occlusion.

2. Retinal Artery Occlusion

Retinal artery occlusion (RAO) represents an ophthalmologic emergency. In 1859, von Graefe first described central retinal artery occlusion (von Graefe, 1859). Retinal artery obstruction may be classified as follows: central (CRAO), affecting the retinal vessel at the optic nerve, hemicentral (occasional, only when one of the two trunks of the CRA is occluded) (Akkoyun et al., 2006; Karagoz et al., 2009; Schmidt & Kramer-Zucker, 2011), branch (BRAO), obstruction distally to the lamina cribrosa of the optic nerve, cilioretinal (CLRAO) and central sparing cilioretinal artery (Hayreh, 2011). Obstructions more proximal to the central retinal artery, in the ophthalmic artery, or even in the internal carotid artery, may produce visual loss as well. More proximal obstructions usually cause a more chronic form of visual problem – the ocular ischemic syndrome often associated with occlusive carotid disease (Kearns & Hollenhorst, 1963).

Central retinal artery occlusion results in sudden visual loss and is therefore one of the most important topics in ophthalmology. Branch retinal artery occlusion causes sudden segmental visual loss and may recur to involve other branch retinal arterioles. Amaurosis fugax is a common transient acute retinal ischemic condition. Acute retinal arterial occlusive disorders together comprise one of the major causes of acute visual loss (Hayreh, 2011). Only anecdotal reports have described spontaneous recovery of vision, and case series have shown only up to 14% of spontaneous recovery (Atebara et al., 1995).

The majority of retinal arterial obstructions are either thrombotic or embolic in nature (an embolus is visible only in 20% of the patients with branch or central retinal artery occlusion)

(Rumelt & Brown, 2003). Arterial occlusions in the eye are almost always due to microembolism and the major source of microemboli is the plaque(s), which may be present with or without any significant carotid artery stenosis. Thus, absence of significant stenosis of the carotid artery does not necessarily rule out the carotid artery as the source of microembolism (Hayreh et al., 2009).

Immediate intervention improves chances of visual recovery, but even then, the prognosis is rather poor, with only 21-35% of eyes retaining useful vision (Jain & Juang, 2009), because it dominantly depends on the type of the occlusion (Hayreh & Zimmerman, 2005). Although restoration of vision is of immediate concern, retinal artery occlusion is a forerunner for other systemic diseases that must be evaluated promptly. Establishing of the cause of obstruction is essential. In case of giant cell arteritis causing occlusion immediate treatment is urgent.

2.1 Epidemiology

Central retinal artery obstruction (CRAO) is a rare event – it has been estimated to account for about 0.85 in 100,000 per year (Jain & Juang, 2009). The mean age at onset is about 60 years, with a range from the first to the ninth decade of life (Duker, 2003). Bilateral obstruction occurs in 1-2% of cases (Brown, 1994). CRAOs account for 58% of acute RAOs, BRAOs for 38%, and cilioretinal artery occlusions (CLRAOs) (Jain & Juang, 2009). There are discrepancies among authors regarding the prevalence of men over women. Some advocate the ratio 2:1 (Duker, 2003) whereas the others found slightly more frequent occurrence in men (Hayreh et al., 2009). A large case series documented that approximately one fourth of patients with CRAO had a form with the cilioretinal sparing (Brown & Shields, 1979). The incidence of CLRA occlusion (CLRAO) varies in different studies from none to 32% (Justice & Lehmann 1976), which would be the most acceptable data, because the incidence was calculated by reviewing stereoscopic color fundus photographs as well as FA; the incidence of CLRAO is in direct proportion with the presence of cilioretinal artery in the population. FA is the most reliable way to ascertain the true incidence because the CLRA dyes concurrently with the filling of the choroid and usually before the start of filling of the CRA. The arteries occurred bilaterally in 14.6% (Justice & Lehmann, 1976).

Multiple studies have shown increased mortality in patients with retinal arterial emboli (Bruno et al., 1995; Ho et al., 2008; Lindley et al., 2009). The frequency of retinal emboli increases with age and are more common in men than in women. Bilateral are rare, although multiple emboli in a single eye may be seen in up to one third of cases. They are associated with the presence of carotid artery disease (CAD), hypertension, smoking, and possibly diabetes (Wong & Klein, 2002). The large Beaver Dam Eye Study calculated the prevalence of retinal arteriolar emboli of 1.3% in the population ranged from 43-86 years, and the 5-year incidence of 0.9%, the 10-year incidence of 1.5% for the same population, and also confirmed a significantly higher hazard of dying from a stroke in people with retinal emboli (Klein et al., 1999; Klein et al., 2003).

Debate exists in the literature on the prevalence and etiology of neovascularization (NV) following CRAO. The reported prevalence varies from 2.5% to 31.6%. Studies have reported prevalence of 18.2% of neovascularization and 15.2% of neovascular glaucoma (NVG) (Duker et al., 1991; Rudkin et al., 2010). In branch retinal artery occlusion, the incidence is even rarer. Neovascularization is more likely to occur in persons with concurrent diseases and not CRAO per se, as with diabetes, severe carotid artery disease or generalized atherosclerosis (Hayreh & Podhajsky, 1982). Clinical cases have been reported in which neovascular glaucoma developed after branch retinal artery occlusion (Brown & Reber, 1986); most probably they are a result of later complete CRAO rather than pure BRAO.

2.2 Pathophysiology and histology

Visual loss from retinal arterial occlusion (RAO) occurs from the loss of blood supply to the inner layer of the retina. Blood supply to the retina originates from the central retinal (CRA) and the cilioretinal (CLRA) artery. The primary source of blood supply to both arteries - the ophthalmic artery (OA), usually the first intracranial branch of the internal carotid artery (ICA), does not always originate from the ICA; the most common abnormal origin is the middle meningeal artery (Hayreh, 2011; Morandi et al., 1998). The central retinal artery arises independently in 37.5% from the ophthalmic artery, in 59.5% by a common trunk with one or another posterior ciliary artery (PCA), and extremely rarely with other branches of the OA. Numerous anastomoses are established by the branches of the CRA with other branches of the OA, mostly pial. The study showed that these pial anastomoses were usually large enough to establish a variable amount of collateral circulation in the eye having an occlusion of the CRA. This was also demonstrated by fluorescein fundus angiography (FA) (Hayreh, 2011; Hayreh & Weingeist, 1980). The central retinal artery supplies the retina as it branches into smaller segments upon leaving the optic disc. The so-called "branch retinal arteries" are in fact arterioles after the first branching in the retina which don't have either an internal elastic lamina or a continuous muscular layer (Hayreh, 2011). A retinal vascular bed does not own any anastomoses; it is end-arterial system. The cilioretinal artery belongs to the PCA system; it usually originates from the peripapillary choroid or directly from one of the PCAs and supplies the part of the macular retina. The CLRA has a characteristic hook-like appearance at its site of entry into the retina at the optic disc margin, usually on the temporal side. Branch retinal artery occlusion (BRAO) occurs when the embolus lodges in a more distal branch of the retinal artery. BRAO typically involves the temporal retinal vessels and usually does not require treatment, unless perifoveolar vessels are threatened (Ho et al., 2008).

Acutely, obstruction of the central retinal artery results in inner retinal layer edema and pyknosis of the ganglion cell nuclei. Ischemic necrosis results and the retina become opacified and yellow-white in appearance. The opacity is most dense in the posterior pole as a result of the increased thickness of the nerve fiber layer and ganglion cells in this region. The opacification takes as little as 15 minutes to several hours before becoming evident and resolves in 4-6 weeks. Furthermore, the foveola assumes a cherry-red spot because of a combination of 3 factors: (i) the intact retinal pigment epithelium and choroid underlying the fovea, (ii) the foveolar retina is nourished by the choriocapillaris, and (iii) the thinnest NFL at this location. The late stage shows a homogenous scar replacing the inner layer of the retina. Pigmentary changes are typically absent since the retinal pigment epithelium remains unaffected (Kearns & Hollenhorst, 1963).

It has been shown experimentally on animal studies that the retinal damage is irreversible after 105 minutes of completely occluded circulation, but may recover at 97 minutes (Hayreh et al., 2004), and the treatment instituted at any time beyond 4h after the onset of

CRAO cannot have any scientific rationale for improvement of vision. However, complete occlusion or retinal artery circulation in humans is rare with retinal artery disease; thus, retinal recovery is possible even after days of ischemia (Brown & Magargal, 1988). Controversy exists regarding the optimal window of treatment in humans, but the conservative approach involves treatment up to 24 hours (Kearns & Hollenhorst, 1963).

The retinal artery could be occluded due to embolism, vasoobliteration (atherosclerotic plaques, giant-cell arteritis and other types of vasculitis) and vascular compression (a retrobulbar mass - hematoma, neoplasm, retrobulbar injections may lead to an optic nerve and central retinal artery compression) (Korner-Stiefbold, 2001), angiospasm, hemodynamic or hydrostatic arterial occlusion (Hayreh, 2011). By far the most common cause of nonarteritic RAO is the embolism. Emboli are usually of three types: cholesterol - Hollenhorst plaque, platelet-fibrin, calcified, and occasionally myxomatous, or bacterial. The incidence is 74%, 15.5% and 10.5% for the first 3 types, respectively (Arruga & Sanders, 1982). They are mostly of carotid and/or cardiac origin (Korner-Stiefbold, 2001). The major source of embolism in the carotid arteries is plaque (66%), whereas a significant carotid stenosis (>50%) accounts for only 30% of cases (Hayreh et al., 2009; Korner-Stiefbold, 2001; Younge, 1989). Statistically, Caucasians, when compared to African Americans, have significantly different incidence of ICA stenosis, which is 41% and 3.4% for the each group, respectively (Ahuja et al., 1999). A significant stenosis of the extracranial internal carotid artery is the most common identified condition associated with retinal and ocular ischemia (Biousse, 1997; Mizener et al., 1997; Sharma et al., 1998). It represents the hemodynamic cause, and, especially if associated with nocturnal arterial hypotension, can lead to transient CRAO (Hayreh & Zimmerman, 2005). The sources of emboli in heart are valvular lesions, patent foramen ovale, myxoma and endocarditis (Mangat, 1995; Reese & Shafer, 1978; Schmidt et al., 2005; Sharma et al., 1997). It must be remembered though, that the absence of any abnormality on color Doppler ultrasound or echocardiography does not exclude carotid artery or the heart as the source of microembolism, because of the test-resolution and location of the plaque/stenosis.

Animal studies have shown that, serotonin in atherosclerotic vessels produces vasospasm of the central retinal artery (CRA) and/or posterior ciliary artery (PCA) in various combinations (but not vasospasm of the arterioles in the retina). It is postulated that in some atherosclerotic individuals this mechanism may play an important role in the development of ischemic disorders of the retina and optic nerve head (ONH), including amaurosis fugax, CRA occlusion and anterior ischemic optic neuropathy, and possibly also glaucomatous optic neuropathy, particularly in normal tension glaucoma (Hayreh, 1999).

Central retinal arterial occlusions could be divided into permanent or transient; arteritic (usually gigantocellular arteritis) or nonarteritic occlusion. The transient is the nonarteritic and could occur due to (i) transient impaction of an embolus, (ii) fall of perfusion pressure in the retinal vascular bed below the critical level (night arterial hypotension, hypovolemic shock, hemodialysis, spasm of CRA, marked carotid artery disease, ocular ischemia, or a rise of intraocular pressure because of orbital swelling, acute angle-closure glaucoma, neovascular glaucoma (NVG) with ocular ischemia), and (iii) vasospasm of the atherosclerotic lesions (induced by the platelet-aggregation plaque secreting serotonin) (Hayreh, 2011).

Branch arterial occlusion is usually due to embolism and occasionally vasculitis. It could be recurrent (Barak et al., 1997; Beiran et al., 1995; Beversdorf et al., 1997; Johnson et al., 1994). Most of these cases probably have Susac's syndrome (autoimmune endotheliopathy leading to encephalopathy, BRAO and hearing loss) (Susac et al., 2007). The etiology of this syndrome is still unknown, but the prognosis is good in most cases. Spontaneous resolution usually occurs, but early treatment minimizes the risk of sequelae (Van Winden & Salu, 2010).

2.3 Causes

Embolism of the carotid artery and the heart are the most common causes of retinal artery obstruction. Carotid artery disease causes retinal arterial occlusion by three mechanisms: embolism, hemodynamic changes in significantly stenosed carotid artery, and arterial spasm. The major source of emboli is plaques in the carotid arteries, and much less frequently stenosis. According to some studies, hemodynamically significant carotid artery stenosis was found in about 18%of patients with acute RAO (Sharma et al., 1998) and as previously mentioned, Hayreh et al. suggest that the presence of plaques on Doppler color imaging is of more value in determining the cause of acute occlusive event rather than the embolus itself (Hayreh, 2005). The probable cause is the microembolism, which may not produce hemodynamically significant stenosis recordable on Doppler color imaging but may indeed account for the retinal artery occlusion. As shown in the study, carotid Doppler and/or angiography showed the presence of plaques in 71% in CRAO and 66% in BRAO (Hayreh et al., 2009). The fluctuation of hemodynamic factors, especially drops in blood pressure in nocturnal hypotension along with significant stenosis of the carotid artery may be responsible for transient retinal artery occlusion (Hayreh & Zimmerman, 2005; McCullough et al., 2004). Based on experimental studies on animals, the investigators have introduced the possible role of serotonin, released by platelet aggregation on atherosclerotic plaques in the carotid artery, causing transient vasospasm of the central retinal artery and thus potentially inducing retinal artery occlusion and retinal ischemic disorders.

Systemic cardiovascular diseases have a well known association with retinal arterial occlusive disease in elderly people (Sharma, 1998). Therefore, a careful history should include identifying the possible underlying causes such as arterial hypertension, diabetes mellitus, hyperlipidemia, carotid artery disease, coronary artery disease, cerebrovascular disease and symptoms suggestive of temporal arteritis. Cigarette smoking has been described significantly more common among these patients than in the general population. In patients with no obvious systemic risk factors and especially in subjects under the age of 40, the other causative options should be considered, which include systemic vasculitis, blood dyscrasias, drug abuse, hypercoagulabile states, infective diseases, migraine and prolonged direct pressure to the globe in unconscious patients (Brown et al., 1981; Graham, 1990; Greven et al., 1995).

Coagulopathies from sickle cell anemia or antiphospholipid antibodies are more common etiologies for CRAO in patients younger than 30 years of age and the proposed mechanisms involve increase in coagulation factor or platelet activity, thrombocytosis, interaction of lupus anticoagulant and anticardiolipin antibodies with phospholipids as well as the deficiencies of protein C and S and resistance to activated protein C (Comp & Esmon, 1984; Love & Santoro, 1990; Palmowski-Wolfe et al., 2007; Vignes et al., 1996). Increased levels of homocysteine have been linked with higher incidence of occlusive vascular incidents damaging the vascular endothelium and thus increasing atherosclerotic changes and the formation of blood cloths. Therefore, in cases of suspected homocystinuria or heterozygosity for homocystinuria an oral methionine loading test may be performed since this state may be preventable by taking appropriate vitamin supplements (Boers et al., 1985; Weger et al., 2002; Wenzler et al., 1993). In cases of clinical suspicion, the HIV testing may be indicated since there have been case reports of CRAO or BRAO associated with HIV infection (Conway et al., 1995). A variety of other diseases, including systemic lupus erythematosus, polyarteritis nodosa, dengue fever, West Nile virus, sickle cell disease, Takayasu's arteritis, after smallpox vaccination, Churg-Strauss syndrome, ocular Behçet's disease, Fabry's disease, Susac'c syndrome, and head injury may present with retinal occlusive disorders. It is necessary to exclude these states if there is a young person with sudden loss of vision, fundoscopic findings of arterial occlusion, central or branch, and no obvious identifiable systemic risk factors as above mentioned. In conclusion, arterial occlusive disease of the retina is the result of either arteriosclerotic thrombosis, embolic impaction (predominantly atheromatous plaques of carotid bifurcation, or the internal carotid artery, but also consisting of different material – fat, parasites, talc, air), vasculitis, vasospasm or systemic hypotension. These numerous potential causes mandate often time-consuming and expensive lab tests, and sometimes a causative management of the underlying disease. The possible causes and underlying states associated with retinal arterial occlusion are incorporated in Table 1.

2.4 Clinical presentation

2.4.1 Symptoms

The main presenting symptom of the arterial occlusive disease is loss of vision, usually monocular, which may be sudden (seconds to minutes) blurring, decrease or total loss of vision. The extent of visual loss depends on the type of the occlusion. In central artery occlusions, visual loss is central and dense. In branch artery occlusions, visual loss may go unnoticed if only a section of the peripheral visual field space is affected. Various types of the retinal artery occlusion have different degree of visual acuity (VA) drop; CRAO characterizes severely decreased VA (counting fingers to light perception); BRAO has VA 20/20 to counting fingers; VA in cilioretinal occlusion ranges from 20/30-20/60; CRAO with cilioretinal sparing has VA 20/30 to hand motion, depending on the amount of the papillomacular bundle supplied by the patent vessel; combined CRAO and CRVO have VA counting fingers to light perception (Rumelt S, Brown GC, 2004). The patients with CRAO without cilioretinal sparing rarely regained any useful vision (Brown & Shields, 1979).

Pain accompanying the visual loss is unusual and usually denotes associated ocular ischemic syndrome (Werner et al. 1994). Rarely, in cases associated with arterial spasm, a relapsing and remitting course of visual loss precedes central retinal artery obstruction. Amaurosis fugax precedes visual loss in about 10% of patients involving transient loss of vision lasting seconds to minutes, but which may last up to 2 hours (Brown, 1999). The vision usually returns to baseline after an episode of amaurosis fugax.

2.4.2 Signs

In CRAO, the first signs are afferent pupillary defect on the affected side and segmental arterial blood flow ("box- carring"), which appear immediately at the occlusion and are accompanied by the various degree of diminished visual acuity. Later signs are retinal opacification and cherry-red spot and optic disc pallor, attenuation of the retinal arteries, arterio-arteriolar collaterals or neovascular glaucoma (as a complication). Von Graefe was the first one who described typical fundoscopic findings associated with occlusion of the central retinal artery: whitish, edematous retina attributable to infarction, especially at the posterior pole where the nerve fibre layer and ganglion cell layer are the thickest (Beatty & Au Eong, 2000). As these layers are absent in the fovea, the underlying choroidal vascular bed can be seen in this area, thus giving rise to the classic cherry-red spot (Fig. 1.). In the presence of a patent cilioretinal artery, the retinal region served by the unobstructed vessel is not involved (Fig. 2.). Disc pallor and retinal vascular narrowing are characteristic of the late stage of CRAO. The characteristic of BRAO is retinal edema in the distribution of the affected vessel only (Fig. 3.). Obstruction of a cilioretinal artery, or even a macular branch arteriole, gives cloudy, edematous appearance of the macula and affects central vision. In acute stage, the arteries appear thin and attenuated while cherry red spot and ground glass appearance may take hours to develop. In severe blockages, both veins and arteries may manifest "box-carring" or segmentation of the blood flow.

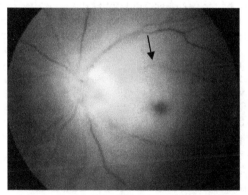

Fig. 1. Central retinal artery occlusion, note foveal cherry red spot and ground glass appearance of the macula (arrow)

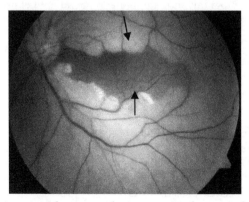

Fig. 2. Cilioretinal sparing central artery occlusion; sparing between the disc and fovea (arrows), representing irrigation area of the cilioretinal artery

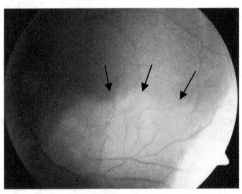

Fig. 3. Branch retinal artery occlusion; note pale, edematous retina in the area of affected vessel (arrows)

Late complication of CRAO is a neovascularization which indicates severe retinal ischemia and is more common at the far periphery and not at the optic disc or the posterior pole, and may complicate with vitreous or preretinal hemorrhage (Duker & Brown, 1989). This is why, in most cases, they are not observed clinically or angiographically with standard angle fundus camera. Only ischemia is usually seen by fluorescein angiography. The typical angiographic finding of neovascularization is the leakage of dye, whereas collateral shunting vessels do not present with such a feature. The fundoscopic findings typically resolve within days to weeks of the acute event, and residual optic atrophy may be the only physical finding. This feature also explains why it is crucial to treat the far periphery of the retina by cryo in addition to treatment by photocoagulation, in cases that the retinal periphery cannot be treated by photocoagulation.

Acute simultaneous obstruction of both the retinal and choroidal circulations is referred to as an ophthalmic artery obstruction. It can be differentiated clinically from central retinal artery obstruction by the following features: severe visual loss — bare or no light perception; intense ischemic retinal whitening that extends beyond the macular area; little to no cherry-red spot; pronounced choroidal perfusion defects on fluorescein angiography; nonrecordable electroretinogram; and late retinal pigment epithelium alterations (Brown et al., 1986). Cases of ophthalmic artery obstruction usually have associated local orbital or systemic diseases: orbital mucormycosis, orbital trauma, retrobulbar anesthesia, depot corticosteroid injection, atrial myxoma, or carotid artery disease (Sullivan et al., 1983). In conjunction with ipsilateral ischemic optic neuropathy, temporal arteritis may produce ophthalmic artery obstruction.

2.5 Evaluation and imaging

To summarize and to choose a rational approach in the workup, it is our opinion that the evaluation should be related to the age group. We recommend the following procedures to be undertaken in the persons over 50 years: the physical examination with complete cardiovascular assessment, ECG, the lab tests including full blood count, erythrocyte sedimentation rate, C reactive protein, fasting blood glucose, lipidogram, urine analysis, Doppler color imaging of the carotid arteries, and transthoracic echocardiography in patients with cardioembolic risk factors.

In the younger patients and those with unidentifiable systemic risk factors these are the proposed investigations: fluorescein angiography, vasculitis screen including anticardiolipin antibodies, antinuclear antibodies, anti-double stranded DNA antibodies, routine coagulation tests (prothrombin time, partial thromboplastin time), specialized clotting factor and platelet activity studies (levels of protein S, protein C, antithrombin III, plasminogen activator, plasminogen activator inhibitor, fibrinogen and resistance to activated protein C) and homocysteine.

Systemic cardiovascular disease
Hypertension, Diabetes mellitus, Atheromatous disease, Cardiac-valvular disease, bacterial endocarditis, myxoma, arrhythmias
Coagulopathies
Antiphospholipid antibodies, Protein C deficiency, Protein S deficiency, Antithrombin III deficiency, Elevation of platelet factor 4, Sickle cell anemia, Homocysteine
Systemic vasculitis
Polyarteritis nodosa, Temporal arteritis, Kawasaki's syndrome, Wegener's granulomatosis, Susac's disease, Systemic lupus erythematosus
Oncologic
Metastatic tumors, Leukemia, Lymphoma
Infective diseases
Syphilis, HIV
Trauma
Direct ocular compression, Penetrating injury, Retrobulbar injection, Orbital trauma, Purtscher's disease
Ocular conditions
Preretinal arterial loops, Optic nerve drusen, Necrotizing herpetic retinitis, Toxoplasmosis
Other causes
Oral contraceptives, Pregnancy, Drug abuse, Migraine

Table 1. Systemic and ocular conditions related to retinal arterial occlusion

It is important to exclude temporal arteritis in older patients, since it follows different clinical course and mandates the prompt administration of systemic corticosteroids. Giant cell arteritis is concerned as approved clinically if two of the three symptoms or signs exist: headache, tenderness over the temple and high sedimentation rate. Biopsy only approves it and treatment should not be deferred for biopsy result. It should be immediately initiated if two or more of the above are present. The purpose of the treatment is to prevent visual loss of the fellow eye, which usually occurs within 10 days of the event in one eye. Apart from the sudden, painless, nonprogressive vision loss in one eye, the patients may have headaches, jaw claudication, scalp tenderness, proximal muscle and joint aches, anorexia, weight loss, or fever.

All patients with acute retinal arterial occlusion must be evaluated for the source of embolism, which is the commonest cause for its development. The imaging techniques are used to confirm the diagnosis in uncertain cases and these are fluorescein angiography, visual field testing, optical coherence tomography and electroretinography.

2.5.1 Fluorescein angiography

Fluorescein angiography is not routinely indicated in the acute phase of arterial occlusive disease. The angiographic findings in both types, CRAO and BRAO (Fig. 4.), include delayed arm-to-retina time which is over 12 seconds (Richard G. et al., 1998), reduced arterial caliber and "cattle-trucking" of the blood column in the branch arteries. Sometimes, it may be minutes before the retinal arterial tree fills with fluorescein. Arteriovenous transit is also delayed, and late staining of the disc is common.

The CLRA dyes concurrently with the filling of the choroid and usually before the start of filling of the CRA (Justice & Lehmann, 1976).

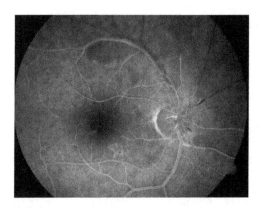

Fig. 4. Superior branch retinal artery occlusion of the right eye. Note the delayed filling of the dye in the superior quadrant of retina

2.5.2 Visual field testing

Visual fields show a remaining temporal island of peripheral vision. In cases of a patent cilioretinal artery, a small intact central island is found as well.

2.5.3 Electroretinography

Electroretinography characteristically shows a decreased to absent b-wave with intact a-wave.

2.5.4 Optical Coherence Tomography (OCT)

Optical coherence findings depend on the duration of the ischemia. Acute stages show increased reflectivity in the inner retinal layers and decreased reflectivity of the photoreceptor layer due to the shadowing effect (Fig. 4.). If involved, the macular region shows cystoid changes with loss of the foveolar contour. Old cases of arterial occlusion are presented with macular thinning with increased reflectivity of the retinal structure denoting ischemia.

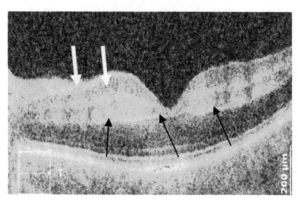

Fig. 5. CRAO – OCT changes, retinal edema in the inner layers (white arrows) denoting ischemia and the shadowing effect in the photoreceptor layer (black arrows)

2.5.5 Color Doppler imaging

Color Doppler imaging is an ultrasonographic evaluation of the blood flow characteristics of the retrobulbar circulation. Color Doppler studies of acute central retinal artery obstruction show diminished to absent blood flow velocity in the central retinal artery, generally with intact flow in the ophthalmic and choroidal branches (Sharma, 1998). Color Doppler imaging can be used to detect calcific emboli at the lamina cribrosa and also may be used to monitor blood flow changes induced by therapy. In addition, carotid artery studies may be carried out concurrently with ocular blood flow determinations to evaluate the possible causes of the central retinal artery obstruction. It is, however, important to determine the presence of plaques in the inspected vessels that are often the source of microemboli responsible for the occlusive event. In doubtful cases, the above-mentioned physical examination and laboratory testing should be carried out, especially in subjects younger than 40 years of age (Table 2).

2.6 Differential diagnosis

Ocular ischemic syndrome

Purtscher's retinopathy

Severe commotio retinae

Inflammatory or infectious retinitis

2.7 Management

Due to the poor prognosis of retinal artery occlusions, several treatment approaches have been attempted. These can be divided into two major categories: (1) conservative treatment, including mechanical (ocular massage and paracentesis), pharmacologic, and other means; and (2) invasive treatment, including catheterization of the proximal ophthalmic artery, usually through the femoral artery with infusion of thrombolytic agents. Any treatment that results in a statistically higher percentage of visual recovery compared with the spontaneous recovery rate and has a low risk for morbidity and mortality could be considered the treatment of choice (Rumelt & Brown, 2003).

2.7.1 Management of central retinal artery occlusion

Conservative treatment

- First step is arterial vasodilatation using sublingval isosorbid dinitrat, or CO_2 rebreathing in the bag;
- Reduction of intraocular pressure (IOP) and improvement of perfusion by means of antiglaucomatous treatment topically (timolol, etc), systemically (manitol), or surgically by paracenthesis;
    - Ocular massage to move embolus further downstream through artery circulation in distant arterioles. Begin ocular massage with 3-mirror contact lens. Press the lens repeatedly for 10 seconds until the appearance of pulsation; or in the absence of pulsation, until collapse of the retinal blood flow. Observation for improvement of retinal blood flow is made through the lens during the ocular massage. If blood supply improves, ocular massage can be stopped and no further steps are required. If the blood flow does not improve, ocular massage should be continued meticulously for approximately 20 minutes. In addition, treatment prior to 24 hours is more highly to be successful and the success depends on the type of the embolus (calcified are the resistant ones). No light perception is also indication to start treatment. Our experience supports the statement of others that even patients with no light perception may recover (this was also seen in cases of orbital compartment syndrome) (Rumelt et al, 1999);
    - During the ocular massage, administer acetazolamide 500 mg IV;
    - During the ocular massage, administer mannitol 20% 1 mg/kg IV or glycerol 1ml/kg PO;
    - Scleral paracenthesis or anterior chamber paracenthesis – anesthetize the limbus with q-tip soaked with lidocaine 4%, and perform anterior chamber paracentesis with 25-G needle withdrawing 0.2 ml of aqueous humor;
- Antiplatelet therapy (streptokinase 750 000 I.U. IV, urokinase), heparin therapy, isovolemic haemodilution, which basically make no sense if there is no circulation in the occluded artery and agents cannot reach the embolus (Hayreh, 2011);
- Pentoxyfilline injection intravenously to reduce red blood cell rigidity;
- Systemic steroids, in case where CRAO is caused by giant cell arteritis;
- yperbaric oxygenation is one of the promising ways of treatment (Weinberger et al., 2002; Bradvica et al., 2009), which can override the time to artery recanalization. However, there is still need for further evaluation because of the lack of greater randomized studies.

Invasive treatment

- Nd:Yag laser arteriotomy and embolectomy (Opremcak et al., 2008), although this rather invasive treatment frequently caused vitreous hemorrhage and need for vitrectomy, so it requires further evaluation;
- Local intraarterial trombolysis, one of the very enthusiastically announced approaches in CRAO therapy, which is suspended due to a high adverse reactions incidence as

reported by the last European Assessment Group for Lysis in the Eye Study (EAGLE) (Schumacher et al., 2010). Probable reason for the high complication rate was the inexperience of some of the participating physicians. The results and complications were much lower when the procedure was performed by one group (Schmidt et al., 1992; Schumacher et al., 1993).

Since the outcome of invasive treatment depends on the experience of the physician and therefore is not applicable to most centers, the best treatment so far is the conservative multi-step treatment that requires the persistence of the physician (Rumelt et al, 1999).

2.7.2 Management of branch retinal artery occlusion

Management of BRAO depends on the type of occlusion; either it is permanent or transient. In permanent BRAO, like in CRAO there are a lot of advocated treatments but none of them has proven efficient. Transient BRAO does not require any treatment at all except a thorough diagnostics to establish the cause of the occlusion and possibly prevent permanent BRAO from occurring. Nonarteritic cilioretinal artery occlusion (CLRAO) can be treated with any of the procedures described in CRAO treatment. Only arteritic CLRAO associated with giant cell arteritis (GCA) has to be treated with a high dose of steroids, i.e. treat GCA to prevent affecting the other eye and total blindness.

It is important that CRAO and BRAO are both emergencies and any procedures leading to recanalization, or improving the outflow, have to be done urgently inside 97 min from the onset of occlusion (Hayreh et al., 2004), and certainly not after 240 min, because after that time the most part of the retinal tissue function is probably destroyed. It has to be emphasized though that these results are valid for experimental models in primates and for complete occlusion and not for humans that usually have partial obstruction. That is probably the reason why the treatment may be successful even more than 24 hours after the occlusion and the onset of symptoms. Therefore, prevention and education of patients to present immediately to an ophthalmologist or emergency care unit may be the one of the measures of improving the chances of treatment in such patients.

3. Retinal Vein Occlusion

Retinal vein occlusion (RVO) has been recognized as an entity since 1855 (Liebreich, 1855) and is one of the most common causes of acquired retinal vascular abnormality in adults as well as the frequent cause of visual loss. However, the pathogenesis and management of this disorder remains somewhat of an enigma. Current treatments for RVO and its sequelae are still evolving.

CRVO and HCRVO are commonly subdivided into nonischemic and ischemic (hemorrhagic) types according to the degree of obstruction. Ischemic type occurs in more severe (complete) obstruction. Such a distinction is relevant to the clinician, since these two types have very different clinical features, visual outcomes, complications, prognosis and management. Nonischemic RVO is a comparatively benign disease, with central scotoma, essentially due to macular edema, as its major complication, with no risk of ocular neovascularization. Ischemic RVO, by contrast, is a seriously blinding disease, since up to two thirds of patients develop the devastating complications of ischemia, and neovascularization that lead to neovascular glaucoma which causes blindness (Hayreh, 1994).

Retinal vein obstruction is divided into central (CRVO), an occlusion of the central retinal vein resulting in four quadrants of retinal involvement; hemi-central retinal vein occlusion (HCRVO) and branch (BRVO) which consists of major BRVO, an occlusion of either a major branch retinal vein draining one quadrant of the retina, macular BRVO (Hayreh, 1994), an occlusion of a macular branch vein draining a portion of the macula, and peripheral BRVO, an occlusion of a branch retinal vein draining a portion of the retinal periphery. According to the most study data, hemicentral (HCRVO) is an anatomic variant of central retinal vein occlusion (CRVO). Thus, HCRVO acts more like CRVO in terms of risk factors, visual outcome, risk of neovascularization, and response to laser treatment (Appiah & Trempe, 1989). CRVO and BRVO have both differences and similarities in pathophysiology, underlying systemic associations, average age of onset, clinical presentation, prognosis (natural history, complication rate) and treatment.

Furthermore, central and hemi-central occlusion are divided into ischemic and nonischemic subtypes each having different clinical implications and ischemic carrying the risk of developing macular edema and devastating consequences regarding the visual function.

3.1 Epidemiology

The worldwide RVO prevalence, according to the meta-analysis which used pooled data from 15 different international studies involving over than 50,000 participants, ranged from 30 to 101 years, has been calculated per 1000 as follows: 5.20 for any RVO, 4.42 for BRVO, and 0.80 for CRVO. On the basis of these rates, projected to the world population, 16.4 million adults are affected by RVO (Rogers et al., 2010). For comparison, more than 171 million adults with diabetes worldwide either have diabetic retinopathy or are at risk of developing this potentially blinding disease, according to a 2005 World Health Organization report (Wild et al., 2004). An estimated 13.9 million people globally are affected by BRVO and 2.5 million by CRVO. Prevalence varied by race/ethnicity and increased with age, but did not have a sex predilection. The age- and sex-standardized prevalence of any RVO was 3.7 per 1000 in whites, 3.9 per 1000 in blacks, 5.7 per 1000 in Asians, and 6.9 per 1000 in Hispanics. Prevalence of CRVO was lower than BRVO in all ethnic populations. Although BRVO prevalence appears to be highest in Asians and Hispanics and lowest in whites, the authors assume this may reflect differences in the prevalence of RVO risk factors, varying methodologies or definitions among reviewed studies (Rogers et al., 2010). Ischemic central retinal vein obstructions account for 20–25% of all central retinal vein obstructions (Klein et al., 2000).

3.2 Pathophysiology

All types of RVO are multifactorial in origin. A whole host of local and systemic factors acting in different combinations and to different extent may produce the vascular occlusion. The role of the various factors may vary, with some as predisposing factors and other as precipitating ones in one group and vice versa in another. Most investigators accept that BRVO and CRVO represent varying degrees of the same underlying disease process. Yet, other clinicians and researchers argue that ischemic and nonischemic types are distinct clinical entities. It is also essential to understand that CRVO and HCRVO are very different from BRVO pathogenetically. In conclusion, it is a mistake to try to explain all types of RVO by one common pathogenetic mechanism (Hayreh, 1994).

3.2.1 Central Retinal Vein Occlusion

The pathogenesis of CRVO is not fully understood and there are marked controversies on the pathogenesis of ischemic and especially nonischemic CRVO. A combination of vascular, anatomic, and inflammatory factors contributes to its pathophysiology.

The occlusive mechanisms in CRVO are mostly these: (i) external mechanical compression of the vein (i.e. by sclerotic adjacent central retinal artery and common adventitia, especially in elderly persons, structural changes in lamina cribrosa, e.g., glaucomatous cupping, inflammatory swelling in optic nerve and orbital disorders) followed by secondary endothelial proliferation; (ii) primary venous wall disease (degenerative or inflammatory); and (iii) hemodynamic disturbances produced by a variety of factors (e.g., hyperdynamic or sluggish circulation, blood dyscrasias, disturbances on the arterial side, etc.). Consequently, a stagnation of the vein flow occurs and a thrombus formation ensues (Hayreh, 1994; Williamson, 1997).

There are multiple anatomic variations of the branching pattern to the central retinal vein. In 20% of eyes there are, as a congenital abnormality, two trunks of the central retinal vein (CRV) in the optic nerve (instead of the usual one), and the merging of the trunks occurs posterior to the lamina cribrosa (Chopdar, 1984; S. S. Hayreh & M. S. Hayreh, 1980). If one of these trunks is occluded, the result is a nonperfusion to superior or inferior retina. Additionally, the venous outflow from the nasal retina may occur via a branch of one of the temporal branches, rather than an independent nasal vein. In an eye with such a branching pattern, an inferior or superior HCRVO may occur if one the venous branches that drain the nasal and temporal retina is occluded (Sanborn & Magargal, 1984). So, considering the various possible scenarios that can result in a HCRVO, a consensus as to whether HCRVO is a variant of BRVO or CRVO still has not been reached.

CRVO is significantly more common in patients with raised intraocular pressure (IOP) and glaucoma (up to 5- to 10-fold increased risk) (Risk factors for central retinal vein occlusion. The Eye Disease Case-Control Study Group, 1996). To maintain the blood flow, the pressure in the CRV at the optic disc has to be higher than the IOP, otherwise a retinal venous stasis and sluggish venous outflow occur (Hayreh, 2005).

There is much more congruence of the data on the pathogenesis of the ischemic CRVO. Most probably ischemic CRVO represents a more extensive (or complete) obstruction while non-ischemic RCVO represents a milder (partial) obstruction. A conception suggests that the vessels are in a tight compartment within limited space for displacement, because of a common adventitial sheath as CRA and CRV exit the optic nerve head and pass through a narrow opening in the lamina cribrosa. This anatomical position *per se* predisposes to thrombus formation in the central retinal vein. But, CRV has multiple tributaries during its course in the optic nerve, pial outside the optic nerve, none in the lamina cribrosa, and only a small one in the prelaminar region. These tributaries establish anastomoses with the surrounding veins. Since the severity of retinal venous stasis depends upon the site of occlusion in the CRV, and the number of available tributaries anterior to it, the site of the occlusion is likely to be much posteriorly to the lamina cribrosa in nonischemic CRVO than in ischemic CRVO (Hayreh, 2005). There is a possibility of changing nonischemic CRVO to ischemic in some patients, probably due to a further precipitous gradual or sudden fall of perfusion pressure (Hayreh, 1994).

Occlusion of the central retinal vein leads to the retention of the blood in the retinal venous system, and increased resistance to venous blood flow subsequently causes a stagnation of the blood and ischemic damage to the retina. It has been postulated that ischemic damage to the retina stimulates increased production of vascular endothelial growth factor (VEGF) in the vitreous cavity. Increased levels of VEGF stimulate neovascularization of the posterior and anterior segment (responsible for secondary complications due to CRVO). Also, it has been shown that VEGF causes capillary leakage leading to macular edema (which is the leading cause of visual loss in both ischemic CRVO and nonischemic CRVO) (Boyd et al., 2002; Noma et al., 2008; Pe'er et al., 1998).

The prognosis of CRVO depends upon the reestablishment of patency of the venous system by recanalization, dissolution of clot, or formation of optociliary shunt vessels.

3.2.2 Combined Retinal Vein and Artery Occlusion

A central retinal artery obstruction combined with central retinal vein obstruction can occur rarely (Richards, 1979), and the mechanism is probably increased pressure on both central retinal artery and vein. The most common cause for combined CRAO and CRVO is retrobulbar anesthetic injection, caused probably by inadvertent injection into the optic nerve sheath (Torres, 2005). If no CRV tributaries are available anterior to the site of occlusion in the CRVO, it converts the circulation into a closed loop and this results in complete hemodynamic block of the retinal circulation, and secondary CRAO. This condition is invariably diagnosed as simultaneous occlusion of CRA and CRV (Hayreh, 2005). Nonischemic CRVO associated with cilioretinal artery occlusion (CLRAO) is usually a result of transient rise i.e. a functional obstruction of the blood pressure in the entire retinal capillary bed due to a sudden blockage of blood flow by a thrombus in the CRV, which, in turn, results in a physiologic block in the CLRA circulation (Theoulakis et al., 2010). Within a day or two, with the development of venous collaterals by the CRV, the blood pressure in the retinal vascular bed falls, and normal cilioretinal filling occurs. However, the severity of retinal ischemia and associated visual loss depends upon the length of time elapsed before the circulation was re-established (Hayreh, 1994).

3.2.3 Branch Retinal Vein Occlusion

Branch retinal vein occlusion is defined as a focal occlusion of a retinal vein at an arterio-venous crossing site. In all but a few rare cases, the BRVO occurs at crossing sites where the artery is passing anteriorly (superficially) to the vein (Duker & Brown, 1989; Weinberg et al., 1990). The upper temporal vascular arcade is more often involved than the lower temporal vascular arcade. Most BRVOs involve the area inside the temporal vascular arcades (macular BRVO), whereas peripheral BRVOs are more rarely seen, partly because they tend to be asymptomatic (Christoffersen & Larsen, 1999).

The arterio-venous crossing plays an important role in the pathogenesis of BRVO, and the anterior position of the arteriole at the crossing somehow renders the underlying vein vulnerable to occlusion. It seems logical to assume that sclerotic retinal arteriole probably compresses the accompanying vein because of a common thickened, adventitial and glial sheath; however, histopathological studies failed to confirm this view. In addition, turbulent flow may injure the vessel wall exposing it for thrombus formation (Hayreh, 1994; Williamson, 1997).

3.3 Causes

Retinal vascular occlusions all have overlapping clinical presentation as well as the similar underlying causes. They are all multifactorial in origin and each patient may have a unique combination of systemic and local factors leading to the occlusive event (Hayreh, 1994). Since the systemic vascular disease is a possible underlying pathophysiological cause, it is important to ask about history of hypertension, diabetes mellitus, any condition predisposing embolic events (endocarditis, atrial fibrillation, atherosclerotic disease, drug and alcohol abuse, hypercoagulabile states) (Klein et al., 2003; Schmidt et al., 2007). Also, the questions regarding possible trauma as well as the undertaken surgical procedures should not be omitted from the medical history since the prolonged pressure to the globe may lead to the ischemic event.

The well-known risk factors contributing to retinal vein occlusions are systemic vascular diseases. The most recognized risk factors for retinal vein occlusion are hypertension, diabetes mellitus, arteriosclerosis and hyperlipidemia. Also, cigarette smoking has been related to increased risk of RVO. They predominately affect the older age group of patients but the younger patients may also develop this type of retinal occlusive disorder and they account for 10-15% of patients with RVO. Mild central retinal vein obstructions in patients younger than 50 years have been referred to as papillophlebitis or optic disc vasculitis. An inflammatory optic neuritis or vasculitis is hypothesized as the cause (Fong, 1992).

According to the recent studies by Hayreh et al. there may be some difference in the risk factors between CRVO and BRVO, with higher prevalence of hypertension, venous disease, peripheral vascular disease and peptic ulcer in the latter (Hayreh et al., 2001). This suggests that it may not be correct to generalize about these underlying causes for the entire group of retinal vein occlusions.

In addition to well-recognized risk factors, new thrombophilic factors have been investigated in these patients. The role of thrombophilic risk factors in RVO is controversial and the studies are showing conflicting results. Hyperhomocysteinemia as well as low levels of vitamin B_6 and folic acid have been identified as independent risk factors (Sofi et al., 2008; Taubert, 2008). Other potential risk factors include elevated factor V Leiden, protein C or S deficiency, anti-cardiolipin antibodies or lupus anticoagulant. Blood dyscrasias and dysproteinemias result in hyperviscosity syndromes, which may appear similar to central retinal vein obstruction but possibly represent curable disease. Hyperviscosity syndromes may produce a bilateral retinopathy similar to central retinal vein obstruction and may, in fact, induce a true central retinal vein obstruction with thrombus formation (Bandello et al., 1994). Simultaneous bilateral disease is an unusual finding in central retinal vein obstructions but occurs more commonly in hypercoagulabile and hyperviscous states. Diseases such as sickle cell disease, polycythemia vera, leukemia, and multiple myeloma are but a few of the possibilities. When there is a patient with bilateral central retinal vein obstructions, especially simultaneous, the medical and laboratory evaluation should include a search for evidence of hyperviscous and hypercoagulabile syndromes (Marcucci et al., 2001) Severe anemia with thrombocytopenia can masquerade as a central retinal vein obstruction, and it is differentiated from a central retinal vein obstruction by a complete blood count with platelets.

In combined central retinal vein occlusion with branch retinal artery occlusion systemic associations other than hypertension and diabetes have not been confirmed. In combination with central retinal artery occlusion associated systemic or local disease is the rule—collagen vascular disorders, leukemia, orbital trauma, retrobulbar injections, and mucormycosis have been implicated (Jorizzo, 1987).

Oral contraceptive use in women may be associated with both thromboembolic disease and central retinal vein obstruction (Stowe et al., 1978). In addition, acute hypertensive retinopathy with disc edema may resemble bilateral central retinal vein obstruction. Obstructive sleep apnea affects more patients with retinal vein obstruction than other disorders and treatment of the sleep apnea may help prevent central vein obstruction (Glacet-Bernard et al., 2010). Other rare associations include closed-head trauma, optic disc drusen, and arteriovenous malformations of retina.

The Eye Disease Case-Control Study Group reported that the risk of CRVO is decreased in men with increased levels of physical activity and increased alcohol consumption (Risk factors for central retinal vein occlusion. The Eye Disease Case-Control Study Group, 1996). The same study group reported a decreased risk of CRVO with the use of postmenopausal estrogens and an increased risk with higher erythrocyte sedimentation rates in women.

An ocular risk factor for the development of central retinal vein occlusion is raised intraocular pressure; the risk of central retinal vein occlusion in glaucoma patients is 5-fold to 10-fold increase (Risk factors for central retinal vein occlusion. The Eye Disease Case-Control Study Group, 1996). Unlike CRVO and HCRVO, glaucoma plays no role in the pathogenesis of BRVO (Hayreh, 1994).

In ischemic CRVO, for example, neovascular glaucoma develops in about 45%. The chronic hypoxia of the retinal tissue induces ocular neovascularization by producing the vasoproliferative factor, which is the proposed mechanism in CRVO whereas in CRAO, there is acute retinal ischemia and infarction responsible for the occlusive event. Also a surprisingly small proportion of patients (2.5%) have the course of illness complicated with neovascular glaucoma (Hayreh, 2011).

3.4 Clinical presentation

3.4.1 Symptoms

Retinal vein occlusion is characterized by painless unilateral loss of vision. It may be subtle in character, with intermittent episodes of blurred vision. In other cases, it may be sudden and dramatic. The nonischemic type is often the more subtle of the two, while the ischemic type is prone to the more acute clinical presentations and may be accompanied by pain.

Ischemic CRVO Acute, markedly decreased visual acuity ranged from 20/200 (6/60) to hand-motion is the usual initial complaint. A prominent afferent pupillary defect is typical. Pain at the time of evaluation may occur if neovascular glaucoma already had developed.

Nonischemic CRVO The majority of patients with central retinal vein obstruction (75–80%) fall into nonischemic form. Patients usually have mild to moderate decreased visual acuity, although this can vary from normal to as poor as the finger counting. Transient visual obscuration may also be a complaint.

Branch retinal vein occlusion is characterized by painless decrease in vision on the affected eye and some patients may have a scotoma.

Combined Retinal Vein and Artery Occlusion Such patients present with acute, severe loss of vision, usually to bare or no light perception. The visual prognosis is generally poor.

3.4.2 Signs

The distinction between the ischemic and nonischemic type is important, because they carry a totally different prognosis regarding visual recovery and potential complication, which may result in permanent visual deterioration.

Both types of central retinal vein obstruction, ischemic and nonischemic, have similar fundoscopic findings—dilated, tortuous retinal veins and retinal hemorrhages in all four quadrants, optic disc swelling, cotton wool spots and macular edema (Fig. 5). Hemorrhages can be superficial, dot and blot, and/or deep. They may vary in severity, covering the whole fundus and sometimes even obscuring retinal and choroidal details, or can be limited to the peripheral fundus only. Vitreous hemorrhage may ensue when bleeding breaks through the internal limiting membrane. The optic disc is usually edematous during the early-stage disease, but the edema may persist in chronic cases (Ehlers & Fekrat, 2011). Many or all of the pathological retinal findings may resolve over the 6–12 months following diagnosis. The resolution of retinal hemorrhages may be complete whereas the optic nerve may appear normal, but optociliary collateral vessels are common finding. In spite the resolution of macular edema, a persistent cystoid macular edema can linger and result in permanent visual loss, often leading to pigmentary changes, epiretinal membrane formation, or subretinal fibrosis.

Ischemic CRVO The presence of cotton-wool spots located around the posterior pole is characteristic of and more common with ischemic CRVO (Fig. 6.). In ischemic CRVO, the ganglion cells in the macular retina are irreversibly damaged by ischemia during the initial stages of the disease; therefore, there is little chance of improvement of visual acuity in such an eye. The distinction between the two types of vein obstructions remains somewhat arbitrary and is based on the total area of nonperfusion on fluorescein angiography. However, dense intraretinal hemorrhage in acute stages may block retinal fluorescence and renders it impossible to determine the extent of retinal nonperfusion. Therefore, it is important to take into account other clinical features such as poor initial visual acuity, the presence of an afferent pupillary defect, neovascularization as well as the functional tests – visual field testing (Goldmann) and electroretinography (ERG) to establish the perfusion status of the retina (Hayreh et al., 2011). In central retinal vein obstruction, perfusion of the inner retina is affected, so that the amplitude of the b-wave is decreased relative to the a-wave; the b-to-a ratio has been shown to be reduced. Some studies indicate that a b-to-a ratio of less than 1 suggests an ischemic central retinal vein obstruction (Matsui et al., 1994). It is only the ischemic CRVO eye which is at risk of developing ocular neovascularization (Hayreh et al., 1983; Natural history and clinical management of central retinal vein occlusion. The Central Vein Occlusion Study Group, 1997). The incidence of anterior segment neovascularization in ischemic central retinal vein obstruction is 60% or higher and has been documented as early as 9 weeks after onset of an occlusive event. The greatest risk of developing anterior segment neovascularization is during the first 7 months, after which the risk of dreaded complication of neovascular glaucoma falls dramatically to minimal. Neovascularization of the optic disc and retinal neovascularization may be seen as well, but they are less common. As with nonischemic central retinal vein obstruction, the findings may decrease or resolve 6–12 months after diagnosis. The anterior segment structures may show signs of ischemia: congestion of the conjunctival and ciliary vessels, corneal edema, iris and anterior chamber angle neovascularization with development of synechial changes predisposing the development of secondary glaucoma.

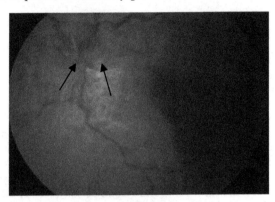

Fig. 6. Central retinal vein occlusion; dilated, tortuous retinal veins and retinal hemorrhages in all four quadrants, optic disc swelling (arrows), cotton wool spots and macular edema

Nonischemic CRVO Neovascularization of either the anterior or posterior segment is rare in a true nonischemic central retinal vein obstruction (less than 2% incidence), although conversion from an initially nonischemic vein obstruction to the ischemic variety is fairly common. The Central Vein Occlusion Study Group noted that 34% of nonischemic central retinal vein occlusions (CRVOs) progressed to become ischemic within 3 years and 15% of the study group converted within the first 4 months (Natural history and clinical management of central retinal vein occlusion. The Central Vein Occlusion Study Group, 1997).

Hemicentral RVO In hemicentral retinal vein obstruction venous outflow from the superior or inferior parts of retina is impaired. Although they involve half of the retina, in terms of visual outcome, the risk of neovascularization, and response to the laser treatment, they resemble the ischemic variant of the disease.

Branch retinal vein occlusion (Fig. 7.) Intraretinal hemorrhages (usually flame shaped), retinal edema, and cotton-wool spots are seen in the distribution of a retinal vessel.

Papillophlebitis The characteristic finding is optic disc edema out of proportion to the retinal findings, cotton-wool spots that ring the optic disc, and occasionally cilioretinal artery obstructions or even partial central retinal artery obstructions. Although spontaneous improvement occurs, the course is not always benign. Approximately 30% of these patients may develop the ischemic type of occlusion, a final visual acuity of 20/200 in nearly 40% of these subjects, and neovascular glaucoma has been reported (Fong, 1992).

Combined Retinal Vein and Artery Occlusion Examination shows a cherry-red spot combined with features of a central retinal vein obstruction, which include dilated, tortuous veins that have retinal hemorrhages in all four quadrants (Fig. 8.). The risk of neovascularization of the iris is about 75%. Exceptionally, a patient may manifest spontaneous improvement (Jorizzo, 1987). Branch retinal artery obstruction combined with simultaneous central retinal vein obstruction has also been reported. This rare entity behaves as a central retinal vein obstruction. Neovascularization of the iris is possible.

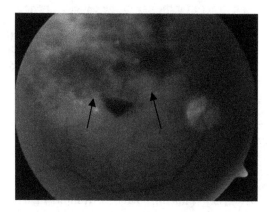

Fig. 7. Branch retinal vein occlusion; note hemorrhages and edema in superior temporal quadrant (arrows)

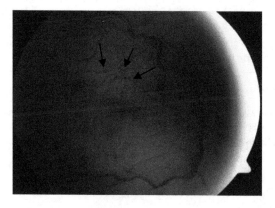

Fig. 8. Combined branch retinal artery occlusion (BRAO) and central retinal vein occlusion (CRVO) of the right eye, ischemia involving superior macular branches (arrows), optic disc swelling, tortuous veins and dot and blot hemorrhages

3.5 Evaluation and imaging

3.5.1 Systemic evaluation

Given the heterogenity of risk factors and their possible interaction in these subjects, the following algorithm of patients with RVO is proposed in the Table 2. As for the arterial occlusive retinal disease, these tests should be performed in younger patients and in doubtful cases.

We feel that, as with the arterial occlusive disease, the stepwise approach to each patient should be tailored, taking into account the age of the patient. Therefore the investigations in the patients older than 50 years of age should consist of: cardiovascular risk assessment, ECG, carotid and vertebral artery Doppler color imaging, echocardiogram; the lab tests including full blood count, erythrocyte sedimentation rate, C reactive protein, fasting blood glucose, lipidogram. The younger patients should be evaluated for thrombophilia, hyperviscosity syndromes, screening for autoimmune diseases and women should be asked about the use of oral contraceptives. Of course, other possible causes of retinal vein occlusions should be considered in cases of normal findings and the investigations should be expanded in stepwise approach, since each case may have a unique combination of risk factors and underlying causes.

Cardiovascular risk factors assessment
(diabetes, hypertension, smoking   habitus, dyslipidemia, BMI)
ECG
Carotid and vertebral artery Doppler color imaging
Echocardiogram
(transthoracic, transesophageal in selected cases)
Lab tests
(complete blood count, fasting glucose, lipidogram, autoimmune screen in
selected cases: ANA, anti ENA, anti DNA; homocysteine level, folic acid,
vitamin B12 and B6, antiphospholipid antibodies)
Thrombophilia assessment in subjects younger than 50 years (factor V Leiden,
antithrombin, protein C, protein S)

Table 2. Proposed systemic work-up in RVO patients

Although most cases are diagnosed straightforward from the fundus appearance, the following ancillary tests may be undertaken to distinguish between ischemic or milder, nonischemic form, which is very important in terms of the treatment options as well as the natural course and visual prognosis of the patients.

3.5.2 Fluorescein angiography

Arteriolar filling is usually normal, but venous filling in the affected vessel is usually delayed in the acute phase. Hypofluorescence caused by hemorrhage and capillary nonperfusion are common findings, and dilated, tortuous veins are seen (Fig. 9a.). The retinal vessels, particularly the vein walls, may stain with fluorescein, especially at the site of the occlusion (Fig.10.). The very important distinction should be made between neovascular fronds, which may show profuse leakage of dye, vs. collateral vessels, which do not leak fluorescein. Cystoid macular edema (Fig. 9b.) appears in the late stage of the angiogram shows typically petaloid pattern and may involve the entire fovea or just several clock hours, depending on the distribution of the obstruction. It is, however, important to emphasize that in early stages the retinal angiograms may be misleading because of the masking by abundant hemorrhages and the fact that retinal capillary obliteration is a progressive phenomenon which takes at least 3-4 weeks or even longer to develop after the occurrence of ischemic CRVO (Hayreh, 1994).

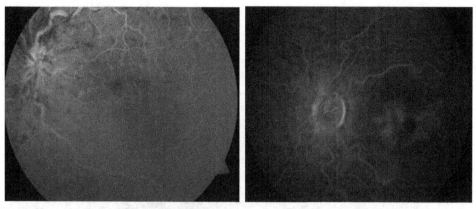

Fig. 9. Fluorescein angiogram of the left eye with central retinal vein occlusion a and b. a) staining of blood vessel walls, disc hyperfluorescence and blockage from intraretinal hemorrhage b) the late stages of angiogram shows leakage of dye in cystoid macular edema, with characteristic "petaloid" appearance.

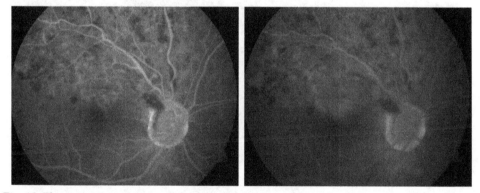

Fig. 10. Fluorescein angiogram of the right eye with superior branch retinal vein occlusion a and b. a) blockage of dye with hemorrhages, mottled areas of intraretinal leakage and microaneurysm formation with vascular teleangiectasia in the upper parts b) the late stages of angiogram shows further diffuse leakage of dye, through all layers of the retina, affecting the macular region as well.

3.5.3 Optical coherence tomography

The optical coherence tomograms show increase in the retinal thickness, which is seen as a loss of macular contour. In the area of edematous retina the presence of cystoids spaces denotes the existence of cystoid macular edema (Fig. 11.). The retinal hemorrhages, subretinal fluid accumulation, cotton wool spots and optic disc edema may also be visualized on OCT. OCT is useful in the management and treatment of the macular edema; it also offers certain advantages over angiograms because it quantifies the macular thickness useful in monitoring the response to treatment and gives valuable data on distribution of the fluid, is not invasive and has no potentially serious side effects. There have been some disputes whether the macular thickness correlates significantly with visual acuity (Nussenblatt et al., 1987). What counts is the improvement in visual functions and not the anatomy. Several factors were predictive of better visual acuity outcomes and more favorable OCT outcomes, including younger age and shorter duration of macular edema, respectively. These factors may assist clinicians in predicting disease course for patients with CRVO and BRVO (Scott et al., 2011). Loss of foveal IS/OS junction line and absence of inner retinal layers in late stage significantly correlated with poorer visual outcome. Macular ischemia by fluorescein angiography shows significant correlation with thinner central subfield thickness, loss of inner retinal layers (Lima, 2011).

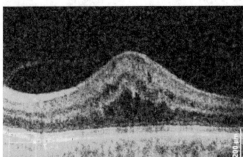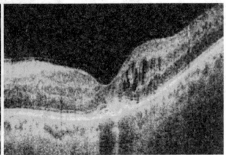

Fig. 11 a and b. Optical coherence tomography (OCT) changes of eye with central retinal vein occlusion a) Cystoid macular edema prior to anti-VEGF injection; b) Cystoid macular edema after anti-VEGF injection treatment Cross-section goes through inferior retina to superior retina, capturing the abnormally thickened retina associated with intracellular edema.

3.6 Differential diagnosis

Hypertensive retinopathy

Diabetic retinopathy

Ocular ischemic syndrome

Juxtafoveal retinal telangiectasia

Radiation retinopathy

Retinal artery occlusion

Retinal detachment

Vitreous hemorrhage

3.7 Management

Some treatments have addressed the venous outflow and the majority the sequelae of the venous occlusion (i.e. cystoid macular edema, neovascularization). In the following text the advocated treatment options are discussed.

3.7.1 Management of branch retinal vein occlusion

Etiology treatment

- Isovolemic hemodilution, used to lower plasma viscosity and to improve retinal perfusion. However, the true benefit of hemodilution has not been established because the published reports have used a combination therapy in the hemodilution groups ;
- Laser chorioretinal venous anastomosis, performed to bypass the occluded site by inducing a communication between the involved branch vein and the choroidal circulation by placing a laser burn directly on the vein and then on the adjacent Bruch's membrane. During the healing process, a chorioretinal anastomosis may form. The technique is studied on CRVO patient, but the small number of BRVO case series were reported (Bavbek et al., 2005; Fekrat et al., 1998);
- Pars plana vitrectomy and arteriovenous sheathotomy. Arteriovenous sheathotomy, in which the retinal vein and artery are surgically separated at the arteriovenous crossing by cutting the common adventitial sheath bare the same idea of improving perfusion. Several small, uncontrolled series have shown good results in improving macular edema and macular perfusion. However, others have reported a lack of efficacy of this procedure (Le Rouic et al., 2001; Cahill et al., 2003).

Sequelae treatment

- Grid laser photocoagulation. The Branch Vein Occlusion Study (BVOS) demonstrated the efficacy of grid laser photocoagulation in the treatment of BRVO-related macular edema. According to the study, grid photocoagulation performed in the first 12 months of onset of the occlusion can, compared to the natural course, improved the response almost twice (Argon laser photocoagulation for macular edema in branch vein occlusion. The Branch Vein Occlusion Study Group, 1984) Argon laser grid or sector treatment result in resolution of the edema but do not improve visual acuity;
- Sector Scatter Retinal Laser Photocoagulation. This treatment was also evaluated during the BVOS study in the ability of preventing the development of neovascularization and vitreous hemorrhage in the BRVO. It is recommended that scatter photocoagulation should be used in BRVO, if and when neovascularization occurs (Argon laser scatter photocoagulation for prevention of neovascularization and vitreous hemorrhage in branch vein occlusion. A randomized clinical trial. Branch Vein Occlusion Study Group, 1986);
- Intravitreal corticosteroids, using a long lasting corticosteroid such as triamcinolone (IVTA), or biodegradable carrier containing dexamethasone to manage macular edema. SCORE study was conducted to compare IVTA versus standard of care, i.e. grid-pattern macular photocoagulation (Scott et al., 2009). The results of this study suggest that both procedures have a similar effect on resolving macular edema and improving visual acuity, but IVTA has more side effects (increasing IOP, cataract progression). In a randomized pilot study of subjects with cystoid macular edema (CME) secondary to BRVO, the increase in visual acuity was significantly greater in those treated with combination of IVTA and grid-pattern laser photocoagulation than in the eyes treated with grid-pattern laser alone, suggesting that IVTA can be effective as an adjunctive treatment to laser (Parodi et al., 2008). Allergan conducted an international study at 167 centers in 24 countries on the effect of intravitreal dexamethasone sustained release delivery system (Ozurdex). The data for the first 6 months was released (Haller et al., 2010). It appears that visual acuity was significantly better in the group of patients who received 0.7 mg dexamethasone implant than in the control group after 60 and 90 days, but is similar 180 days after the treatment. Ozurdex received FDA approval for treatment of macular edema

secondary to BRVO in 2009. An implantable fluocinolone acetonide (Retisert, Bausch and Lomb, Rochester, NY), at present being registered for the intravitreal treatment of chronic non-infectious uveitis, is also being evaluated for the treatment of BRVO and CRVO. The beneficial effect of intravitreal corticosteroids is limited in time and repeated treatment is associated with the accumulation of the complications including steroid-induced glaucoma, cataract, endophthalmitis and retinal detachment. IOP sparing corticosteroids may only prevent glaucoma but not the other side-effects;

- Intravitreal Anti-Vascular Endothelial Growth Factor. It was noticed that VEGF plays a substantial role in the development of CME and neovascular complication in RVO patients. The first intravitreally used drug was bevacizumab, originally developed for the intravenous treatment of colorectal carcinoma metastases, but widely used for treating RVO complications and other retinal disorders (e.g. diabetic macular edema, age related macular degeneration). Several studies have reported a decrease in retinal thickness and improved visual acuity after receiving bevacizumab (Kreutzer et al., 2008; Kriechbaum et al., 2008; Pai et al., 2007). Visual acuity usually increased to maximum in 3-6 weeks after the injections (Stahl et al., 2007). A subsequent decrease in visual acuity appeared to be closely related to an increase in CME. Early recurrence of CME should prompt consideration for retreatment. The most appropriate timing interval between injections is still unclear. The other anti-VEGF agents on the market are pegaptanib, the first FDA approved intravitreal agent (for the treatment of neovascular age-related macular degeneration - ARMD) and ranibizumab, the first FDA approved agent for the treatment of not only ARMD but also macular edema caused by BRVO, based on the results of BRAVO study. Results of phase III BRAVO study show us that after six monthly intravitreal injections of ranibizumab 55% (0.3mg group), and 61% (0.5mg group) gain more than 15 letters, compared to 28.8% in the control group. Also a central foveal thickness decreased by 158 microns in the control group versus 337 microns in the 0.3 mg group and by 345 microns in the 0.5 mg group. Adverse events are rare - one retinal detachment in the 0.3 mg group, one endophthalmitis and one myocardial infarction in 0.5 mg group, and one stroke in the control group. According to our experience as well as numerous other authorities it is doubtfull that myocardial infarction and stroke are caused by the local treatment with anti-VEGF, since they are most prominent in the older population which is prone to these conditions (Rosenfeld, 2006). After six months the control group received intravitreal ranibizumab on as needed basis; i.e. if macular edema occurs. Therefore, the long-term results remain unknown. We can say that, according to this data, the use of anti-VEGF agents become an important option in macular edema treatment secondary to BRVO;

- Pars plana vitrectomy with removal of the posterior hyaloid is effective in resolving CME (only if the traction is the cause of retinal edema and usually if the duration of the edema is less than 6 months) and improving visual acuity (Figueroa et al., 2004). Due to complications associated with these procedures, such as vitreous hemorrhage, intraoperative retinal tears, rhegmatogenous retinal detachment and cataract development, they are not often in use.

3.7.2 Management of central retinal vein occlusion

Etiology treatment

- Isovolemic hemodilution. Several studies have suggested the presence of abnormal blood viscosity in CRVO patients. Based on that assumption, some authors have advocated the use of hemodilution in CRVO, but other (Hayreh, 2003) claim that there is little scientifically valid evidence of beneficial effects of this therapy;

- Anticoagulant and antiplatelet therapy. Although no clear ocular benefit of antithrombotic drugs has been demonstrated, antiplatelet drugs (e.g. aspirin) are prescribed for many patients, including CRVO patients. Hayreh (Hayreh, 2002) claims that this therapy as well as the anticoagulant therapy, such as recombinant tissue plasminogen activator (rt-PA), is contraindicated and even harmful for CRVO patients. Some authors have tried local application of rt-PA into retinal branch vein but the results are controversial and complication rate (haemophtalmus, neovascular glaucoma, retinal detachment, eye phthysis) is unacceptably high; rt-PA should penetrate the retina to exert its activity
- Chorioretinal venous anastomosis. The techniques explained earlier may create an anastomosis, but also carry significant risks. Given the variable success rate, these techniques are rarely employed;
- Surgical decompression of the retinal vein. Proposed procedures can be divided into two mayor types; the first is the vitrectomy with radial optic neurotomy, in which a surgeon's approach is from inside the globe, and the second is optic nerve sheet decompression using orbital "outer" approach. Because of the danger and invasiveness of the procedures and the lack of scientific explanation (Hayreh et al., 2002), there is a need for a larger study to eventually find a place for these procedures in the management of CRVO.

Treatment directed at sequelae

- When speaking of sequelae treatment, we have to add an antiglaucomatous treatment as needed if increase of IOP occurs. Local medical therapy such as, β-blocker (timolol 0,5%), α-2 agonists (brimonidine 0'1-0,2%), carbonic anhydrase inhibitor (acetazolamide, dorzolamide) and panretinal photocoagulation. If failed, the other method of treatment has to be applied such as (i) trabeculectomy with antimetabolites as a first step when there is potential to improve state, (ii) aqueous shunt implants as a second step, and (iii) diode laser cyclophotocoagulation or retinal cryoablation , and in the worst case, with no vision and the patient suffering from great pain, (iv) evisceration or enucleation should be considered (Sivak-Callcott et al., 2001);
- Grid-pattern laser photocoagulation. According to CVOS study, these procedures have no beneficial effect on the visual outcome in macular edema due to CRVO, either ischemic or non-ischemic;
- Scatter panretinal laser photocoagulation. It has been almost universally accepted that prophylactic panretinal photocoagulation (PRP) is the treatment of choice to prevent neovascular glaucoma or treat neovascular glaucoma itself in ischemic CRVO. CVOS study revealed that there is no benefit of the prophylactic PRP in the eyes with ischemic CRVO. These results have led to the recommendation that PRP should be applied promptly after the identification of intraocular neovascularization in eyes with ischemic CRVO to minimize the risk of the development of neovascular glaucoma;
- Corticosteroids. Steroids reduce vascular permeability and stabilize the blood-retina barrier. The mechanism for these effects involves inhibition of the production of inflammatory mediators and vascular permeability factors (e.g. VEGF) as well as the stabilization of the vascular endothelial cell tight junctions. The inhibition of VEGF production may further help prevent neovascular sequelae. Some authors have proposed for some patients the systemic use of corticosteroids (Hayreh, 2010) in high

oral doses of about 80 mg of prednisone to control macular edema, which is the main cause of visual loss. Most of the patients with CRVO according to the SCORE study respond to intravitreal triamcinolone application of either 1 or 4 mg doses compared to the standard care in terms of improving visual acuity of more than 15 letters. As far as the safety is concerned, there are more complications such as cataract formation and IOP elevation in the triamcinolone group. Complications rate is higher in the group with higher dose (4 mg) (Ip et al., 2009). Although triamcinolone is a long lasting corticosteroid, it appears that it is not enough and it leads to the development of sustained corticosteroid delivery devices, which release the drug longer. One of them is Retisert which has good results in chronic refractory CME (Ramchandran et al., 2008), with the best results 12 month after injection. However, the complication rates are very high - all phakic eyes developed visually significant cataracts, and 92% have had an elevation of IOP that needed intervention. Allergan conducted an international study on dexamethasone sustained delivery devices (Ozurdex) and the six month results have been published. In CRVO subgroup of patients a significantly better result in gaining visual acuity (more than 15 letters) has been recorded in the group which received 0.7 mg implant compared with control group at 30 and 60 days control point, and not significantly better at 90 and 180 days point. There were no significant differences in cataract formation between groups and ocular hypertension occurred in only 4% of patients receiving an implant. In 2009 FDA gave approval for the Ozurdex in the treatment of macular edema secondary to CRVO;

- Intravitreal anti vascular endothelial growth factor (anti-VEGF). As VEGF plays a key role in the pathophysiology of CRVO, several anti-VEGF treatments have been developed to decrease VEGF and block vascular permeability and angiogenic activity (bevacizumab, ranibizumab, pegaptanib). According to the results of CRUISE study, FDA released approval of intravitreal ranibizumab for the treatment of CRVO (Brown et al., 2010);

- In cases of refractory CME secondary to CRVO with no resolution after bevacizumab or IVTA individually, a combination treatment with both agents may result in resolution of CME and significant recovery of visual acuity (Ehlers & Fekrat, 2011; Ekdawi & Bakri, 2007). These results suggest that for some patients, the complementary actions of bevacizumab and IVTA on VEGF and inflammation may be more effective than either therapy used alone in the treatment of RVO. Further studies examining multi-modal therapy are needed to answer these questions regarding optimal therapy. Probably a combined treatment or new drugs will have a better efficacy.

4. Ocular Ischemic Syndrome

Obstructions more proximal to the central retinal artery usually cause a more chronic form of visual problem – the ocular ischemic syndrome. Ocular ischemic syndrome (OIS) is a condition that has a variable spectrum of signs and symptoms that result from chronic ocular insufficiency, usually secondary to severe carotid artery disease (CAD). Moreover, they may be the first manifestations of CAD (Dugan & Green, 1991). OIS was firstly described in 1963 and named *venous stasis retinopathy* (Hedges, 1963; Kearns & Hollenhorst, 1963).

4.1 Epidemiology

The OIS occurs at a mean age of 65 years and generally does not develop before 50 years of age. Men outnumber women by a ratio of 2:1, because of the higher incidence of atherosclerosis in men (Brown & Magargal, 1988). No racial predilection exists. Bilaterally OIS occurs up to 22% of cases (Mendrinos et al., 2010). The incidence of OIS is not known precisely, but is estimated at 7.5 cases per million people annually (Sturrock & Mueller, 1984).

Different studies found various incidence of OIS development in patients with hemodynamically significant CAD, which is 4%, 18%, and 1.5% respectively (Kearns & Hollenhorst, 1963; Kearns et al., 1978; Klijn et al., 2002). Ipsilateral transient monocular visual loss is the hallmark of carotid insufficiency and occurs in 30-40% of patients with CAD. CAD on the one common (CCA) or internal carotid artery (ICA) is often accompanied by occlusion or stenosis of the opposite carotid artery (Mendrinos et al., 2010).

4.2 Pathophysiology and causes

Both stenosis and occlusion of the common or internal carotid arteries are responsible for ipsilateral ocular signs and symptoms that may herald a devastating cerebral infarction (Biousse, 1997). The decreased vascular perfusion results in tissue hypoxia and increased ocular ischemia, leading to neovascularization (Leibovitch et al., 2009; Kahn et al., 1986; Takaki et al., 2008).

Patients who develop OIS show decreased blood flow in the retrobulbar vessels and reversal of blood flow in the ophthalmic artery (OA) (Mendrinos et al., 2010). OA shunts blood flow away from the eye to the low-resistance intracranial circuit. This blood steal leads to further reduction of retrobulbar blood flow, hypoperfusion, and subsequently ocular ischemia.

OIS develops especially in patients with poor collateral circulation between the internal and external arterial systems or between the two ICAs. The occurrence of cerebral infarctions and poor neurologic prognosis could also be explained by the insufficient collateral circulation.

4.3 Clinical presentation

Ocular ischemic syndrome encompasses a spectrum of ocular signs and symptoms that are the result of ocular hypoperfusion caused by severe carotid artery obstruction.

4.3.1 Symptoms

The presenting symptom is a variable degree of visual loss often accompanied by pain caused either by ischemia of the globe or elevated intraocular pressure in neovascular glaucoma. The natural course of the ischemic syndrome is generally poor, although there is certain proportion of cases with milder clinical picture retaining the visual function.

4.3.2 Signs

The anterior segment signs are often present: neovascularization of the iris in approximately two thirds of eyes at the time of initial examination; corneal edema and striae usually concurrent with increased pressure from neovascular glaucoma. Although the iris neovascularization is the presenting sign in large percentage of patients with ischemic syndrome, only one third of cases develop secondary neovascular glaucoma. This may be due to a lower arterial supply of the ciliary body causing hypotony or normal pressure in spite neovascular changes in the iridocorneal angle. There may be signs of mild anterior chamber reaction in 20% of these eyes with flare being a more prominent feature than the cellular response (Kahn et al., 1986). Advanced lens opacification may also be present in the late stages of this syndrome. The fundoscopic findings may mimic other vascular retinal disorders and involutive changes seen in elderly population: constriction, straightening and narrowing of the arteries, dilated retinal veins, but without accentuated tortuosity commonly seen in vein occlusions. Venous beading may resemble features of proliferative diabetic retinopathy. In the majority of cases there are dot and blot retinal hemorrhages distributed diffusely around the periphery, but they can spread onto the posterior pole. The other features of retinal ischemia may also be present: cherry red spot appearance, cotton wool exudates, optic atrophy and edema.

4.4 Evaluation and imaging

A careful clinical examination and lab tests (ESR, CRP) must be undertaken to exclude possible temporal arteritis, which may resemble this clinical entity and mandates different diagnostic and therapeutic approach, which may prevent further visual loss and potentially blindness.

4.4.1 Fluorescein and indocyanine green angiography

Besides clinical examination, fluorescein angiography (FA) can help to establish the diagnosis of ocular ischemic syndrome. Prolonged choroidal filling time is the most specific angiographic sign of ocular ischemic syndrome (Mendrinos et al., 2010). Patchy filling of the choroid that lasts more than 5 seconds is seen in about 60% of eyes affected by ocular ischemic syndrome (Brown & Margargal, 1998). Staining of the retinal vessels, both the major vessels and its branches, is another sign seen in 85% of eyes with ocular ischemic syndrome. Demonstration of a well-demarcated leading edge of fluorescein dye within a retinal artery is a typical sign of OIS. Other findings on fluorescein angiography include an increased arteriovenous transit time (over 11 seconds), macular edema, retinal capillary nonperfusion, and evidence of microaneurysms (especially in the periphery) (Richard et al., 1998).

Indocyanine green angiography (ICG) shows signs of choroidal hypoperfusion – occlusion of choriocapillaries with filling defects in the posterior pole or the mid-periphery. There is also prolonged arm to choroid (over 10 seconds) and intrachoroidal circulation time (over 5-6 seconds). Another characteristic finding is slow filling of the watershed zones of the choroids) (Richard et al., 1998).

4.4.2 Electroretinography

Electroretinography demonstrates a decrease in both a and b waves in these eyes, which is in contrast to the sparing of the a wave found in central retinal artery occlusions (Brown et al., 1982).

It is of paramount role to assess the carotid artery function since the endarterectomy procedure reduces the risk of stroke as life threatening consequence and there is some evidence of improvement in retinal function viewed through the improvement of a and b waves in electroretinography, as well as the normalization of preoperative retrograde ophthalmic artery flow shown on Doppler color imaging (Kawaguchi et al., 2001; Story et al., 1995).

4.4.3 Duplex carotid ultrasonography

Duplex carotid ultrasonography combines B-mode ultrasound and Doppler ultrasound providing the morphologic imaging and flow velocity data. It is the most commonly used noninvasive method in evaluation of carotid artery obstruction.

Color Doppler imaging is a noninvasive tool for assessing the velocity of blood flow in the retrobulbar circulation. Diminished velocities of the blood flow in the central retinal artery, choroidal vessels, and ophthalmic artery are typical. There may be a reversal of flow in the ophthalmic artery, as well. Color Doppler imaging may assess the carotid arteries simultaneously.

4.4.4 Invasive diagnostics

If noninvasive carotid artery evaluation is unremarkable in an eye that shows signs suggestive of ocular ischemia, conventional carotid arteriography or digital subtraction angiography may be required to detect possible chronic obstruction of the ophthalmic artery (Wardlaw et al., 2006).

The new minimally invasive methods, magnetic resonance angiography and computed tomographic angiography are evolving and improving as adjunctive diagnostic tests in evaluating the patients with carotid occlusive disease.

4.5 Differential diagnostic

Diabetic retinopathy

Nonischemic central retinal venous occlusions

Giant cell arteritis

Takayasu arteritis

Ischemic optic neuropathy

Retinal artery occlusion

Neovascular glaucoma

4.6 Management

Management of OIS is basically multidisciplinary and the task of the ophthalmologist is to treat ocular condition, recognize the possible cause of OIS and refer the patient to a cardiologist, neurologist or other specialists, where they can get proper treatment of the cause of OIS.

Ophthalmology treatment consists of increased IOP control, management of neovascularization and control of anterior segment inflammation.

- Anterior segment inflammation is usually treated with topical steroids and long acting cycloplegic agents;
- Increased IOP, usually controlled with topical β-adrenergics blockers, ɑ-agonists and topical or oral carbonic anhydrase inhibitors to reduce aqueous production; prostaglandins (could increase ocular inflammation) and pilocarpin should be avoided;

- Ocular neovascularization following carotid occlusive disease is usually managed with panretinal photocoagulation and can prevent neovascular glaucoma (Carter, 1984; Chen et al., 2001). If PRP is not possible due to media opacities or refractory miosis, other modalities such as transconjunctival cryotherapy of peripheral retina or transscleral diode laser retinopexy should be considered to prevent neovascularization. In any case, PRP works effectively and reduces the iris neovascularization in only 36% of patients with OIS (Sivalingam et al., 1991). In other cases it can even get worse (Turut & Malthieu, 1986), which suggests that uveal ischemia can induce neovascularization, as it is shown on animal model (Hayreh & Baines, 1973). Therefore, in the cases where there is retinal ischemia, prophylactic PRP is advisable. Neovascularization and macular edema caused by OIS can be also treated with intravitreal bevacizumab (Amselem et al., 2007). In this case report neovascularization regressed, but there was no improvement in VA or IOP. Macular edema can also be treated with triamcinolone intravitreally, reducing macular edema and improving visual acuity (Klais & Spaide, 2004). Further investigation with a more reliable sample is needed to establish the role of this therapy in IOS patient. Additionally, we have to mention that when neovascular glaucoma occurs it is usually refractory to medical therapy and if panretinal photocoagulation failed the other method of treatment has to be applied, such as (i) trabeculectomy with antimetabolites as a first step when there is potential to improve state, (ii) aqueous shunt implants as a second step, and (iii) diode laser cyclophotocoagulation or retinal cryoablation, and in the worst case, with no vision and the patient suffering from great pain (iv) evisceration or enucleation should be considered (Sivak-Callcott et al., 2001).

Medical treatment includes conservative treatment by other specialists in order to manage associated systemic diseases or states such as coronary artery disease, hiperlipidemia, hypertension, diabetes mellitus etc.

Some of the surgical treatment is advocated to manage carotid stenosis and to improve ocular ischemia (Costa et al. 1999; Chaer & Makaroun, 2008; Sivalingam et al., 1991), such as carotid artery endarterectomy (CEA), carotid artery stenting (CAS) or extracranial-intracranial arterial bypass surgery (EC-IC), but without sufficient evidence to claim improvement of the ocular state with this treatment, except for CEA, where studies show some beneficial effect on the patient who has mild ocular ischemia and less effect on the patient with a greater degree of ocular ischemia, where retinal damage has probably become irreversible.

In conclusion, we can say that the ocular ischemic syndrome is a rare, vision-threatening condition and since the ophthalmologists may be the first to deal with such patients, they should be aware of the clinical presentation of OIS and recognize it early enough to start treating the condition when visual acuity is preserved enough and when prognosis is better. The continuing improvements in the diagnostic techniques, medical management and surgical treatment of carotid artery occlusive disease make the role of ophthalmologists increasingly important in the early detection and management of the OIS and its comorbidity.

5. Conclusion

Retinal vascular occlusions are an important cause of visual loss, particularly in elderly patients with multifactorial pathophysiological arms uniquely intertwined in each patient. They are often referred to as a „stroke"in the eye due to symptoms and clinical picture, often dramatic in its presentation. It also emphasizes the tremendous influence on patient's quality of life.

Apart from the similar clinical symptoms of visual loss there are some distinctive features that direct the clinician towards the diagnosis of arterial or venous occlusion. A thorough examination should assess the degree of vision loss by testing visual acuity, the presence of afferent pupillary defect, visual field testing, slit lamp examination of both anterior and posterior segments of the eye as well as ERG, which along with afferent pupillary defect and visual field testing provides the most sensitive diagnostic test in distinguishing between ischemic and non ischemic types of the occlusive disease (Hayreh, 2005). Visual acuity alone is not sufficient to validate peripheral retinal function but solely central vision. Therefore, it has been advocated by some authors to combine morphologic and functional tests in order to establish the type of the occlusion which has tremendous impact on the clinical course, prognosis and management of each case. The oxymetry (Gehlert et al., 2010) offers new possible tool in evaluating the perfusion status of the retina as this is extremely important prognostic factor when deciding which diagnostic and therapeutic algorithm should be undertaken in patient with occlusive disorder.

In conclusion we can say that retinal vascular occlusions are very common ocular diseases and the causes of visual loss with poor perspectives in the past, but recent studies on various medications and treatment modalities raise hope between a patient and ophthalmologist for establishing the proper treatment. Although we still cannot foresee, prevent, or causatively and successfully treat occlusive diseases of the retina, there are promising, recently introduced novel options focused on the management of visually deteriorating complications. Intravitreal agents, especially anti-VEGF medications and intravitreal corticosteroid implants have drastically changed the visual outcome for the affected patients. The perspective looks brighter as the development of the most effective treatment regimens and their combinations is evolving. Probably a combined therapy will better act than a single one. Developing new drugs is warranted.

6. Acknowledgement

Authors would like to thank Zoran Pletikosa, MD on providing them with useful medical sources from some databases unavailable to them in a time of writing this chapter.

7. References

Ahuja, R. M., Chaturvedi, S., Eliott, D., Joshi, N., Puklin, J. E., & Abrams, G. W. (1999). Mechanisms of retinal arterial occlusive disease in African American and Caucasian patients. *Stroke, 30*(8), 1506-1509.

Akkoyun, I., Baskin, E., Caner, H., Agildere, M. A., Boyvat, F., & Akova, Y. A. (2006). [Hemicentral retinal artery occlusion associated with moyamoya syndrome]. *Ophthalmologe, 103*(10), 888-891.

Amselem, L., Montero, J., Diaz-Llopis, M., Pulido, J. S., Bakri, S. J., Palomares, P., et al. (2007). Intravitreal bevacizumab (Avastin) injection in ocular ischemic syndrome. *Am J Ophthalmol, 144*(1), 122-124.

Appiah, A. P., & Trempe, C. L. (1989). Differences in contributory factors among hemicentral, central, and branch retinal vein occlusions. *Ophthalmology, 96*(3), 364-366.

Argon laser photocoagulation for macular edema in branch vein occlusion. The Branch Vein Occlusion Study Group. (1984). *Am J Ophthalmol, 98*(3), 271-282.

Argon laser scatter photocoagulation for prevention of neovascularization and vitreous hemorrhage in branch vein occlusion. A randomized clinical trial. Branch Vein Occlusion Study Group. (1986). *Arch Ophthalmol, 104*(1), 34-41.

Arruga, J., & Sanders, M. D. (1982). Ophthalmologic findings in 70 patients with evidence of retinal embolism. *Ophthalmology, 89*(12), 1336-1347.

Atebara N. H., Brown, G. C., & Cater, J. (1995). Efficacy of anterior chamber paracentesis and Carbogen in treating acute nonarteritic central retinal artery occlusion. *Ophthalmology* 102:2029-2034.

Bandello, F., Vigano D'Angelo, S., Parlavecchia, M., Tavola, A., Della Valle, P., Brancato, R., et al. (1994). Hypercoagulability and high lipoprotein(a) levels in patients with central retinal vein occlusion. *Thromb Haemost, 72*(1), 39-43.

Barak, N., Ferencz, J. R., Freund, M., & Mekori, Y. (1997). Urticaria in idiopathic bilateral recurrent branch retinal arterial occlusion. *Acta Ophthalmol Scand, 75*(1), 107-108.

Bavbek, T., Yenice, O., & Toygar, O. (2005). Problems with attempted chorioretinal venous anastomosis by laser for nonischemic CRVO and BRVO. *Ophthalmologica, 219*(5), 267-271.

Beatty, S., & Au Eong, K. G. (2000). Acute occlusion of the retinal arteries: current concepts and recent advances in diagnosis and management. *J Accid Emerg Med, 17*(5), 324-329.

Beiran, I., Dori, D., Pikkel, J., Goldsher, D., & Miller, B. (1995). Recurrent retinal artery obstruction as a presenting symptom of ophthalmic artery aneurysm: a case report. *Graefes Arch Clin Exp Ophthalmol, 233*(7), 444-447.

Beversdorf, D., Stommel, E., Allen, C., Stevens, R., & Lessell, S. (1997). Recurrent branch retinal infarcts in association with migraine. *Headache, 37*(6), 396-399.

Biousse, V. (1997). Carotid disease and the eye. *Curr Opin Ophthalmol, 8*(6), 16-26.

Boers, G. H., Smals, A. G., Trijbels, F. J., Fowler, B., Bakkeren, J. A., Schoonderwaldt, H. C., et al. (1985). Heterozygosity for homocystinuria in premature peripheral and cerebral occlusive arterial disease. *N Engl J Med, 313*(12), 709-715.

Boyd, S. R., Zachary, I., Chakravarthy, U., Allen, G. J., Wisdom, G. B., Cree, I. A., et al. (2002). Correlation of increased vascular endothelial growth factor with neovascularization and permeability in ischemic central vein occlusion. *Arch Ophthalmol, 120*(12), 1644-1650.

Bradvica, M., Barać, J., Benašić, T., Kalajdžić Čandrlić, J., Štenc Bradvica, I., & Biuk, D. (2009). Treatment of occlusion of the central retinal artery with hyperbaric oxygenation - our experience on eight patients. *Medicinski Glasnik, 6*(1), 4.

Brown, D. M., Campochiaro, P. A., Singh, R. P., Li, Z., Gray, S., Saroj, N., et al. (2010). Ranibizumab for macular edema following central retinal vein occlusion: six-month primary end point results of a phase III study. *Ophthalmology, 117*(6), 1124-1133 e1121.

Brown, G. C. (1994). Retinal artery obstructive disease. In S. J. Ryan (Ed.), *Retina* (2 ed., Vol. 2, pp. 1361-1377). St. Louis: Mosby.

Brown, G. (1999). Retinal arterial occlusive disease. In D. Guyer (Ed.), *Retina-Vitreous-Macula* (Vol. 1, pp. 271-285).

Brown, G. C., Magargal, L. E., Shields, J. A., Goldberg, R. E., & Walsh, P. N. (1981). Retinal arterial obstruction in children and young adults. *Ophthalmology, 88*(1), 18-25.

Brown, G. C., Magargal, L. E., & Sergott, R. (1986). Acute obstruction of the retinal and choroidal circulations. *Ophthalmology, 93*(11), 1373-1382.

Brown, G. C., & Magargal, L. E. (1988). The ocular ischemic syndrome. Clinical, fluorescein angiographic and carotid angiographic features. *Int Ophthalmol, 11*(4), 239-251.

Brown, G. C., & Reber, R. (1986). An unusual presentation of branch retinal artery obstruction in association with ocular neovascularization. *Can J Ophthalmol, 21*(3), 103-106.

Brown, G. C., & Shields, J. A. (1979). Cilioretinal arteries and retinal arterial occlusion. *Arch Ophthalmol, 97*(1), 84-92.

Bruno, A., Jones, W. L., Austin, J. K., Carter, S., & Qualls, C. (1995). Vascular outcome in men with asymptomatic retinal cholesterol emboli. A cohort study. *Ann Intern Med, 122*(4), 249-253.

Cahill, M. T., Kaiser, P. K., Sears, J. E., & Fekrat, S. (2003). The effect of arteriovenous sheathotomy on cystoid macular oedema secondary to branch retinal vein occlusion. *Br J Ophthalmol, 87*(11), 1329-1332.

Carter, J. E. (1984). Panretinal photocoagulation for progressive ocular neovascularization secondary to occlusion of the common carotid artery. *Ann Ophthalmol, 16*(6), 572-576.

Chaer, R. A., & Makaroun, M. S. (2008). Evolution of carotid stenting: indications. *Semin Vasc Surg, 21*(2), 59-63.

Chen, K. J., Chen, S. N., Kao, L. Y., Ho, C. L., Chen, T. L., Lai, C. C., et al. (2001). Ocular ischemic syndrome. *Chang Gung Med J, 24*(8), 483-491.

Chopdar, A. (1984). Dual trunk central retinal vein incidence in clinical practice. *Arch Ophthalmol, 102*(1), 85-87.

Christoffersen, N. L., & Larsen, M. (1999). Pathophysiology and hemodynamics of branch retinal vein occlusion. *Ophthalmology, 106*(11), 2054-2062.

Comp, P. C., & Esmon, C. T. (1984). Recurrent venous thromboembolism in patients with a partial deficiency of protein S. *N Engl J Med, 311*(24), 1525-1528.

Conway, M. D., Tong, P., & Olk, R. J. (1995). Branch retinal artery occlusion (BRAO) combined with branch retinal vein occlusion (BRVO) and optic disc neovascularization associated with HIV and CMV retinitis. *Int Ophthalmol, 19*(4), 249-252.

Costa, V. P., Kuzniec, S., Molnar, L. J., Cerri, G. G., Puech-Leao, P., & Carvalho, C. A. (1999). The effects of carotid endarterectomy on the retrobulbar circulation of patients with severe occlusive carotid artery disease. An investigation by color Doppler imaging. *Ophthalmology, 106*(2), 306-310.

Dugan, J. D., Jr., & Green, W. R. (1991). Ophthalmologic manifestations of carotid occlusive disease. *Eye (Lond), 5* (Pt 2), 226-238.

Duker, J. S. (2003). Retinal Arterial Obstruction. In M. Yanoff, J. S. Duker & A. J. James (Eds.), *Ophthalmology* (2nd ed.). St. Louis: Mosby.

Duker, J. S., & Brown, G. C. (1989a). Anterior location of the crossing artery in branch retinal vein obstruction. *Arch Ophthalmol, 107*(7), 998-1000.

Duker, J. S., & Brown, G. C. (1989b). Neovascularization of the optic disc associated with obstruction of the central retinal artery. *Ophthalmology, 96*(1), 87-91.

Duker, J. S., Sivalingam, A., Brown, G. C., & Reber, R. (1991). A prospective study of acute central retinal artery obstruction. The incidence of secondary ocular neovascularization. *Arch Ophthalmol, 109*(3), 339-342.

Ehlers, J. P., & Fekrat, S. (2011). Retinal vein occlusion: beyond the acute event. *Surv Ophthalmol, 56*(4), 281-299.

Ekdawi, N. S., & Bakri, S. J. (2007). Intravitreal triamcinolone and bevacizumab combination therapy for macular edema due to central retinal vein occlusion refractory to either treatment alone. *Eye (Lond), 21*(8), 1128-1130.

Fekrat, S., Goldberg, M. F., & Finkelstein, D. (1998). Laser-induced chorioretinal venous anastomosis for nonischemic central or branch retinal vein occlusion. *Arch Ophthalmol, 116*(1), 43-52.

Figueroa, M. S., Torres, R., & Alvarez, M. T. (2004). Comparative study of vitrectomy with and without vein decompression for branch retinal vein occlusion: a pilot study. *Eur J Ophthalmol, 14*(1), 40-47.

Fong, A. C., Schatz, H., McDonald, H. R., Burton, T. C., Maberley, A. L., Joffe, L., et al. (1992). Central retinal vein occlusion in young adults (papillophlebitis). *Retina, 12*(1), 3-11.

Gehlert, S., Dawczynski, J., Hammer, M., & Strobel, J. (2010). Haemoglobin Oxygenation of Retinal Vessels in Branch Retinal Artery Occlusions over Time and Correlation with Clinical Outcome. *Klin Monbl Augenheilkd, 227*(12), 976-980.

Glacet-Bernard, A., Leroux les Jardins, G., Lasry, S., Coscas, G., Soubrane, G., Souied, E., et al. (2010). Obstructive sleep apnea among patients with retinal vein occlusion. *Arch Ophthalmol, 128*(12), 1533-1538.

Graham, E. M. (1990). The investigation of patients with retinal vascular occlusion. *Eye (Lond), 4* (Pt 3), 464-468.

Greven, C. M., Slusher, M. M., & Weaver, R. G. (1995). Retinal arterial occlusions in young adults. *Am J Ophthalmol, 120*(6), 776-783.

Haller, J. A., Bandello, F., Belfort, R., Jr., Blumenkranz, M. S., Gillies, M., Heier, J., et al. (2010). Randomized, sham-controlled trial of dexamethasone intravitreal implant in patients with macular edema due to retinal vein occlusion. *Ophthalmology, 117*(6), 1134-1146 e1133.

Hayreh, S. S. (1994). Retinal vein occlusion. *Indian J Ophthalmol, 42*(3), 109-132.

Hayreh, S. S. (1999). Retinal and optic nerve head ischemic disorders and atherosclerosis: role of serotonin. *Prog Retin Eye Res, 18*(2), 191-221.

Hayreh, S. S. (2002). t-PA in CRVO. *Ophthalmology, 109*(10), 1758-1761; author reply 1761-1753.

Hayreh, S. S. (2003). Management of central retinal vein occlusion. *Ophthalmologica, 217*(3), 167-188.

Hayreh, S. S. (2005). Prevalent misconceptions about acute retinal vascular occlusive disorders. *Prog Retin Eye Res, 24*(4), 493-519.

Hayreh, S. S. (2010). Central Retinal Vein Occlusion from webeye.ophth.uiowa.edu/dept/crvo/

Hayreh, S. S. (2011). Acute retinal arterial occlusive disorders. *Prog Retin Eye Res, 30*(5), 359-394.

Hayreh, S. S., & Baines, J. A. (1973). Occlusion of the vortex veins. An experimental study. *Br J Ophthalmol, 57*(4), 217-238.

Hayreh, S. S., & Hayreh, M. S. (1980). Hemi-central retinal vein occulsion. Pathogenesis, clinical features, and natural history. *Arch Ophthalmol, 98*(9), 1600-1609.

Hayreh, S. S., Opremcak, E. M., Bruce, R. A., Lomeo, M. D., Ridenour, C. D., Letson, A. D., et al. (2002). Radial optic neurotomy for central retinal vein obstruction. *Retina, 22*(3), 374-377; author reply 377-379.

Hayreh, S. S., & Podhajsky, P. (1982). Ocular neovascularization with retinal vascular occlusion. II. Occurrence in central and branch retinal artery occlusion. *Arch Ophthalmol, 100*(10), 1585-1596.

Hayreh, S. S., Podhajsky, P. A., & Zimmerman, M. B. (2009). Retinal artery occlusion: associated systemic and ophthalmic abnormalities. *Ophthalmology, 116*(10), 1928-1936.

Hayreh, S. S., Podhajsky, P. A., & Zimmerman, M. B. (2011). Natural history of visual outcome in central retinal vein occlusion. *Ophthalmology, 118*(1), 119-133 e111-112.

Hayreh, S. S., Rojas, P., Podhajsky, P., Montague, P., & Woolson, R. F. (1983). Ocular neovascularization with retinal vascular occlusion-III. Incidence of ocular neovascularization with retinal vein occlusion. *Ophthalmology, 90*(5), 488-506.

Hayreh, S. S., & Weingeist, T. A. (1980). Experimental occlusion of the central artery of the retina. I. Ophthalmoscopic and fluorescein fundus angiographic studies. *Br J Ophthalmol, 64*(12), 896-912.

Hayreh, S. S., Zimmerman, B., McCarthy, M. J., & Podhajsky, P. (2001). Systemic diseases associated with various types of retinal vein occlusion. *Am J Ophthalmol, 131*(1), 61-77.

Hayreh, S. S., & Zimmerman, M. B. (2005). Central retinal artery occlusion: visual outcome. *Am J Ophthalmol, 140*(3), 376-391.

Hayreh, S. S., Zimmerman, M. B., Kimura, A., & Sanon, A. (2004). Central retinal artery occlusion. Retinal survival time. *Exp Eye Res, 78*(3), 723-736.

Hedges, T. R., Jr. (1963). Ophthalmoscopic findings in internal carotid artery occlusion. *Am J Ophthalmol, 55*, 1007-1012.

Ho, T. Y., Lin, P. K., & Huang, C. H. (2008). White-centered retinal hemorrhage in ocular ischemic syndrome resolved after carotid artery stenting. *J Chin Med Assoc, 71*(5), 270-272.

Ip, M. S., Scott, I. U., VanVeldhuisen, P. C., Oden, N. L., Blodi, B. A., Fisher, M., et al. (2009). A randomized trial comparing the efficacy and safety of intravitreal triamcinolone with observation to treat vision loss associated with macular edema secondary to central retinal vein occlusion: the Standard Care vs Corticosteroid for Retinal Vein Occlusion (SCORE) study report 5. *Arch Ophthalmol, 127*(9), 1101-1114.

Jain, N., & Juang, P. S. C. (2009, Jun 30, 2009). Retinal Artery Occlusion. Retrieved Jun 12, 2011, from http://emedicine.medscape.com/article/799119-overview

Johnson, M. W., Thomley, M. L., Huang, S. S., & Gass, J. D. (1994). Idiopathic recurrent branch retinal arterial occlusion. Natural history and laboratory evaluation. *Ophthalmology, 101*(3), 480-489.

Jorizzo PA, K. M., Shults WT, Linn ML. (1987). Visual recovery in combined central retinal artery and central retinal vein occlusion. *Am J Ophthalmol, 104*, 358-363.

Justice, J., Jr., & Lehmann, R. P. (1976). Cilioretinal arteries. A study based on review of stereo fundus photographs and fluorescein angiographic findings. *Arch Ophthalmol, 94*(8), 1355-1358.

Kahn, M., Green, W. R., Knox, D. L., & Miller, N. R. (1986). Ocular features of carotid occlusive disease. *Retina, 6*(4), 239-252.

Karagoz, B., Ayata, A., Bilgi, O., Uzun, G., Unal, M., Kandemir, E. G., et al. (2009). Hemicentral retinal artery occlusion in a breast cancer patient using anastrozole. *Onkologie, 32*(7), 421-423.

Kawaguchi, S., Okuno, S., Sakaki, T., & Nishikawa, N. (2001). Effect of carotid endarterectomy on chronic ocular ischemic syndrome due to internal carotid artery stenosis. *Neurosurgery, 48*(2), 328-332; discussion 322-323.

Kearns, T. P., & Hollenhorst, R. W. (1963). Venous-Stasis Retinopathy of Occlusive Disease of the Carotid Artery. *Proc Staff Meet Mayo Clin, 38,* 304-312.

Kearns, T. P., Siekert, R. G., & Sundt, T. M. (1978). The ocular aspects of carotid artery bypass surgery. *Trans Am Ophthalmol Soc, 76,* 247-265.

Klais, C. M., & Spaide, R. F. (2004). Intravitreal triamcinolone acetonide injection in ocular ischemic syndrome. *Retina, 24*(3), 459-461.

Klein, R., Klein, B. E., Jensen, S. C., Moss, S. E., & Meuer, S. M. (1999). Retinal emboli and stroke: the Beaver Dam Eye Study. *Arch Ophthalmol, 117*(8), 1063-1068.

Klein, R., Klein, B. E., Moss, S. E., & Meuer, S. M. (2000). The epidemiology of retinal vein occlusion: the Beaver Dam Eye Study. *Trans Am Ophthalmol Soc, 98,* 133-141; discussion 141-133.

Klein, R., Klein, B. E., Moss, S. E., & Meuer, S. M. (2003). Retinal emboli and cardiovascular disease: the Beaver Dam Eye Study. *Arch Ophthalmol, 121*(10), 1446-1451.

Klijn, C. J., Kappelle, L. J., van Schooneveld, M. J., Hoppenreijs, V. P., Algra, A., Tulleken, C. A., et al. (2002). Venous stasis retinopathy in symptomatic carotid artery occlusion: prevalence, cause, and outcome. *Stroke, 33*(3), 695-701.

Korner-Stiefbold, U. (2001). [Central retinal artery occlusion--etiology, clinical picture, therapeutic possibilities]. *Ther Umsch, 58*(1), 36-40.

Kreutzer, T. C., Alge, C. S., Wolf, A. H., Kook, D., Burger, J., Strauss, R., et al. (2008). Intravitreal bevacizumab for the treatment of macular oedema secondary to branch retinal vein occlusion. *Br J Ophthalmol, 92*(3), 351-355.

Kriechbaum, K., Michels, S., Prager, F., Georgopoulos, M., Funk, M., Geitzenauer, W., et al. (2008). Intravitreal Avastin for macular oedema secondary to retinal vein occlusion: a prospective study. *Br J Ophthalmol, 92*(4), 518-522.

Le Rouic, J. F., Bejjani, R. A., Rumen, F., Caudron, C., Bettembourg, O., Renard, G., et al. (2001). Adventitial sheathotomy for decompression of recent onset branch retinal vein occlusion. *Graefes Arch Clin Exp Ophthalmol, 239*(10), 747-751.

Leibovitch, I., Calonje, D., & El-Harazi, S. M. (2009, May 13, 2009). Ocular Ischemic Syndrome *The Medscape from WebMD Journal of Medicine* Retrieved June 11, 2011, from http://emedicine.medscape.com/article/1201678-overview

Liebreich, R. (1855). Ophthalmoskopische Notizen: Ueber die Farbe des Augengrundes. *Albrecht Von Graefes Arch Ophthalmol, 1,* 333-343.

Lima, V. C., Yeung, L., Castro, L.C., Landa, G. & Rosen, R. B. (2011). Correlation between spectral domain optical coherence tomography findings and visual outcomes in central retinal vein occlusion. *Clin Ophthalmol, 5*:299-305.

Lindley, R. I., Wang, J. J., Wong, M. C., Mitchell, P., Liew, G., Hand, P., et al. (2009). Retinal microvasculature in acute lacunar stroke: a cross-sectional study. *Lancet Neurol, 8*(7), 628-634.

Love, P. E., & Santoro, S. A. (1990). Antiphospholipid antibodies: anticardiolipin and the lupus anticoagulant in systemic lupus erythematosus (SLE) and in non-SLE disorders. Prevalence and clinical significance. *Ann Intern Med, 112*(9), 682-698.

Mangat, H. S. (1995). Retinal artery occlusion. *Surv Ophthalmol, 40*(2), 145-156.

Marcucci, R., Bertini, L., Giusti, B., Brunelli, T., Fedi, S., Cellai, A. P., et al. (2001). Thrombophilic risk factors in patients with central retinal vein occlusion. *Thromb Haemost, 86*(3), 772-776.

Matsui, Y., Katsumi, O., Sakaue, H., & Hirose, T. (1994). Electroretinogram b/a wave ratio improvement in central retinal vein obstruction. *Br J Ophthalmol, 78*(3), 191-198.

McCullough, H. K., Reinert, C. G., Hynan, L. S., Albiston, C. L., Inman, M. H., Boyd, P. I., et al. (2004). Ocular findings as predictors of carotid artery occlusive disease: is carotid imaging justified? *J Vasc Surg, 40*(2), 279-286.

Mendrinos, E., Machinis, T. G., & Pournaras, C. J. (2010). Ocular ischemic syndrome. *Surv Ophthalmol, 55*(1), 2-34.

Mizener, J. B., Podhajsky, P., & Hayreh, S. S. (1997). Ocular ischemic syndrome. *Ophthalmology, 104*(5), 859-864.

Morandi, X., Le Bourdon, E., Darnault, P., Brassier, G., & Duval, J. M. (1998). Unusual origin of the ophthalmic artery and occlusion of the central retinal artery. *Surg Radiol Anat, 20*(1), 69-71.

Natural history and clinical management of central retinal vein occlusion. The Central Vein Occlusion Study Group. (1997). *Arch Ophthalmol, 115*(4), 486-491.

Noma, H., Funatsu, H., Mimura, T., & Hori, S. (2008). Changes of vascular endothelial growth factor after vitrectomy for macular edema secondary to retinal vein occlusion. *Eur J Ophthalmol, 18*(6), 1017-1019.

Nussenblatt, R. B., Kaufman, S. C., Palestine, A. G., Davis, M. D., & Ferris, F. L., 3rd. (1987). Macular thickening and visual acuity. Measurement in patients with cystoid macular edema. *Ophthalmology, 94*(9), 1134-1139.

Opremcak, E., Rehmar, A. J., Ridenour, C. D., Borkowski, L. M., & Kelley, J. K. (2008). Restoration of retinal blood flow via translumenal Nd:YAG embolysis/embolectomy (TYL/E) for central and branch retinal artery occlusion. *Retina, 28*(2), 226-235.

Pai, S. A., Shetty, R., Vijayan, P. B., Venkatasubramaniam, G., Yadav, N. K., Shetty, B. K., et al. (2007). Clinical, anatomic, and electrophysiologic evaluation following intravitreal bevacizumab for macular edema in retinal vein occlusion. *Am J Ophthalmol, 143*(4), 601-606.

Palmowski-Wolfe, A. M., Denninger, E., Geisel, J., Pindur, G., & Ruprecht, K. W. (2007). Antiphospholipid antibodies in ocular arterial and venous occlusive disease. *Ophthalmologica, 221*(1), 41-46.

Parodi, M. B., Iacono, P., & Ravalico, G. (2008). Intravitreal triamcinolone acetonide combined with subthreshold grid laser treatment for macular oedema in branch retinal vein occlusion: a pilot study. *Br J Ophthalmol, 92*(8), 1046-1050.

Pe'er, J., Folberg, R., Itin, A., Gnessin, H., Hemo, I., & Keshet, E. (1998). Vascular endothelial growth factor upregulation in human central retinal vein occlusion. *Ophthalmology, 105*(3), 412-416.

Ramchandran, R. S., Fekrat, S., Stinnett, S. S., & Jaffe, G. J. (2008). Fluocinolone acetonide sustained drug delivery device for chronic central retinal vein occlusion: 12-month results. *Am J Ophthalmol, 146*(2), 285-291.

Reese, L. T., & Shafer, D. (1978). Retinal embolization from endocarditis. *Ann Ophthalmol, 10*(12), 1655-1657.

Richard, G., Saubrane, G., & Yanuzzi, L. A. (1998). *Fluorescein and ICG Angiography: Textbook and atlas.* (2 Rev Exp ed.). New York, N.Y. U.S.A. : Thieme.

Richards, R. D. (1979). Simulataneous occlusion of the central retinal artery and vein. *Trans Am Ophthalmol Soc, 77*, 191-209.

Risk factors for central retinal vein occlusion. The Eye Disease Case-Control Study Group. (1996). *Arch Ophthalmol, 114*(5), 545-554.

Rogers, S., McIntosh, R. L., Cheung, N., Lim, L., Wang, J. J., Mitchell, P., et al. (2010). The prevalence of retinal vein occlusion: pooled data from population studies from the United States, Europe, Asia, and Australia. *Ophthalmology, 117*(2), 313-319 e311.

Rudkin, A. K., Lee, A. W., & Chen, C. S. (2010). Ocular neovascularization following central retinal artery occlusion: prevalence and timing of onset. *Eur J Ophthalmol, 20*(6), 1042-1046.

Rosenfeld, P. J., Rich, R. M., & Lalwani, G. A. (2006). Ranibizumab: Phase III clinical trial results. *Ophthalmol Clin North Am, 19*(3), 361-372.

Rumelt, S., Dorenboim, Y., & Rehany, U. (1999). Aggressive systematic treatment for central retinal artery occlusion. *Am J Ophthalmol, 128*(6), 733-738.

Rumelt, S., & Brown, G. C. (2003). Update on treatment of retinal arterial occlusions. *Curr Opin Ophthalmol* 14 - (3):139-141.

Rumelt, S., & Brown, G. C. (2004). A systematic approach to evaluate and treat retinal arterial occlusions. Handouts for a course on retinal arterial occlusions for the American Academy of ophthalmology Meetings.

Sanborn, G. E., & Magargal, L. E. (1984). Characteristics of the hemispheric retinal vein occlusion. *Ophthalmology, 91*(12), 1616-1626.

Schmidt, D., Schumacher, M., & Wakhloo, A. K. (1992). Microcatheter urokinase infusion in central retinal artery occlusion. *Am J Ophthalmol, 113*(4), 429-434.

Schmidt, D., Hetzel, A., & Geibel-Zehender, A. (2005). Retinal arterial occlusion due to embolism of suspected cardiac tumors -- report on two patients and review of the topic. *Eur J Med Res, 10*(7), 296-304.

Schmidt, D., Hetzel, A., Geibel-Zehender, A., & Schulte-Monting, J. (2007). Systemic diseases in non-inflammatory branch and central retinal artery occlusion--an overview of 416 patients. *Eur J Med Res, 12*(12), 595-603.

Schmidt, D., & Kramer-Zucker, A. (2011). [Hemicentral Retinal Artery Occlusion due to Oral Contraceptives.]. *Klin Monbl Augenheilkd.*

Schumacher, M., Schmidt, D., & Wakhloo, A. K. (1993). Intra-arterial fibrinolytic therapy in central retinal artery occlusion. *Neuroradiology, 35*(8), 600-605.

Schumacher, M., Schmidt, D., Jurklies, B., Gall, C., Wanke, I., Schmoor, C., et al. (2010). Central retinal artery occlusion: local intra-arterial fibrinolysis versus conservative treatment, a multicenter randomized trial. *Ophthalmology, 117*(7), 1367-1375 e1361.

Scott, I. U., Ip, M. S., VanVeldhuisen, P. C., Oden, N. L., Blodi, B. A., Fisher, M., et al. (2009). A randomized trial comparing the efficacy and safety of intravitreal triamcinolone with standard care to treat vision loss associated with macular Edema secondary to branch retinal vein occlusion: the Standard Care vs Corticosteroid for Retinal Vein Occlusion (SCORE) study report 6. *Arch Ophthalmol, 127*(9), 1115-1128.

Scott, I. U., VanVeldhuisen, P. C., Oden, N. L., Ip, M. S., Blodi, B. A., Hartnett, M. E., & Cohen, G. (2011). Baseline predictors of visual acuity and retinal thickness outcomes in patients with retinal vein occlusion: Standard Care Versus COrticosteroid for REtinal Vein Occlusion Study report 10. *Ophthalmology 118* (2):345-52.

Sharma, S. (1998). The systemic evaluation of acute retinal artery occlusion. *Curr Opin Ophthalmol, 9*(3), 1-5.

Sharma, S., Pater, J. L., Lam, M., & Cruess, A. F. (1998). Can different types of retinal emboli be reliably differentiated from one another? An inter- and intraobserver agreement study. *Can J Ophthalmol, 33*(3), 144-148.

Sharma, S., Sharma, S. M., Cruess, A. F., & Brown, G. C. (1997). Transthoracic echocardiography in young patients with acute retinal arterial obstruction. RECO Study Group. Retinal Emboli of Cardiac Origin Group. *Can J Ophthalmol, 32*(1), 38-41.

Sivak-Callcott, J. A., O'Day, D. M., Gass, J. D., & Tsai, J. C. (2001). Evidence-based recommendations for the diagnosis and treatment of neovascular glaucoma. *Ophthalmology, 108*(10), 1767-1776; quiz1777, 1800.

Sivalingam, A., Brown, G. C., & Magargal, L. E. (1991). The ocular ischemic syndrome. III. Visual prognosis and the effect of treatment. *Int Ophthalmol, 15*(1), 15-20.

Sofi, F., Marcucci, R., Bolli, P., Giambene, B., Sodi, A., Fedi, S., et al. (2008). Low vitamin B6 and folic acid levels are associated with retinal vein occlusion independently of homocysteine levels. *Atherosclerosis, 198*(1), 223-227.

Stahl, A., Agostini, H., Hansen, L. L., & Feltgen, N. (2007). Bevacizumab in retinal vein occlusion-results of a prospective case series. *Graefes Arch Clin Exp Ophthalmol, 245*(10), 1429-1436.

Story, J. L., Held, K. S., Harrison, J. M., Cleland, T. P., Eubanks, K. D., & Brown, W. E., Jr. (1995). The ocular ischemic syndrome in carotid artery occlusive disease: ophthalmic color Doppler flow velocity and electroretinographic changes following carotid artery reconstruction. *Surg Neurol, 44*(6), 534-535.

Stowe, G. C., 3rd, Zakov, Z. N., & Albert, D. M. (1978). Central retinal vascular occlusion associated with oral contraceptives. *Am J Ophthalmol, 86*(6), 798-801.

Sturrock, G. D., & Mueller, H. R. (1984). Chronic ocular ischaemia. *Br J Ophthalmol, 68*(10), 716-723.

Sullivan, K. L., Brown, G. C., Forman, A. R., Sergott, R. C., & Flanagan, J. C. (1983). Retrobulbar anesthesia and retinal vascular obstruction. *Ophthalmology, 90*(4), 373-377.

Susac, J. O., Egan, R. A., Rennebohm, R. M., & Lubow, M. (2007). Susac's syndrome: 1975-2005 microangiopathy/autoimmune endotheliopathy. *J Neurol Sci, 257*(1-2), 270-272.

Takaki, Y., Nagata, M., Shinoda, K., Tatewaki, S., Yamada, K., Matsumoto, C. S., et al. (2008). Severe acute ocular ischemia associated with spontaneous internal carotid artery dissection. *Int Ophthalmol, 28*(6), 447-449.

Taubert, M., Dowd, T. C., & Wood, A. (2008). Malnutrition and bilateral central retinal vein occlusion in a young woman: a case report. *J Med Case Reports, 2*, 77.

Theoulakis, P. E., Livieratou, A., Petropoulos, I. K., Lepidas, J., Brinkmann, C. K., & Katsimpris, J. M. (2010). Cilioretinal artery occlusion combined with central retinal vein occlusion - a report of two cases and review of the literature. *Klin Monbl Augenheilkd, 227*(4), 302-305.

Torres, R. J., Luchini, A., Weis, W., Frecceiro, P. R., & Casella, M. (2005). Combined central retinal vein and artery occlusion after retrobulbar anesthesia--report of two cases. *Arq Bras Oftalmol, 68*(2):257-61.

Turut, P., & Malthieu, D. (1986). [Failure of laser photocoagulation in ischemic retinopathy associated with carotid occlusion]. *Bull Soc Ophtalmol Fr, 86*(11), 1297-1299.

Van Winden, M., & Salu, P. (2010). Branch retinal artery occlusion with visual field and multifocal erg in Susac syndrome: a case report. *Doc Ophthalmol* 121(3):223-9.

Vignes, S., Wechsler, B., Elmaleh, C., Cassoux, N., Horellou, M. H., & Godeau, P. (1996). Retinal arterial occlusion associated with resistance to activated protein C. *Br J Ophthalmol, 80*(12), 1111.

von Graefe, A. (1859). Ueber Embolie der Arteria centralis retinae als Ursache plotzlicher Erblindung. *Albrecht Von Graefes Arch Ophthalmol, 5*, 136-157.

Wardlaw, J. M., Chappell, F. M., Best, J. J., Wartolowska, K., & Berry, E. (2006). Non-invasive imaging compared with intra-arterial angiography in the diagnosis of symptomatic carotid stenosis: a meta-analysis. *Lancet, 367*(9521), 1503-1512.

Weger, M., Stanger, O., Deutschmann, H., Leitner, F. J., Renner, W., Schmut, O., et al. (2002). The role of hyperhomocysteinemia and methylenetetrahydrofolate reductase (MTHFR) C677T mutation in patients with retinal artery occlusion. *Am J Ophthalmol, 134*(1), 57-61.

Weinberg, D., Dodwell, D. G., & Fern, S. A. (1990). Anatomy of arteriovenous crossings in branch retinal vein occlusion. *Am J Ophthalmol, 109*(3), 298-302.

Weinberger, A. W., Siekmann, U. P., Wolf, S., Rossaint, R., Kirchhof, B., & Schrage, N. F. (2002). [Treatment of Acute Central Retinal Artery Occlusion (CRAO) by Hyperbaric Oxygenation Therapy (HBO)--Pilot study with 21 patients]. *Klin Monbl Augenheilkd, 219*(10), 728-734.

Wenzler, E. M., Rademakers, A. J., Boers, G. H., Cruysberg, J. R., Webers, C. A., & Deutman, A. F. (1993). Hyperhomocysteinemia in retinal artery and retinal vein occlusion. *Am J Ophthalmol, 115*(2), 162-167.

Werner, M. S., Latchaw, R., Baker, L., & Wirtschafter, J. D. (1994). Relapsing and remitting central retinal artery occlusion. *Am J Ophthalmol, 118*(3), 393-395.

Wild, S., Roglic, G., Green, A., Sicree, R., & King, H. (2004). Global prevalence of diabetes: estimates for the year 2000 and projections for 2030. *Diabetes Care, 27*(5), 1047-1053.

Williamson, T. H. (1997). Central retinal vein occlusion: what's the story? *Br J Ophthalmol, 81*(8), 698-704.

Wong, T. Y., & Klein, R. (2002). Retinal arteriolar emboli: epidemiology and risk of stroke. *Curr Opin Ophthalmol, 13*(3), 142-146.

Younge, B. R. (1989). The significance of retinal emboli. *J Clin Neuroophthalmol, 9*(3), 190-194.

4

Retinitis Pigmentosa in Northern Sweden – From Gene to Treatment

Irina Golovleva and Marie Burstedt
*University Hospital of Umeå, Umeå,
Sweden*

1. Introduction

Blindness is a loss of vision resulting in the inability to continue with a normal lifestyle. The prevalence of blindness varies from country to country and from region to region within the same country. An average estimate of the number of blind people in industrialized countries is 1–2 per 2000, compared to 5–10 per 1000 in developing countries. According to World Health Organisation estimates, there are between 27 and 35 million blind people in the world today.

Retinal dystrophies and degenerations represent a heterogeneous group of disorders affecting the function of the retina. They are characterized by degeneration of photoreceptors or adjacent cells such as retinal pigment epithelium or Müller cells. Retinitis pigmentosa (RP), hereditary maculopathies, and age-related macular degeneration (AMD) are representative of these diseases. RP as well as macular degeneration can be part of syndromes with symptoms from other organs or organ systems, for example, Usher syndrome with RP and deafness. More than 190 loci for different retinal diseases have been localized, and 140 genes have been identified (http://www.sph.uth.tmc.edu/Retnet/).

In northern Sweden the presence of all hereditary disorders is higher than in the southern part of the country. Explanations offered include a low migration rate in the sixteenth to nineteenth centuries and a certain number of marriages among relatives, which influenced the presence of autosomal recessive disorders. Furthermore, a disposition to a genetic abnormality in a geographically restricted area gave rise to a 'founder' effect, which influenced the presence of autosomal dominant disorders. These factors are taken into consideration in studies of all hereditary disorders, including those affecting vision.

2. Retinitis pigmentosa

Retinitis pigmentosa is a genetically and clinically heterogeneous group of hereditary retinopathies characterized by a degeneration of photoreceptors (rods primary) with a progressive loss of peripheral vision. This leads to night blindness, 'tunnel vision', and eventually, complete blindness. Typical signs of the disease, except for night blindness and progressive loss of the peripheral visual field, are typical pigment deposition in the retina, attenuation of the retinal blood vessels, and optic disc pallor. The diagnosis is confirmed by an abnormal or extinguished electroretinogram (ERG). RP can be nonsyndromic, syndromic, or systemic, when multiple tissues are affected. Nonsyndromic RP can be inherited in autosomal dominant (15–25%), autosomal recessive (5–20%), and X-linked (5–15%) manners (Daiger & Pagon, 2000). However, an inheritance pattern is still unknown in many cases. So-called simplex usually represents an isolated case without any family history. Due to different degrees of penetrance and expressivity of RP genes, the phenotype can vary between families and even within the same family (Shintani et al., 2009).

The prevalence in the United States and Europe is approximately 1/3500 to 1/4000, and the disorder is the most common cause of blindness among young adults. In Denmark the lifetime risk of developing RP is 1/2500 (Haim et al., 2002), and in Sweden it is 1/2000 (Burstedt et al., 1999). Similar frequencies can be expected in other populations, but they have not been well documented. Frequency of RP in certain isolated or consanguineous populations might be higher due to mutations in particular genes (Daiger & Pagon, 2000). Among known loci and genes there are 57 identified for autosomal dominant RP and autosomal recessive RP. Many genes associated with RP encode proteins functioning as photoreceptor transcription factors; others are involved in phototransduction and the visual cycle or photoreceptor structure (Phelan & Bok, 2000; Fig. 1). Despite many retinal diseases having been mapped to specific chromosomal regions, the genes and their functions still have not been identified in all cases.

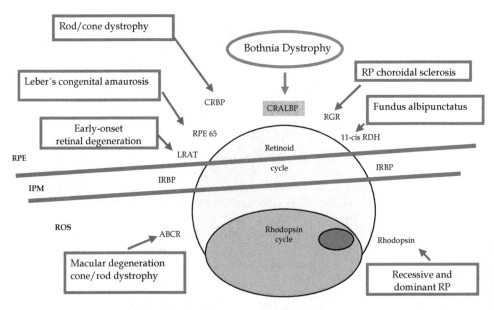

Fig. 1. Visual cycle proteins cause retinal degenerations. CRBP = cellular retinol binding protein, RPE65 = retinal pigment epithelium-specific protein 65kDa, LRAT = lecithin retinol acyltransferase, IRBP = interphotoreceptor retinoid-binding protein, RPE = retinal pigment epithelium, IPM = interphotoreceptor matrix, ROS = rod outer segment, ABCR = retina-specific ATP-binding cassette transporter, CRALBP = retinaldehyde-binding protein 1, RGR = retinal G protein coupled receptor, 11-cis RDH = retinol dehydrogenase 5 (11-cis/9-cis).

In Västerbotten County of northern Sweden 160 RP cases were identified and genetic defects were found in 66%, representing 79 patients with autosomal recessive RP of Bothnia type and 27 patients with autosomal dominant RP. However, genetic mechanisms of RP are still unknown in patients from other counties of northern Sweden. In this chapter we will focus on a disease with characteristic phenotype common in northern Sweden form of autosomal recessive RP, Bothnia dystrophy.

2.1 Autosomal recessive RP, Bothnia Dystrophy (BD)

Examination of medical records for patients with RP in Västerbotten County in northern Sweden has shown an accumulation of cases with a unique phenotype of RP called Bothnia dystrophy. Bothnia is the region in northern Sweden west of the Gulf of Bothnia, historically known as Bothnia Occidentalis (Fig. 2). Affected individuals showed night blindness with onset in early childhood, retinitis punctata albescens (RPA) at some stage of the disease, macular degeneration, and markedly elevated dark adaptation (DA) thresholds.

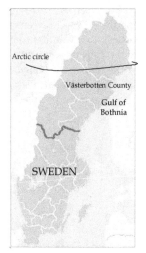

Fig. 2. The map shows the location of Västerbotten County in Scandinavia.

2.1.1 Genetic cause of BD

Initially, twenty patients from seven families originating from the same geographic area were included in the linkage analysis study aimed at identifying a disease-causing gene (Burstedt et al., 1999). All affected individuals had a nonsyndromic type of retinal degeneration inherited in an autosomal recessive way (Fig. 3). By statistical two-point lod (logarithm [base 10] of odds) score analysis, which is used to determine the linkage between trait and a chromosome marker, BD was mapped between the markers D15S526 and FES on chromosome 15q26.1. The D15S116, located near the *RLBP1* gene showed a maximum lod score of 7.79. Since lod score greater than 3 is considered evidence for linkage, the *RLBP1* gene was a strong candidate to cause the BD. Mutation analysis showed that all patients were homozygous for a cytosine (C) to thymine (T) change in exon 7 of the *RLBP1* gene, resulting in a substitution of a conservative arginine to tryptophan at position 234 (c.700C>T, p.R234W) in encoded cellular retinaldehyde-binding protein (Burstedt et al., 1999). No homozygotes for the c.700C>T mutation were found among 33 unaffected control subjects who underwent ophthalmologic examinations or 92 anonymous blood donors.

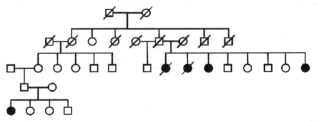

Fig. 3. A pedigree demonstrating autosomal recessive inheritance of BD in one of the families used for linkage analysis study.

2.1.2 Compound heterozygosity in BD

Sixty-nine BD cases homozygous for the c.700C>T were identified amongst patients with retinal dystrophies. In addition, 10 patients with similar to BD phenotype were heterozygous. Further screening for known mutations causing autosomal recessive RP revealed a second *RLBP1* mutation, a thymine (T) to adenine (A) change, resulting in a substitution of a methionine to lysine, c.677 T>A, p.M226K (Köhn et al., 2008). R234W and M226K were shown to be allelic and the patients were compound heterozygotes, c.[677T>A]+[700C>T] (Fig. 4).

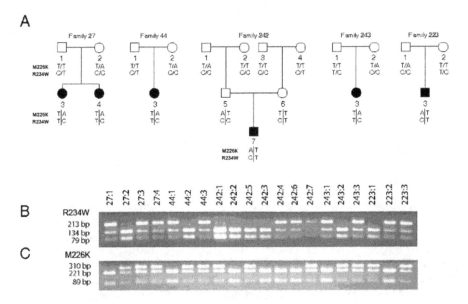

Fig. 4. Pedigrees of compound heterozygotes (A) and segregation analysis of *RLBP1* c.700C>T (B) and c.677T>A (C) performed by polymerase chain reaction and restriction fragment length polymorphism. (Figure published in Invest Ophthal Vis Sci, 2008;49(7):3172–3177).

Frequency of c.677 T>A allele in a matched control population was 0.0021. Among RP patients from northern Sweden two were homozygotes for p.M226K mutation. Based on allele frequency of R234W (3/250) and M226K (1/466), we believe that R234W was the first mutation to appear in northern Sweden, resulting in expected disease incidence of 1.5 per 10,000 in a population of 257,000 inhabitants.

Notably, one *RLBP1* compound heterozygote BD patient tested for 848 mutations in 29 genes causing autosomal dominant RP was shown to be a carrier of a mutation in carbonic anhydrase IV (CAIV), known to be associated with autosomal dominant retinitis pigmentosa RP17 (Rebello et al., 2004; Yang et al., 2005). Presence of this sequence variant in 6 out of 143 blood donors from a control Swedish population (4%) and phenotype undistinguishable from the other BD patients casts doubt on the pathogenic role of the CAIV (Köhn et al., 2008), though modifier genes switching off the mutant CAIV protein or other factors resisting its function in carriers of Swedish origin remain to be investigated.

2.1.3 *RLBP1* mutations in RP

To date, at least 12 mutations representing single nucleotide changes, in addition to small and one gross deletion have been reported (http://www.hgmd.cf.ac.uk). First homozygous *RLBP1* mutation was found in a consanguineous family of Indian origin and in one of consanguineous kindred from Saudi Arabia, both diagnosed with retinitis punctata albescens (Maw et al., 1997; Katsanis et al., 2001). Three additional mutations in the *RLBP1* gene were identified in the patients of European ancestry with recessively inherited RPA (Morimura et al., 1999), and in patients of Newfoundland origin with a severe rod cone dystrophy two splice junction mutations were detected (Eichers et al., 2002). The reported cases of retinal degeneration associated with *RLBP1* mutations were either homozygous or compound heterozygous (Demirci et al., 2004; Eichers et al., 2002; Fishman et al., 2004; Morimura et al., 1999; Nakamura et al., 2005). One of the compound heterozygotes, a Japanese patient with RPA, carried the c.700C>T mutation on one allele (Nakamura et al., 2005). Finally, changes involving single nucleotides are not the only type of mutation that affects the *RLBP1* gene. A large homozygous deletion was described in a RPA patient (Humbert et al., 2006).

2.1.4 Cellular retinaldehyde-binding protein (CRALBP)

RLBP1 gene mapped to chromosome 15q26 (Rosenfeld & Dryja, 1995) encodes the human cellular retinaldehyde-binding protein (CRALBP) expressing in outer epithelium of the iris, ciliary body pigment epithelium, cornea, optic nerve, pineal gland, Müller cells of the retina, and retinal pigment epithelium (RPE) (Bridges et al., 1987; Bunt-Milan & Saari, 1983; Eisenfeldt et al., 1985; Futterman & Saari, 1977; Saari et al., 1997; Sarthy, 1996). In the RPE, CRALBP functions as a carrier protein for endogenous retinoids, such as 11-cis-retinol, participating in the visual cycle. 11-cis-retinol can either be stored as an ester in the RPE or become oxidized to 11-cis-retinal by 11-cis-retinol dehydrogenase for visual pigment regeneration, and consecutively recycled back to the outer segment of photoreceptor cells of the retina (Saari, 1990). In vitro studies indicate that the presence of CRALBP diminishes the esterification and enhances oxidation of 11-cis-retinol (Saari et al., 1994).

A missense mutation of a conserved residue arginine at position 150 of CRALBP abolished binding to 11-cis-retinaldehyde. The mutation was shown to be associated with an atypical form of autosomal recessive RP in a small consanguineous Indian family (Maw et al., 1997).

We evaluated binding activities for two recombinant mutant proteins causing BD (Golovleva et al., 2003). M226K mutation completely abolished binding of the recombinant protein with 11-cis retinaldehyde, while the R234W, in contrast, increased binding activity of the recombinant CRALBP (Fig. 5). Double mutant M226K + R234W showed less solubility than the wild type rCRALBP (Köhn et al., 2008).

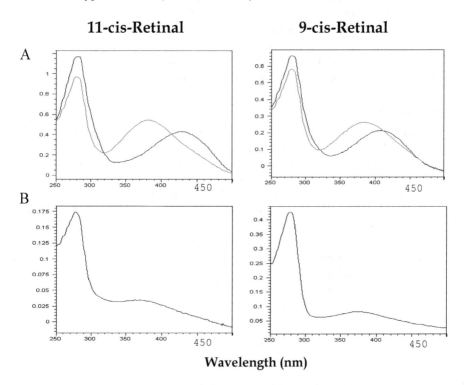

Fig. 5. Retinoid binding analysis of CRALBP mutants R234W (A) and M226K (B). UV-visible absorption spectra are shown before and after exposure to bleaching illumination following retinoid labelling with either 11-cis- or 9-cis-retinal. Spectra from wild-type rCRALBP (black line) and mutant R234W (red line) are indistinguishable and reflect stoichiometric binding of 11-cis- and 9-cis-retinal. The absorption spectra from mutant M226K show no chromophore absorbance at 425 nm or 400 nm, indicating no bound retinoid (Figure published in J Biol Chem, 2001;278:14,12397–12402).

We also analysed *RLBP1* promoter by sequencing 4kb in the upstream region in two BD compound heterozygotes. Seven single nucleotide polymorphisms (SNP) were identified; six had been reported previously and one was unique (cytosine to thymine change at position 2614, C2614T). Haplotype was constructed for BD patients. R234W and C2614T were both associated with BD phenotype. In experiments with reporter gene expression, decrease of expression level was shown when using either the entire 'affected' promoter haplotype or only C2614T (Golovleva, personal communication).

Thus, M226K mutation resulted in loss of functional CRALBP, which is true even for R234W mutant, since gene expression was decreased due to sequence variant in promoter.

2.2 Phenotype of retinitis pigmentosa of Bothnia type

All 79 patients originating from Västerbotten County, with a population of 257,000 inhabitants, present the phenotype caused by loss of CRALBP function.

2.2.1 Clinical findings and effects of age

The BD phenotype is characterized by central and peripheral degeneration of the retina with a unique expression of retinitis pigmentosa. All BD patients from the north of Sweden being homozygous for either the c.700C>T (p.R234W) (n = 67) or for the c.677T>A (p.M226K) (n = 2), and compound heterozygous [c.677T>A]+[c.700C>T] (p.M226K+p.R234W) (n = 10), have a clinical expression of the disease with a progression of retinal degeneration. The progressive maculopathy in BD presents an overall decrease of the visual acuity (VA) with age, leading to legal blindness in early adulthood (Fig. 6; Burstedt et al., 2001).

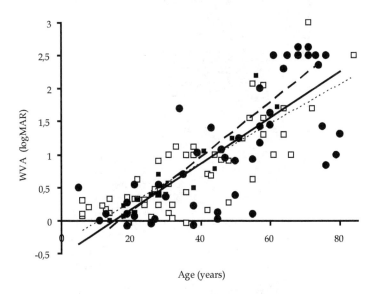

Fig. 6. Scatterplot of BD patients showing the relation of weighted distance logMAR visual acuity (WVA) with age. (●) Single observations of WVA vs. age in homozygotes c.700C>T (p.R234W); n = 49, (y = 0.035 × -0.53). (□) Retrospective recordings of WVA vs. age in compound heterozygotes [c.677T>A] + [c.700C>T] (p.M226K + p.R234W); n = 10 (y = 0.04 × −0.7), and homozygotes c.677T>A (p.M226K) (■); n = 2 (y = 0.03 × -0.32). Trendlines are drawn.

Notably, testing of monocular low-contrast VA using Sloan letter logarithmic translucent contrast charts (10% and 2.5%, Precision Vision®) allowed recording of measurable results, predominantly in the younger patients (Burstedt et al., 2005).

The retinal findings in BD patients show distinct maculopathy with central pigment deposits in the teens, and areolar maculopathy is observed in the younger adults (Burstedt et al., 1999, 2001, 2010). In the peripheral retina the pigmentations are similar to a 'salt and pepper' pattern and round retinal atrophies develop paracentrally and/or peripherally with age. The areolar atrophies are the most common peripheral findings in BD fundus as the degeneration progresses, though discrete pigmentations with an appearance similar to bone spicules may occasionally be found. No premature cataract of significance is observed in BD, and in advanced cases narrowing of the retinal vessels and pale optic disc are not typical findings (Fig. 7).

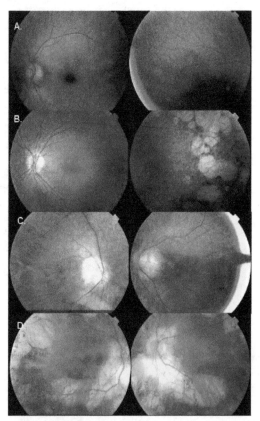

Fig. 7. Fundus photography. (A) 16-year-old girl, discrete central maculopathy and peripheral mottling, (WVA, weighted visual acuity, 0.00 logMAR). (B) 25-year-old woman with maculopathy and peripheral areolar atrophies (WVA 0.5 logMAR). (C) 41-year-old woman with central maculopathy and central RPA changes (WVA 0.3 logMAR). (D) 52-year-old woman with maculopathy, pigmentary changes (WVA 1.2 logMAR), and advanced retinal degeneration with retinal atrophies.

2.2.2 Morphological changes in BD found with ocular computed tomography

A generalized early decrease of the central foveal thickness (Ø 1 mm) and the inner ring of the retina (Ø 3 mm) are shown with optical coherence tomography (Burstedt et al., 2010). In the outer ring (Ø 6 mm), the generalized thinning is seen predominately in the inferior regions of the OCT measurement and a trend of more preserved areas of the retinal thickness of the superior and nasal regions are observed. The total macular volumes in all ages of BD patients are low compared with those of controls. Comparisons of macular thickness in each region of the BD patients and age-matched controls are presented in Fig. 8.

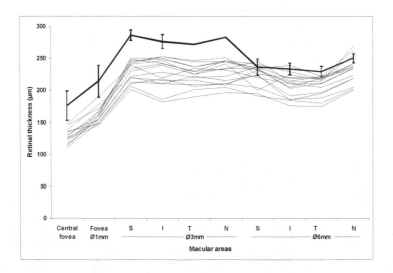

Fig. 8. Optical coherence tomography (OCT) macular thickness measurements of 9 areas in young BD patients (age 9–34 years, n = 8) and controls (in bold), using a Stratus OCT, model 3000 (Carl Zeiss Meditec AG, Jena, Germany): the central foveal, the foveal (Ø 1mm), the inner ring (Ø 3mm), and the outer ring (Ø 6 mm) with Superior area (S), Inferior area (I), Temporal area (T), and Nasal areas (N). The controls are presented with standard deviation shown on the graph. (Figure was published in Arch Ophthalmol. 2010;128(8); 989–995).

The cross-sectional morphology visualized by OCT presents a general thinning of cell layers and a reduced outer nuclear layer (ONL) in the youngest BD patients (9–34 years). Also, a third high-reflectance band, (3rd HRB), found in the younger cases, diminished in younger adults with BD, possibly representing the loss of the outer segment length of photoreceptors, predominately the cones in the fovea measured with OCT (Burstedt et al., 2010; Costa et al., 2004; Sandberg et al., 2005). This finding probably indicates an affection of the cone photoreceptors, and a possible degeneration of the outer segments of cones early in the course of the BD disease. The decreased retinal thickness and degenerative signs in the outer retinal layer were detected early in the course of the disease reported in a compound heterozygous patient with mutations in the RLBP1 gene (R103W/R234W) (Nakamura et al., 2005). Similar to BD, prominent photoreceptor loss in the foveal and extrafoveal retina even in the youngest patients studied (6–17 years), with relative preservation localized in the superior–temporal and temporal pericentral retina and the ONL, were demonstrated in the patients with Leber congenital amaurosis, another retinal degenerative disease caused by mutations in *RPE65* gene encoding for a protein active in the visual cycle (Jacobson et al., 2008). How can an early foveal thinning, suggesting early degeneration of cone photoreceptors in BD patients possibly be explained? Studies show that not only the rods but the cones also incorporate 11-*cis* retinoids, derived from the rod and cone visual cycles, in their visual pigments, and when examining the visual cycle in the *RPE-65* and *LRAT* knock-out mice, diseases affecting the visual cycle, a key role for cell survival, was found to be 11-*cis*-retinal bound to cone opsins, important for retinal protein sorting, transport, and targeting (Collery et al., 2008; Zhang et al., 2008).

2.2.3 Morphological findings of retinitis punctata albescens (RPA)

The subretinal white lesions, retinitis punctata albescens, were initially observed in the teens with BD phenotype (Burstedt et al., 1999, 2001, 2010). The RPA spots often dominate in the macula area and adjacent to the arcades, varying from single to multiple generalized white lesions scattered over the posterior pole of the retina. Notably, these changes fade as the progressive retinal degeneration advances (Fig. 9).

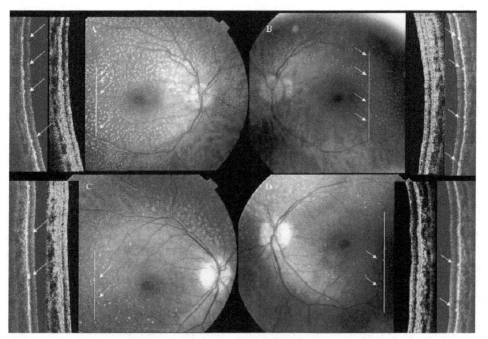

Fig. 9. Colour fundus photo and OCT. Top: 23-year-old man; below: 30-year-old woman. The vertical line of the binocular fundus photo with multiple generalized RPA traversing the retina at the temporal area of the macula between the arcades represents the scan lines of the corresponding OCT image presenting cross-sectional, visualized RPA (marked with arrows). (Figure published in Arch Ophthalmol. 2010;128(8);989–995).

RPA or subtle white lesions of the fundus have previously been described in several autosomal recessive RP cases with *RLBP1* mutations, and also in other progressive degenerative diseases, for example, the rhodopsin-related RP (Demirci et al., 2004; Eichers et al., 2002; Fishman et al., 2004; Katsanis et al., 2001; Nakamura et al., 2005; Souied et al., 1996). The localization of RPA lesions and their appearance may resemble more commonly known retinal lesions like drusen in age-related macular degeneration. However, the RPA lesions in BD do not present elevation, disruption, or detachment of RPE. Another finding in AMD is an accumulation of drusen between the retina and choriocapillaris that is shown to interfere with the exchange of nutrients and products close to the drusen, inducing RPE or neural retinal damage with overlaying photoreceptor cell layer thinning, predominately the photoreceptor outer segment affection (Holz et al., 2004; Pauleikhoff et al., 1990; Schumann et al., 2009). Since similar thinning or compression of the ONL overlaying the RPA lesions is observed in BD, a possible cause could be an accumulation of products in the RPE, possibly due to the higher affinity and impaired 11-*cis*-retinal release in the visual cycle in the BD phenotype shown in previous studies (Golovleva et al., 2003; He et al., 2009; Saari, 1990).

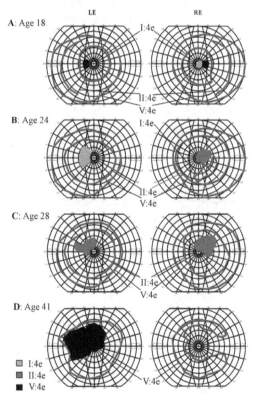

Fig. 10. Progression of visual field defects in a BD case. (A) Small central scotoma is noted in one eye at the age of 18. (B, C) Deeper and larger central-paracentral scotomas develop in young adulthood. (D) In middle age absolute central-paracentral scotomas are present and expanded, finally affecting the peripheral border. (Figure published in Arch Ophthalmol. 2001;119(2):260–267).

2.2.4 Psychophysical findings

Significant foveal depression was found early in BD by testing foveal threshold with Humphrey SITA standard 24-2. The mean deviations in all younger cases show significant loss, indicating an overall depression and/or loss of the central parts of the visual field in BD. Goldmann perimetries are unaffected in the BD cases under the age of 10, and relative parafoveal scotoma and/or ring scotoma is found in the teens, with additional large, deep to absolute central scotomas in both eyes, accompanied by a decrease in visual acuity in adulthood. The visual fields and the development of defects, registered over a time period of 23 years, are presented in Fig. 10.

In the fifth decade, extensive scotomas are present and only peripheral islets of the visual fields remain in middle age.

2.2.5 Angiographic findings

The fundus fluorescein angiograms in the early arteriovenous phase show a diffuse hyperfluorescence in the anatomic macular area, and locally, in the centre of the fovea, also presenting an early retinal thinning. As well as outside the arcades, corresponding to the atrophic areas in the colour fundus photograph, a general hyperfluorescence of granular type appears, indicating a gross atrophy of the pigment epithelium of the entire retina as a common clinical finding in this retinal degeneration (Burstedt et al., 2001).

2.3 Dark adaptometry and electrophysiological findings

2.3.1 Dark adaptometry and electrophysiological findings during standard dark-adapted conditions

Recovery of dark adaptation shows abnormalities of both rod and cone function (Fig. 11).

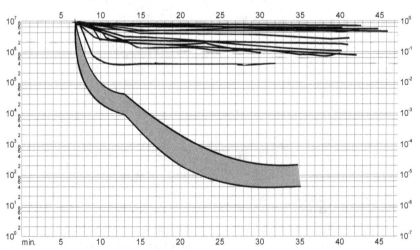

Fig. 11. Results of dark adaptometry in 14 cases aged 8–59 years. The grey area indicates the normal range of recovery of cone and rod sensitivity during dark adaptation for corresponding ages. (Figure published in Arch Ophthalmol. 2001;119(2):260–267).

In the younger patients the rod function is severely affected or absent and the cone adaptation often shows an extremely high, elevated final threshold, with the final dark-adapted sensitivity about four log units higher than a normal range. In elderly affected cases an even more pronounced cone dysfunction is found (Burstedt et al., 2001, 2003).

Full-field, single flash, and flicker electroretinograms (ERGs), including the oscillatory potentials (OPs) are recorded (UTAS-E 2000 LKC Technologies Inc., Gaithersburg, MD) using Burian-Allen bipolar electrodes during standard dark-adapted conditions, according to the recommendations of ISCEV (International Society for Clinical Electrophysiology of Vision). The outcome of the ERGs in all BD cases is subnormal or with non-recordable amplitudes of the rod-isolated b-waves with peak times either within the normal range or prolonged compared to controls (Burstedt et al., 2001, 2003, 2008). Representative full-field ERGs from five individuals from one family are presented in Fig. 12. The mixed rod-cone b-waves amplitudes are subnormal/non-recordable with comparatively short peak times in the younger cases. The amplitudes of the mixed rod-cone a-waves are found to be within the normal range in younger patients and subnormal to non-recordable with a prolonged peak time in adulthood. The amplitudes of the cone b-waves are better preserved and are within the normal range at the very young age, with peak times within the normal range, but prolonged in young adulthood and thereafter. Most of the younger patients had normal amplitudes and implicit times of the 30-Hz flicker ERGs that are within the normal limits, but already in early adulthood subnormal and delayed. The summed amplitudes of the individual oscillatory peaks, representing the Ops, show subnormal values at young age, decreasing with age and becoming non-recordable in BD cases older than 40 years of age.

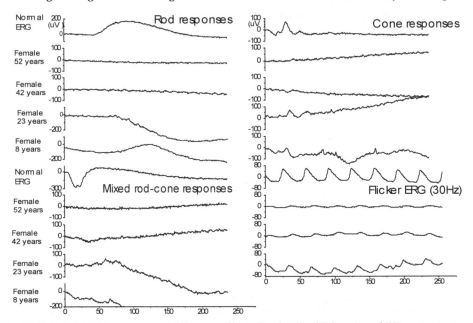

Fig. 12. Full-field ERG responses of the nonaffected individual (above) and BD patients, two elderly, and two younger women (52, 42, 23, and 8 years of age, respectively) from the same family. (Figure published in Arch Ophthalmol. 2001;119(2):260–267).

The ERGs recorded under standard conditions show that the rod and mixed rod-cone b-wave responses are relatively more affected than the mixed a-wave. The cone b-wave and the 30 Hz flicker amplitudes are significantly better preserved than the b-wave amplitudes of the rod and mixed rod-cone responses as well as the a-wave amplitude of the mixed rod-cone response, indicating later disturbance of the cones compared with the rods. At the same time the glial and inner retinal cell types seem to be affected at a relatively early stage in retinal degenerative disease (Burstedt et al., 2003).

2.3.2 Dark adaptometry and electrophysiology findings during 24 h prolonged dark-adaptation conditions

It has been shown that after illumination, the rhodopsin regeneration, 11-*cis*-retinal production, and dark adaptation are delayed by >10-fold in the visual cycle in *RLBP1* knockout mice (Saari et al., 2001). This could also be observed in humans, in six younger adults with BD, examined with a standardized Goldmann-Weekers adaptometer during an extremely prolonged dark adaptation of 24 hours (Burstedt et al., 2003). The extremely slow DA reaches steady state within 5 to 12 hours (Fig. 13); however, the final visual sensory thresholds do not return to normal levels after 24 hours of DA in most of the cases studied, probably affected by the disturbance in the normal function of CRALBP and lack of regeneration of 11-*cis* retinal in the RPE. An apparent plateau of recovery in the dark is observed, and duration for about 1 to 4 hours possibly represents a removal of bleached pigments, which has been suggested to occur in other retinal diseases affecting visual cycle function (Cideciyan et al., 1997). The 11-*cis*-retinal has been estimated to range from about 3.5% to 8% of that in normal subjects (Lamb & Pugh, 2004), with an average level of about 6% in the RPE in the BD phenotype.

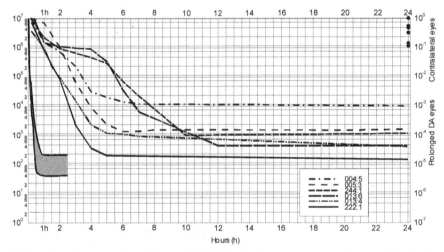

Fig. 13. Results of extremely prolonged (24 h) dark-adaptometry examinations in single eyes in BD patients, n = 6 (age 12–47 years). The final thresholds after 24 h were measured in both the patched single eye and in the unpatched contralateral eye. The values of the unpatched contralateral eye are indicated as filled symbols (•). The shaded area indicates normal range for corresponding age groups. (Figure published in Vision Research 2003:43(24):2559–2571).

Full-field ERGs after 24 hours of extremely prolonged DA were performed to evaluate the capacity of recovery of the whole retinal area and different cell types in BD disease. Six young cases (age 15–30 years) underwent full-field ERGs after 24 hours of DA in one eye and standard DA in the fellow eye. The results could be compared with the effect of the ERG after 10 hours' prolonged DA from a previous study (Burstedt et al., 2003, 2008). Enhanced rod-isolated b-wave after extremely prolonged DA (24 h) shows a sufficient number of rods able to function, generating responses of normal amplitudes even in young BD patients, although still with prolonged peak times (Fig. 14). Since the b-wave of the ERG is a glial response reflecting a depolarization of the Müller cells (Miller & Dowling, 1970), these findings may be correlated to an affected CRALBP function in the Müller cells of the retina or possibly a reversible effect on the second-order ON-bipolar cell function, as a consequence of a change in photoreceptor function.

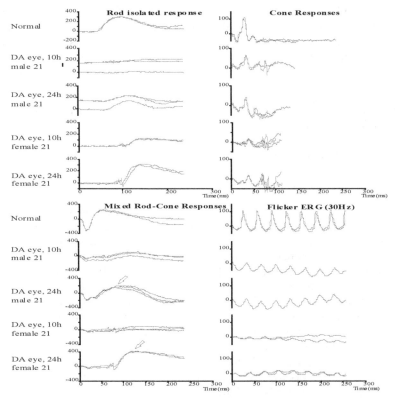

Fig. 14. Full-field electroretinograms of one eye, recorded after prolonged DA (10 h) and after extremely prolonged DA (24 h) in two BD patients (both 21 years old). A 'second', comparatively slowly rising positivity was observed in the mixed rod-cone response (arrows). For comparison, recordings of a normal subject are shown. (Figure published in Doc Ophthalmol. 2008;116(3):193–205).

The mixed rod-cone b-wave amplitude created by depolarization of the Müller and ON-bipolar cells in the inner retina is increased but still subnormal in the majority of patients.

After extended (24 h) DA, the mixed rod-cone a-wave response increases in amplitude to normal values in 4/5 cases with normal or somewhat delayed peak times. As the mixed a-wave shows normalized responses in the majority of the young BD cases examined, and the leading edge of the a-wave mainly represents a light-evoked hyperpolarization of the photoreceptors (Brown, 1968; Jamison et al., 2001; Robson et al., 2003; Tomita, 1965), these data suggest an additional, extremely slow regeneration of photopigments occurring even after 10 h DA. No obvious recovery of the cone b-wave is noted after the extremely prolonged DA (24 h); therefore, a relatively early damage to the cone system in BD patients cannot be excluded. Even though regeneration of opsin photopigments has been demonstrated in cone-dominant retinas, suggesting an interaction between Müller cells and cones in the recycling of visual chromophore (Mata et al., 2002), these electrophysiological results cannot confirm these findings.

In three younger BD patients a late evolvement in the mixed rod-cone response is observed (Fig. 14, arrows). The amplitudes are within the normal range of a mixed rod-cone b-wave, but the peak is extremely delayed (115 ms) compared to normal. This can be related to an enhanced scotopic activity associated with the slow and disturbed regeneration of photopigments. However, the exact origin of this late positive potential observed in BD patients is not known.

In summary, the continuous but slow regeneration of rod photopigments in *RLBP1* mutants presents an additional capacity for recovery of rod function and gain in activity in the inner retinal layers with extremely prolonged dark adaptation, possibly as a consequence of a change in photoreceptor function (Burstedt et al., 2003, 2008).

2.4 Outcome of visual function

Visual loss is an early sign of the BD disease, and individuals of working age may experience important socioeconomic consequences and interference with education as a result of their visual impairment. To provide insight into the perceived visual function of retinitis pigmentosa of Bothnia type, measurements of visual function were associated with the patients' self-assessment of their total self-reported visual function and health-related quality of life, measured with a questionnaire in 49 BD cases (Burstedt et al., 2010). Significant correlation was found between objective visual functions studied, and the subjective visual function. Almost 70% of the variability of the composite score could be explained by WVA and age alone. BD patients' responses to a majority of the questionnaire subscales significantly correlated with several of the clinical vision measures, especially those depending on central vision. Notably, the progressive declines in visual field area did not seem to affect significantly the self-perceived quality of life in patients with this phenotype. This finding might be an indication of ability to adapt to this type of gradual progressive visual field area loss, probably due to use of paracentral preserved areas. The expression of the disease has a significant impact on multiple domains of daily living, but there are no signs of worsening depression related to the increasing visual impairment.

2.5 Tinted contact lenses in BD

Could visual function be improved in BD? With the knowledge of an extremely prolonged dark adaptation (5–12 h) and even further gain of the ERG responses up to more than 12 h in this phenotype, outcome of wearing of tinted contact lenses during daylight was tested (Jonsson et al., 2007).

Twelve patients with BD were fitted with soft contact lenses tinted dark brown. Outcome of visual parameters, and visual-function questionnaire, were tested before the contact lens fitting and after one month. Visual function was improved by dark-tinted contact lenses, and it was observed that the BD cases with the lowest visual acuity described the most obvious improvement of their visual function and preferred the darker tinted contact lenses; the majority of BD cases from this study have also chosen to continue wearing the brown-tinted contact lenses for several years following the study, possibly indicating a continuous benefit in their daily life over time (authors' comments).

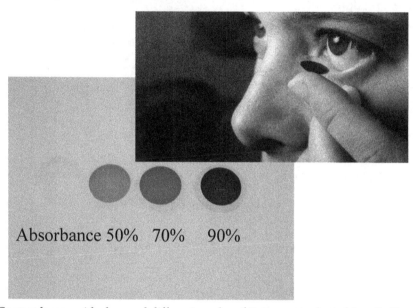

Fig. 15. Contact lenses with clear and different grades of tint were evaluated in retinitis pigmentosa of Bothnia type.

3. Conclusions

The RP population of northern Sweden has given us a unique opportunity to evaluate and compare the phenotypical expression of different *RLBP1* mutations over time. Despite genetic heterogeneity, the clinical expression of different *RLBP1* mutations in northern Sweden presents a unique phenotype of the retinal disease, clearly directing the molecular diagnosis and search for *RLBP1* mutations. It became possible to offer genetic testing among the families related to BD patients and also to the patients with a hereditary form of the recessive form of RP. In BD families we can offer risk assessment to future generations, providing genetic counselling based on molecular testing and clinical findings. There are several approaches to treatment of RP patients, although there are no established standards. Several drugs and nutritional supplements such as vitamin A palmitate, ascorbic acid, docosahexaenoic acid and others were evaluated with contradictory outcomes in different studies. Vitamin A palmitate, the most-used nutritional supplement, is shown to slow the rate of retinal degeneration, but this type therapy is not without controversy (Shintani et al., 2009). Gene therapy, which replaces or turns off the mutant disease-causing gene, represents another option for treatment. Several years of basic research of *RPE65*-Lebers congenital amaurosis, a retinal disease affecting the visual cycle, by several independent research groups, resulted in clinical trials of human gene therapies during recent years, demonstrating short-term evidence of visual gain (Jacobson & Cideciyan, 2010; Musarella & MacDonald, 2011). Therefore, we suggest that for treatment of BD patients, gene therapy is the most promising option among other concepts in the treatment of retinitis pigmentosa.

4. Acknowledgments

We acknowledge all BD patients and their families for their participation in all our studies. The authors express their thanks to all collaborators, and especially to Dr. Sandgren, for being a source of initiative and interest, and an engine in valuable discussions. This research was supported by funding from Crown Princess Margaretha's Foundation for Vision Research (KMA), the Swedish Medical Research Council, and grants from the County Council of Västerbotten.

5. References

Bridges, CDB., Foster, RG., Landers, RA., & Fong, S-L. (1987). Interstitial retinol-binding protein and cellular retinal-binding protein in the mammalian pineal. *Vis Res*, Vol. 27, No. 12, pp. 2049-2060, PMID: 3447356

Brown, KT. (1968). The electroretinogram: its components and their origins. *Vision Research*, Vol. 8, No. 6, (Jun), pp. 633–677, PMID: 4978009

Bunt-Milan, A., & Saari, J. (1983). Immunocytochemical localization of two retinoid-binding proteins in vertebrate retina. *J Cell Biol*, Vol. 97, Vol. 3, (Sep), pp. 703-712, PMID: 6350319

Burstedt, MSI., Sandgren, O., Holmgren, G., & Forsman-Semb, K. (1999). Bothnia dystrophy caused by mutations in the cellular retinaldehyde-binding protein gene (*RLBP1*) on chromosome 15q26. *Invest Ophthalmol Vis Sci*, Vol. 40, No. 5, (Apr), pp. 995-1000, PMID: 10102298

Burstedt, MSI., Forsman-Semb, K., Golovleva, I., Janunger, T., Wachtmeister, L., & Sandgren, O. (2001). Ocular phenotype of Bothnia Dystrophy, an autosomal recessive retinitis pigmentosa associated with an R234W mutation in the *RLBP1* gene. *Arch Ophthalmol*, Vol. 119, No. 2, (Feb), pp. 260-267, PMID: 11176989

Burstedt, MSI., Golovleva, I., Sandgren, O., & Wachtmeister, L. (2003). Retinal function in Bothnia Dystrophy. An electrophysiological study. *Vision Research*, Vol. 43, No. 24, (Apr), pp. 2559-2571, PMID: 12536144

Burstedt, MSI., Mönestam, E., & Sandgren, O. (2005). Association between specific measures of vision and Vision-Related Quality of Life in patients with Bothnia Dystrophy, a defined type of Retinitis Pigmentosa. *Retina*, Vol. 25, No. 3, (Apr-May), pp. 317-323, PMID: 15805909

Burstedt, MSI., Sandgren, O., & Wachtmeister, L. (2008). Effects on electrophysiological functions in the electroretinogram of extremely prolonged dark adaptation in patients with Retinitis Pigmentosa of Bothnia type. *Doc Ophthalmol*, Vol. 116, No. 3, (May), pp. 193-205. Epub 2007 Oct 6. PMID: 17922155

Burstedt, MSI., & Mönestam, E. (2010). Vision-related quality of life in patients with Bothnia Dystrophy, a defined type of Retinitis Pigmentosa. *Clin Ophthal*, Vol. 4, (Mar), pp. 147-154, PMID: 20390035

Burstedt, MSI., & Golovleva, I. Central retinal findings in retinitis pigmentosa of Bothnia type caused by *RLBP1* mutation. *Arch Ophthalmol*, Vol. 128, No. 8, pp. 989-995, (Aug), PMID: 20696998

Cideciyan, AV., Pugh, EN Jr., Lamb, TD., Huang, Y., Jacobson, SG. (1997). Rod plateaux during dark adaptation in Sorsby's fundus dystrophy and vitamin A deficiency. *Invest Ophthalmol Vis Sci*, Vol. 38, No. 9, (Aug), pp. 1786-1794. PMID: 9286267

Costa, RA., Calucci, D., Skaf, M., Cardillo, JA., Castro, JC., Melo, LA., Martins, MC., & Kaiser, PK. (2004). Optical coherence tomography 3: automatic delineation of the outer neural retinal boundary and its influence on retinal thickness measurements. *Invest Ophthalmol Vis Sci*, Vol. 45, No. 7, (Jul), pp. 2399–2406, PMID: 15223823

Collery, R., McLoughlin, S., Vendrell, V., Finnegan, J., Crabb, JW.,Saari, JC., & Kennedy, BN. (2008). Duplication and divergence of zebrafish CRALBP genes uncovers novel role for RPE- and Muller-CRALBP in cone vision. *Invest Ophthalmol Vis Sci*, Vol. 49, No. 9,(Sept), pp. 3812–3820, PMID: 18502992

Demirci, FY., Rigatti, BW., Mah, TS., Gorin, MB. (2004). A novel compound heterozygous mutation in the cellular retinaldehyde-binding protein gene (RLBP1) in a patient with retinitis punctata albescens. *Am J Ophthalmol*, Vol. 138, No. 1, (Jul), pp. 171-173, PMID: 15234312

Eichers, ER., Green, JS., Stockton, DW., Jackman, CS., Whelan. J., McNamara, JA., Johnson, GJ., Lupski, JR., & Katsanis, N. (2002). Newfoundland rod–cone dystrophy, an early-onset retinal dystrophy, is caused by splice-junction mutations in RLBP1. *Am J Hum Genet*, Vol. 70, No. 4, (Apr), pp. 955–964, PMID: 11868161

Eisenfeldt, AJ., Bunt-Milam, AH., & Saari, JC. (1985). Localization of retinoid-binding proteins in developing rat retina. *Exp Eye Res*, Vol. 41, No. 3, (Sep), pp. 299-304, PMID: 3905423

Fishman, GA., Roberts, MF., Derlacki, DJ., Grimsby, JL., Yamamoto, H., Sharon, D., Nishiguchi, KM., & Dryja, TP. (2004). Novel mutations in the cellular retinaldehyde-binding protein gene (RLBP1) associated with retinitis punctata albescens: evidence of interfamilial genetic heterogeneity and fundus changes in heterozygotes. *Arch Ophthalmol*, Vol. 122, No. 1, (Jan), pp. 70–75, PMID: 14718298

Futterman, S., & Saari JC. (1977). Occurrence of 11-cis-retinal-binding protein restricted to the retina. *Invest Ophthalmol Vis Sci*, Vol. 16, No. 8, (Aug), pp. 768-771, PMID: 560359

Golovleva, I., Battacharya, S., Wu, Z., Shaw, N., Yang, Y., Andrabi, K., West, KA., Burstedt, MSI., Forsman, K., Holmgren, G., Sandgren, O., Noy, N., Qin, J., &Crabb, JW. (2003). Disease causing mutations in the cellular retinaldehyde- binding protein tighter and abolish ligand interactions. *J Biol Chem*, Vol. 278, No, 14, (Apr), pp. 12397-12402. Epub 2003 Jan 20. PMID: 12536144

Haim, M. (2002). Epidemiology of retinitis pigmentosa in Denmark. *Acta Ophthalmol Scand Suppl.*, Vol. 80, pp. 1–34

He, X., Lobsiger, J., & Stocker, A. (2009). Bothnia dystrophy is caused by domino-like rearrangements in cellular retinaldehyde-binding protein mutant R234W. *PNAS*, Vol. 106, No. 44, (Nov), pp. 18545-18550. Epub 2009 Oct 21. PMID: 19846785

Humbert, G., Delettre, C., Senechal, A., Bazalgette, C., Barakat, A., Bazalgette, C., Arnaud, B., Lenaers, G., & Hamel, CP. (2006). Homozygous deletion related to Alu repeats in RLBP1 causes retinitis punctata albescens. *Invest Ophthalmol Vis Sci*, Vol. 47, No. 11, (Nov), pp. 4719-4724, PMID: 17065479

Jacobson, SG., Cideciyan, AV., Aleman, TS., Sumaroka, A., Windsor, EA., Schwarz, SB., Heon, E., & Stone, EM.(2008). Photoreceptor layer topography in children with Leber congenital amaurosis caused by RPE65 mutations. *Invest Ophthalmol Vis Sci*, Vol. 49, No. 10, (Oct), pp. 4573-4577. Epub 2008 Jun 6. PMID: 18539930

Jacobson SG.,& Cideciyan, AV. (2010). Treatment possibilities for retinitis pigmentosa. *N Engl J Med.*, Vol. 363, No. 17, (Oct), pp. 1669-1671, PMID: 20961252

Jamison, JA., Bush, RA., Lei, B., & Sieving, PA. (2001). Characterization of the rod photoresponse isolated from the dark-adapted primate ERG. *Vis Neurosci*, Vol. 18, (May-Jun), pp. 445-455, PMID: 11497421

Holz, FG., Pauleikhoff, D., Klein, R., & Bird, AC. (2004). Pathogenesis of lesions in late age-related macular disease. *Am J Ophthalmol*, Vol. 137, Vol. 3, (Mar), pp. 504-510, PMID: 15013875

Jonsson, Å., Sandgren, O., & Burstedt, MSI. (2007). Evaluation of dark tinted lenses i Bothnia Dystrophy, a defined type of retinitis pigmentosa. *Acta Ophthalmol Scand*, Vol. 85, No. 5, (Aug), pp. 534-539. Epub 2007 Mar 22. PMID: 17376191

Katsanis, N., Shroyer, NF., Lewis, RA., Cavender, JC., Al-Rajhi, AA., Jabak, M., & Lupski, JR. (2001). Fundus albipunctatus and retinitis punctata albescens in a pedigree with an R150Q mutation in RLBP1. *Clin Genet*, Vol. 59, No. 6, (Jun), pp. 424-429. PMID: 11453974

Köhn, L., Burstedt, M., Jonsson, F., Kadzhev, K., Haamere, E., Sandgren, O., & Golovleva, I. (2008). Carrier of R14W in carbonic anhydrase IV presents Bothnia Dystrophy phenotype caused by two allelic mutations in RLBP1. *Invest Ophthal Vis Sci*, Vol. 49, No. 7, (Jul), pp. 3172-3177, PMID: 11453974

Lamb, TD., & Pugh, EN, Jr. (2004). Dark adaptation and the retinoid cycle of vision. *Prog Retin Eye Res*, Vol. 23, No. 3, (May), pp. 307-380, PMID: 15177205

Mata, NL., Radu, RA., Clemmons, RC., & Travis, GH. (2002) Isomerization and oxidation of vitamin A in cone-dominant retinas: a novel pathway for visual-pigment regeneration in daylight. *Neuron*, Vol. 36, No. 1, (Sep), pp. 69-80, PMID: 12367507

Maw, MA., Kennedy, B., Knight, A., Bridges, R., Roth, KE., Mani, EJ., Mukkadan, JK., Nancarrow, D., Crabb, JW., & Denton, MJ. (1997). Mutation of the gene encoding cellular retinaldehyde-binding protein in autosomal recessive retinitis pigmentosa. *Nat Genet.* Vol. 17, No. 12, (Oct), pp. 198-200, PMID: 9326942

Miller, RF., & Dowling, JE. (1970) Intracellular responses of the Müller (glial) cells of mudpuppy retina: their relation to b-wave of the electroretinogram. *J Neurophysiol*, Vol. 33, No. 3, (May), pp. 323-341, PMID: 5439340

Morimura, H., Berson, EL., & Dryja, TP. (1999). Recessive mutations in the *RLBP1* gene encoding cellular retinaldehyde-binding protein in a form of retinitis punctata albescens. *Invest Ophthalmol Vis Sci*, Vol. 40, No. 5, (Apr), pp. 1000-1004, PMID: 10102299

Musarella, MA., & Macdonald, IM. (2011). Current concepts in the treatment of retinitis pigmentosa. *J Ophthalmol.* Epub 2010 Oct 11, doi: 10.1155/2011/753547, PMID: 21048997

Nakamura, M., Lin, J., Ito,Y., & Miyake, Y. (2005). Novel mutation in RLBP1 gene in a Japanese patient with retinitis punctata albescens. *Am J Ophthalmol,* Vol. 139, No. 6, (Jun), pp. 1133–1135, PMID: 15953459

Pauleikhoff, D., Harper, CA., Marchall, J., & Bird, AC. (1990). Aging changes in Bruch´s membrane: a histochemical and morphologic study. *Ophthalmology,* Vol. 97, No. 2, (Feb), pp. 171–178, PMID: 1691475

Phelan, JK., & Bok, D. (2000). A brief review of retinitis pigmentosa and the identified retinitis pigmentosa genes. *Mol Vis,* Vol. 6, (Jul), pp. 116–124, PMID: 10889272

Rebello, G., Ramesar, R., Vorster, A., Roberts, L., Ehrenreich, L., Oppon, E., Gama, D., Bardien, S., Greenberg, J., Bonapace, G., Waheed, A., Shah, GN., & Sly, WS. (2004) Apoptosis-inducing signal sequence mutation in carbonic anhydrase IV identified in patients with the RP17 form of retinitis pigmentosa. *Proc Natl Acad Sci U S A,* Vol. 101, No. 17, (Apr), pp. 6617-6622. Epub 2004 Apr 16. PMID: 15090652

Robson, JG., Saszik, SM., Ahmed, J., & Frishman, LJ. (2003). Rod and cone contributions to the a-wave of the electroretinogram of the macaque. *J Physiol,* Vol. 547, Pt. 2, (Mar), pp. 509–530, Epub 2003 Jan 24. PMID: 12562933

Rosenfeld, PJ., & Dryja, TP. (1995). Molecular genetics of retinitis pigmentosa and related retinal degenerations, In: *Molecular Genetics of Ocular Disease.* pp. 99-126, New York, Wiley-Liss

Saari, JC. (1990). Enzymes nd proteins of the mammilian visual cycle. In: *Progress in Retinal Research,* Osborn, N., & Chader, G., editors, pp. 363-381, Oxford, England: Pergamon Press

Saari, JC., Bredberg, L., & Noy, N. (1994). Control of substrate flow at a branch in the visual cycle. *Biochemistry,* Vol. 33, No. 10, (Mar), pp. 3106-3112, PMID: 8130225

Saari, JC,. Huang, J., Possin, DE., Fariss, RN., Leonard, J., Garwin, GG., Crabb, JW., & Milam, AH. (1997). Cellular retinaldehyde-binding protein is expressed by oligodendrocytes in optic nerve and brain. *Glia,* Vol. 21, No. 3, (Nov), pp. 259-268, PMID: 9383035

Saari, JC., Nawrot, M., Kennedy, BN., Garwin, GG., Hurley, JB., Huang, J., Possin, DE., & Crabb, JW. (2001). Visual impairment in cellular retinaldehyde binding protein (CRALBP) knockout mice results in delayed dark adaptation. *Neuron,* Vol. 29, No. 3, (Mar), pp. 739-748, PMID: 11301032

Sandberg, MA., Brockhurst, RJ., Gaudio, AR., & Berson, EL. (2005). The association between visual acuity and central retinal thickness in retinitis pigmentosa. *Invest Ophthalmol Vis Sci,* Vol. 46, No. 9, (Oct), pp. 3349–354, PMID: 16123439

Sarthy, V. (1996). Cellular retinaldehyde-binding protein localization in cornea. *Exp Eye Res,* Vol. 63, No. 6, (Dec), pp. 759-762, PMID: 9068383

Shintani, K., Shechtman, DL., & Gurwood, AS. (2009). Review and update: current treatment trends for patients with retinitis pigmentosa. *Optometry,* Vol. 80, No. 7, (Jul), pp.384-401, PMID: 19545852

Schuman, SG., Koreishi, AF., Farsiu, S., Jung, S., Izatt, JA., & Toth, CA. (2009). Photoreceptor layer thinning over drusen in eyes with age-related macular degeneration imaged in vivo with spectral-domain optical coherence tomography.*Ophthalmology*, Vol. 116, No. 3, (Mar), pp. 488-496. Epub 2009 Jan 22. PMID: 19167082

Souied, E., Soubrane, G., Benlian, P., Coscas, GJ., Gerber, S., Munnich, A., & Kaplan, J. (1996). Retinitis punctata albescens associated with the Arg135Trp mutation in the rhodopsin gene. *Am J Ophthalmol*, Vol. 121, No. 1, (Jan), pp. 19–25, PMID: 8554077

Tomita, T. (1965). Electrophysiological study of the mechanisms subserving color coding in the fish retina. *Cold Spring Harb Symp Quant Biol*, Vol. 30, pp. 559-566, PMID:5219504

Zhang, H., Fan, J., Li, S., Karan, S., Rohrer, B., Palczewski, K., Frederick, JM., Crouch, RK., & Baehr, W. (2008). Trafficking of membrane-associated proteins to cone photoreceptor outer segments requires the chromophore 11-cis-retinal. *J Neurosci*, Vol. 28, No. 15, (Apr), pp. 4008–4014, PMID: 18400900

Yang, Z., Alvarez, BV., Chakarova, C., Jiang, L., Karan, G., Frederick, JM., Zhao, Y., Sauve, Y., Li, X., Zrenner, E., Wissinger, B., Hollander, AI., Katz, B., Baehr, W., Cremers, FP., Casey, JR., Bhattacharya, SS., & Zhang K. (2005) Mutant carbonic anhydrase 4 impairs pH regulation and causes retinal photoreceptor degeneration. *Hum Mol Genet*, Vol. 14, No. 2, (Jan), pp. 255-265. Epub 2004 Nov 24. PMID: 15563508

5

A Novel Artificial Vitreous Substitute – Foldable Capsular Vitreous Body

Qianying Gao

State Key Laboratory of Ophthalmology, Zhongshan Ophthalmic Center,
Sun Yat-sen University, Guangzhou,
China

1. Introduction

The natural vitreous is a transparent, gelatinoid structure occupying four-fifths of the volume of the eye. It has a thin, membrane-like structure corresponding to the vitreous cortex that extends from the ora serrata to the posterior pole.[1] It is somewhat spherical but slightly flattened meridionally, and it has a cup-shaped depression in its anterior side. It consists of about 99% water by weight, collagen fibers (types II, V/XI, VI, and IX), hyaluronic acid, opticin, fibrillin, and hyaluronan, which can maintain a certain spatial relationship with dipolar water molecules.[1,2] However, very few cells are found in the vitreous body. These cells are mostly phagocytes that clear useless cellular debris and hyalocytes mainly found at the periphery and that produce hyaluronic acid and collagen. In human adults, the vitreous body has an approximate weight of 4 g, a density of 1.0053–1.0089g cm[-3], a refractive index of 1.3345–1.3348, and a PH range of 7.0–7.4. [3-5]

The physiological function of the vitreous body involves supporting adjacent posterior segment structures, providing an ocular refractive medium, and acting as a cell barrier to inhibit cell migration from the retina to the vitreous cavity.[6] With age, the natural vitreous body gradually shrinks and collapses during the course of syneresis. This phenomenon may eventually lead to posterior vitreous detachment and can play a crucial role in the formation of retinal breaks which result in rhegmatogenous retinal detachment if untreated.[7,8]

The removal of diseased vitreous bodies using pars plana vitrectomy combined with artificial vitreous substitutes can restore vision in many patients. These individuals include those affected by proliferative diabetic retinopathy, proliferative vitreoretinopathy, and endophthalmitis or patients otherwise regarded as hopeless.[9-11]

The vitreous body cannot regenerate, so the vitreous cavity must be filled with suitable artificial vitreous substitutes that will keep the retina in place and prevent phthisis bulbi. Artificial vitreous substitutes are one of the most interesting and challenging topics of research in ophthalmology.[2] A number of artificial vitreous substitutes, such as gas, silicone oil, heavy silicone oil, and hydrogels, have been used.[2,12]

There are three major categories of currently available gas vitreous substitutes: air substitutes, expansile gas substitutes, and Xenon. Gases are used for pneumatic retinopexy and post-operative endotamponade. However, they are suitable only as short-term vitreous substitutes (Table 1).[13]

G	Molecular Weight	Purity (mol%)	Expansion Coefficient	Duration* (day)	Expansion Concentration (%)
Air	29	--	0	5-7	-
Xenon	131	99.995	0	1	-
SF6	146	99.9	1.9-2.0	10-14	18
C2F6	88	99.7	1.9	10-14	-
C4F8	138	99.9	3.3	30-35	16+
C3F8	188	99.7	4	55-65	14

Table 1. Physical characteristics of gases as vitreous substitutes

In 1969, Norton et al. highlighted the advantages of clinical management with intravitreal air for the treatment of giant retinal tears.[14] However, the intravitreal longevity of air is only a few days[15] due to diffusion across the retina. The refractive index of the air (1.0008) is also incompatible with optically important tissues. Therefore, these issues limit the use of air. To date, air is mainly used in liquid–air exchanges during vitrectomy procedures.[16]

In 1973, Norton first experimented with sulphur hexafluoride (SF6) and found that the persistence of the gas and its expansile characteristics are superior to air. SF6 expands to twice its volume by dissolving nitrogen, oxygen, and carbon dioxide from the blood. It also stays in the vitreous cavity for about two weeks.[17] In 1980, Lincoff et al. proposed the use of perfluorocarbon gases[18]. These gases expand after intravitreal injection because of the diffusion of other gases from the blood stream. Perfluoropropane expands to four times its original volume by the fourth day after injection. It is also absorbed at a much slower rate than air or sulphur hexafluoride. To date, C3F8 is the agent of choice. Expansile gases last longer in the vitreous chamber than air, but they are spontaneously absorbed in 6 to 80 days and replaced by aqueous humor. Therefore, postsurgical removal is avoided if they cause certain concomitant complications.[19] However, they may induce lens opacification and usually result in a high intraocular pressure (IOP).[20,21] As with air, the refractive indices of gases are also lower (w1.17).[22]

Xenon was tested in rabbit eyes to evaluate its longevity in the vitreous cavity.[23] It is considered as the most promising gas with successful retinal reattachment in all cases. However, the major drawback is its rapid disappearance; almost 90% of Xenon disappears 3 h after introduction.[24]

Silicone oil is hydrophobic, viscous, transparent, and stable. It has a specific gravity of 0.97 g/mL and a refractive index of 1.4. Its viscosity is measured in centistokes and linearly varies with chain lengths and molecular weight. The 1,000 and 5,000 centistoke varieties are commonly used in clinics. The surface tension is approximately 40 mN/m. Introduced by Cibis in 1962,[25] silicone oil has been the most important adjunct for internal tamponade in the treatment of complicated retinal or choroidal detachment for the past five decades. It is commonly applied for the treatment of superior retinal detachment through buoyancy force and high interfacial tension. It is the only substance currently accepted as a long-term vitreous substitute and is the preferred choice in complex retinal detachments, such as long-standing rhegmatogenous retinal detachment, traction retinal detachment, giant retinal tears, proliferative diabetic retinopathy, and severe endoophthalmitis involving the posterior segment.

However, the use of silicone oil has not always been successful. An anatomic success rate of around 70% has been reported,[19] with complications including cataract, keratopathy, anterior chamber oil emulsification, and glaucoma.[26] Several reports have demonstrated the migration of silicone oil droplets into the retina and the optic nerve. Others have shown the widespread loss of myelinated optic nerve fibers due to the oil's free-fluid characteristics within the eye.[27, 28]

Heavy oil, a solution of perfluorohexyloctane and silicone oil prepared as internal tamponade, has recently been used in retinal detachment surgery. However, it causes complications, such as emulsification and inflammatory reaction.[29] Some very recent results are encouraging,[30] but most clinicians are awaiting results from ongoing heavy silicone oil trials.[12]

Hydrogels and smart hydrogels seem to remain as the best candidates as long-term vitreous substitutes because they show excellent transparency and good biocompatibility. They can act as viscoelastic shock-absorbing materials, thereby closely mimicking the behavior of natural vitreous bodies. Hydrogels are networks of polymer chains that can contain over 99.9% water so they are hydrophilic and not flowable. Currently, a number of cross-linked polymeric hydrogels have been proposed, such as poly (vinyl alcohol) (PVA), poly poly (1-vinyl-2-pyrrolidone), poly (acrylamide) (PAA), and poly (ethylene glycol) (PEG).[2,12,31-34] Among these, the PVA and PAA hydrogels are the most promising candidates for long-term vitreous body replacement and are highly recommended for use. They show excellent biocompatibility, are biodegradable, and can closely mimic the physico-mechanical properties of natural vitreous bodies.[2] PEG is a synthetic water-soluble polymer that has been approved by the Food and Drug Administration (FDA) for use in a wide range of biomedical applications, including injectable hydrogels.[35] However, issues such as retinal toxicity, increased IOP, and formation of opacities still need to be addressed.[36] Fragmentation and changes in viscoelastic properties and resiliency after injection through a small-gauge needle have also been found in some types of hydrogels.[36, 37]

Smart hydrogels are a relatively new class of stimuli-sensitive hydrogels. They possess the common properties of conventional hydrogels, and they can respond to a variety of signals, including PH, temperature, light, pressure, electric fields, or chemicals.[38] Temperature-sensitive hydrogels, such as poly(N-isopropylacrylamide), the most extensively studied one, undergo sharp hydrophilic-hydrophobic transition in aqueous media at a lower critical solution temperature of 32 °C, which is close to the body temperature.[39] Generally, smart hydrogels appear promising, but they are still at an early experimental stage, and their long-term toxicity is unknown.[12] Therefore, despite half a century of research efforts to replace the vitreous body of the eye, an ideal and permanent vitreous body replacement has yet to be found.[40,41]

Current research on artificial vitreous bodies aims to determine ideal materials that are nontoxic and inert, thin and transparent, and have good water and oxygen permeability, high compatibility, and good elasticity[46] in order to mimic the natural vitreous perfectly. The materials must be hydrophilic and can form a gel within the vitreous cavity.[35] However, directly injected vitreous substitutes, like silicon oil and heavy silicon oil, often result in severe complications, such as intraocular toxicity, retinal cell proliferation, leakage into the anterior chamber, and difficulty of complete removal if emulsified with time, among others.

Inspired by the structure of the natural vitreous, we postulated a novel foldable capsular vitreous body (FCVB) to restore the shape and function of the natural vitreous body. The FCVB consisted of a capsule, drain tube, and valve. The capsule exactly mimicked the vitreous body using a computer. The intra-capsule pressure can be adjusted from the valve with a syringe, and there is a slice of anti-penetrating metal in the valve. Figure 1 and Table 2 show the images and parameters of the FCVB, respectively.[50] Silicone rubber elastomer has been used for tissue augmentation for many years, [43-45] so it was utilized to manufacture the capsule of FCVB. It showed good oxygen permeability, good mechanical and optical properties (Shore A hardness: 37.4˚, tensile intensity: >5.86 MPa, elongation ratio: >1200%, tear intensity: 34KN/m, transmittance: 93%, Hazes<1%),[46] and good biocompatibility as shown in stable extracts experiment (no significant fever, good genetic safety, and no structural abnormality or apoptosis in the cornea, ciliary body, and retina over a six-month observation period).[50] After pars plana vitrectomy, the seamlessly connected FCVB was triple-folded and inserted into the vitreous cavity through a 3 mm × 1 mm scleral incision without air fluid exchange. Then an injectable medium, such as balanced salt solution (BSS) or silicone oil, can be injected into the capsule and inflated to support the retina. Through the tube–valve system, IOP can be adjusted by the volume of the injected medium. Similar to the glaucoma valve, the valve can be fixed onto the sclera surface. [46]

Component parts		Dimension (mm)	Permissible deviation (mm)
Capsule	Diameter	20.00	±2.00
	Rise of arch	2.00	±0.20
	Radius of curvature of fovea lentis	6.00	±0.50
	Chord length of fovea lentis	9.50	±0.50
	Optic part thickness	0.06	±0.02
Drain tube	Outside diameter	1.50	±0.20
	Inner diameter	1.20	±0.20
	Tube length	4.00	±0.50
	Vertical distance from the open end to the principal axis	7.99	±0.20
Drain valve	Top diameter	4.00	±0.20
	Bottom diameter	6.00	±0.20
	Total thickness	3.50	±0.20
	Puncture part thickness	2.00	±0.20
	Location hole diameter	0.50	±0.05

FCVB, foldable capsular vitreous body; BSS, balanced salt solution.
Note: The FCVB consisted of capsule, drain tube, and valve. The capsule was mimicking the vitreous body exactly by computer, and BSS was injected through the tube-valve system to inflate the capsule.

Table 2. Standard dimensions of the components of the human FCVB

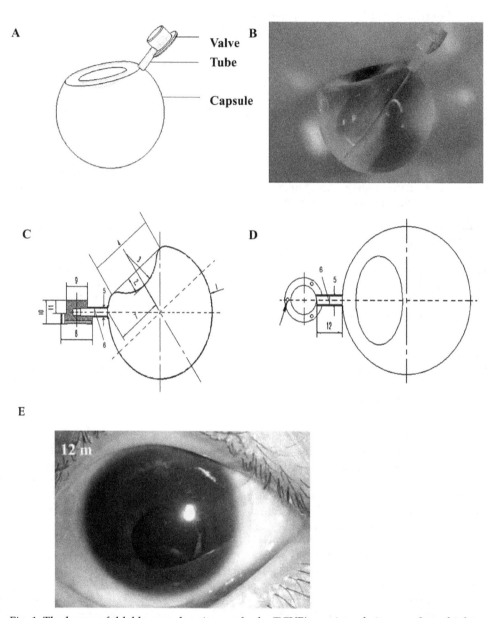

Fig. 1. The human foldable capsular vitreous body (FCVB) consists of vitreous-shape high molecular capsule, tube, and valve. The intra-capsule pressure can be adjusted from the valve with a syringe and there is a slice of anti-penetrating metal in the valve; the designed parameters finely mimic the vitreous shape of a human. (A) Illustration of FCVB. (B) Final sample of the FCVB (Outside the eye). (C) Side view of varied parameters. (D) Vertical view of varied parameters. (E) FCVB inside the eye (Twelve months after implantation).

Theoretically, a new artificial vitreous has the following advantages. First, it does not flow into the anterior chamber and subretinal regions or other sites. Second, it does not emulsify or damage the media over time nor cause it to be isolated in the capsule. Third, it has the capability to support discretionary retina using a 360-degree solid arc.

Developing an irregular vitreous-shaped thin capsule and smoothly connecting it to a very thin diameter tube and a pressure-control valve are very difficult. According to this hypothesis, a mirror steel mold is specially designed to fabricate FCVB using an injection-forming technology that would make the capsule, drainage tube, and valve of the FCVB seamlessly connected. The mold consists of an upper composite die, a lower composite die, and a core.[47] The core shape can be manipulated using a computer to match the human vitreous parameters. The capsular film is 60 μm thick, only one-third the thickness of the retina. In its natural shape, the human FCVB is somewhat spherical, but it is slightly flattened meridionally and has a cup-shaped depression anteriorly.

In the rabbit model of severe retinal detachment, the BSS-filled FCVB was found to mimic the morphology of the natural vitreous very closely and to restore its physiological functions, such as support, refraction, and cellular barriers, during a three-month observation period and without obvious complications. By contrast, the silicone oil control group showed obvious lens opacity, significant hyperopic shift, recurrent retinal detachment, preretinal membrane formation, and vitreoretinal traction.[48] The FCVB capsule can provide the detached retina with a platform to form a flat scar and a barrier to block cell migration from the retina to the vitreous cavity.

Interestingly, the BSS-filled FCVB very slightly changes the refraction compared with silicone oil and heavy silicone oil based on Gullstrand–Emsley and Liou–Brennan schematic eyes.[49] Reports from the State FDA in China show that FCVB has suitably mechanical, optical, and biocompatibility properties.[50] Its optical characteristics indicate that FCVB has high light transmission and laser irradiation stability.

In the early development of breast implants in plastic surgery, similar to current clinical vitreous substitutes, directly injectable materials were used. In fact, hydrophilic polyacrylamide gel (PAAG) was directly injected into the breast. This procedure was practiced widely in China and Eastern Europe in the 1990s. The breast implantation procedure was analogous to the use of silicone oil to replace the vitreous body. However, the injected PAAG was gradually found to induce severe complications, such as inflammation and infection, multiple indurations, hematoma, painful masses, and mastalgia. Currently, the direct injection of PAAG is prohibited, and it has been replaced with the use of capsule-like implants whose fluid substitute is contained in a thin, elastic capsule. This approach to implantation has shown clinical success.[51] In case of severe complications, as mentioned above, the implant can be completely removed without leaving behind residual fluid substitute. Apparently, the development of both artificial vitreous and breast substitutes shared a similar path, and both have suffered setbacks from the direct injection of the fluid substitute into the organ. Therefore, similar lessons can be learned, and the use of a capsule-type implant may be a good replacement for the use of the vitreous body.[46]

The use of FCVBs in the eyes is not yet a common practice worldwide. Therefore, an exploratory study of our new treatment for severe retinal detachment was conducted. The detachment cannot be easily reattached with silicone oil tamponade, such as posterior scleral ruptures with large disruptions of the retina or severe scleral ruptures with retinal and choroidal detachments. It may also have rigid retinal redetachments or inferior holes occurring after silicone or heavy oil tamponade had been attempted. At Zhongshan Ophthalmic Center, 11 patients were implanted with FCVBs filled with BSS,[52] whereas 3 patients were implanted with FCVBs filled with silicone oil.[53] Patients with serious eye inflammation, with only one eye remaining, with silicone oil-filled eyes, with serious heart, lung, liver, or kidney dysfunctions, or have other diseases that make them unsuitable for inclusion were excluded from the research. Retinal reattachments were found by B-scan in 8 (73%) of the 11 eyes at the end of the three-month treatment time; leakage of FCVB caused failure in three eyes. The production method of FCVB was correspondingly revised, and this addressed the problem. No obvious inflammation was observed in any eye after FCVB implantation, and UBM showed that the FCVB did not crush the ciliary body. There was no obvious difference between the FCVB's spectral transmittance before implantation and after removal.[52] Overall, the results showed that FCVB is an effective and safe artificial vitreous body for severe retinal detachments. It can help avoid the complications induced by silicone oil, such as glaucoma, corneal keratopathy, and silicone oil emulsification during a 12-month implantation time.[53]

Current data have demonstrated the theoretical advantages of using FCVBs, as mentioned above. Even if an ideal injectable material can be found, the use of FCVB is necessary to the artificial vitreous body. It acts as a transporter that can be injected with media, such as BSS, silicone oil, heavy oil, and hydrogels. In the present research, BSS was injected into the capsule of FCVB after PPV, and it was demonstrated as a flexible, effective, and safe vitreous substitute over a three-month implantation period.[52] Further multiple-central clinical trials are in progress in China, and the encapsulation of silicone oil, heavy oil, or hydrogels in PPV eyes will be attempted. Some common substances are active, such as collagen, hyaluronic acid, water, and the natural vitreous that consists of approximately 99% water and 1.0% inorganic salts, organic lipids, and hyaluronan[1], so these are not recommended as encapsulated tamponades in PPV eyes.

In addition, tiny (300 nm) apertures (Fig.2)[54] exist in the capsule, so the FCVB can release dexamethasone sodium phosphate and Protein kinase Cα. It can also be used as an intravitreal drug delivery system in addition to serving as a vitreous substitute.[54,55] Therefore, without the need to change its chemical properties, FCVB may provide a common vehicle for different drug releases, including antibiotics, anti-proliferative agents, and vascular endothelial growth factor antagonists.

The present exploratory clinical study was not large enough to provide a definitive conclusion. Further, the effects of FCVB on the lens should be further evaluated because 10 of 11 eyes were aphakic, and only one eye was phakic.[52] Based on this trial, a nine-hospital clinical trial is currently in progress in China to ascertain FCVBs' safety and efficacy as a vitreous substitute. The FCVB produced by Guangzhou Vesber Co. Ltd. is still in the stage of clinical trial, so it is not commercially available.

FCVBs have some similarities to thin elastic capsule breast implants and tissue expander systems used in plastic surgery. However, they also have differences, which are as follows. (1) Production methods: FCVBs are formed by injection forming technology and have a US patent, whereas capsule breast implants and tissue expander systems are made by dip forming for large balloons. (2) Sample size: Producing an irregular vitreous-shaped thin capsule and smoothly connecting it to a 1.2 mm diameter tube and a pressure-control valve are major challenges. However, capsule breast implants and tissue expander systems are large and easily made. (3) Implantation site: FCVBs are implanted into the vitreous cavity and come into contact with very tender tissues, such as the retina, ciliary body, lens, and anterior chamber. However, capsule breast implants and tissue expander systems directly come into contact with adipose tissues. Therefore, there are a number of safety issues in the use of FCVBs, which have to be addressed.

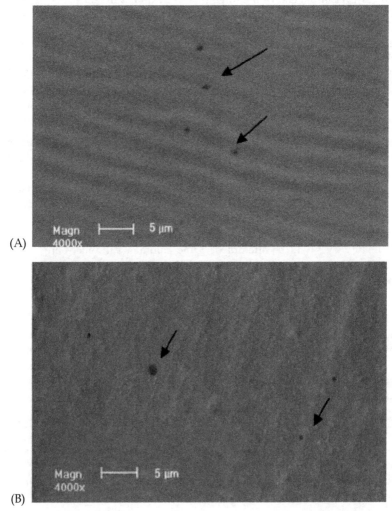

Fig. 2. Scanning electron microscope images of the capsule of the FCVB. Before implantation (**A**) and at the end of the observation time (**B**) 300-nm-mili apertures in the capsule were observed (*arrows*).

In conclusion, a new paradigm for the fabrication of a vitreous body substitute using FCVB was proposed in the current work. FCVB was established as an acceptable replacement as it closely mimics the morphology and restores the physiological function of the vitreous body. This idea provided us with a novel approach in researching on a new therapy strategy mimicking the natural vitreous that has been used for nearly half a century.

2. Acknowledgments

This study was supported by the National Nature Science Foundation of China (30973258) and National High-tech R&D Program of China (863 Program, 2009AA2Z404). I would like to thank my postgraduates, Shuyi Mai, Peijuan Wang, Ting Wang, Xuyuan Sun and Zhen Huang, for collecting the data.

3. References

[1] Green WR, Sebag J. Vitreoretinal interface. In: Ryan SJ, eds. Retina. 4th ed. Philadelphia, USA: Elsevier Mosby, 2006:1921-1989.

[2] Baino F. Towards an ideal biomaterial for vitreous replacement: Historical overview and future trends. Acta Biomater 2011; 7: 921-935.

[3] Gloor BP. The vitreous. In: Moses RA, Hart WM, editors. Adler's physiology of the eye. St. Louis: CV Mosby Co.; 1987: 246-267.

[4] Sebag J. Macromolecular structure of the corpus vitreus. Prog Polym Sci 1998; 23: 415-446.

[5] Chirila TV, Hong Y. The vitreous humour. In: Black J, Hastings GW, editors. Handbook of biomaterial properties. London: Chapman & Hall; 1998: 125-31.

[6] Goff MM Le, Bishop PN. Adult vitreous structure and postnatal changes. Eye. 2008; 22: 1214-1222.

[7] Byer NE. Natural history of posterior vitreous detachment with early management as the premier line of defense against retinal detachment. Ophthalmology. 1994;101:1503-1514.

[8] Los LI, Van Der Vorp RJ, Van Luyn MJA, Hooymans JMM. Age-related liquefaction of vitreous body: LM and TEM evaluation of the role of proteoglycans and collagen. Invest Ophthalmol Vis Sci 2003; 44: 2828-2833.

[9] Castellarin A, Grigorian R, Bhagat N, Del Priore L, Zarbin MA. Vitrectomy with silicone oil infusion in severe diabetic retinopathy. Br J Ophthalmol 2003; 87: 318-321.

[10] Quiram PA, Gonzales CR, Hu W, et al. Outcomes of vitrectomy with inferior retinectomy in patients with recurrent rhegmatogenous retinal detachments and proliferative vitreoretinopathy. Ophthalmology 2006; 113: 2041-2047.

[11] Yoon YH, Lee SU, Sohn JH, Lee SE. Result of early vitrectomy for endogenous Klebsiella pneumoniae endophthalmitis. Retina 2003; 23: 366-370.

[12] Kleinberg TT, Tzekov RT, Stein L, Ravi N, Kaushal S. Vitreous substitutes: a comprehensive review. Surv Ophthalmol. 2011; 56: 300-323

[13] 13. Ryan SJ, 4th edition, Retina, London, England: Elsevier/Mosby 127: 2137-2149.

[14] 14. Norton EWD, Aaberg T, Fung W and Curtin VT. Giant retinal tears. I. Clinical management with intravitreal air. Trans Am Ophthalmol Soc. 1969; 67: 374-393.

[15] 15. Marcus DM, D'Amico DJ, Mukai S. Pneumatic retinopexy versus scleral buckling forrepair of primary rhegmatogenous retinal detachment. Int Ophthalmol Clin. 1994; 34: 97-108.

[16] 16. Brinton DA, Wilkinson CP. Retinal detachment-principles and practice. Oxford, UK: Oxford University Press; 2009.

[17] 17. Norton EWD. Intraocular gas in the management of selected retinal detachments. Trans Am Acad Ophthalmol Otolaryngol. 1973; 77: 85-98.

[18] 18. Lincoff HA, Mardirossian J, Lincoff A, Ligget P, Iwamoto T, Jakobiec F. Intravitreal longevity of three perfluorocarbon gases. Arch Ophthalmol. 1980; 98:1610-1611.

[19] 19. Azen SP, ScottIU, Flynn HW Jr, et al.Silicone oil in the repair of complex retinal detachments. A prospective observational multicenter study. Ophthalmology. 1998;105(9):1587-1597.

[20] 20. Lee DA, Wilson MR, Yoshizumi MO,et al. The ocular effects of gases when injected into the anterior chamber of rabbit eyes. Arch Ophthalmol.1991;109(4):571-575.

[21] 21. Wilkinson C, Rice T. Instrumentation, materials, and treatment alternatives,in Craven L (ed) Michels Retinal Detachment.St.Louis, MO, Mosby,ed 21996,pp 391--461.

[22] 22. Yaws CL, Braker W. Matheson Gas Data Book. Appendix18, Refractive index, dipole moment and radius of gyration. New York, McGraw--Hill Professional, 2001, ed7, p919.

[23] 23. Lincoff A, Lincoff H, Solorzano C, Iwamoto T. Selection of Xenon gas for rapidly disappearing retinal tamponade. Arch Opthalmol. 1982; 100: 996-997.

[24] 24. Lincoff H, Kreissig I. Applications of Xenon gas to clinical retinal detachment. Arch Ophthalmol. 1982; 100:1083-1085.

[25] 25. Cibis PA, Becker B, Okun E, Canaan S. The use of liquid silicone in retinal detachment surgery. Arch Ophthalmol. 1962; 68: 590-599.

[26] 26. Soman N, Banerjee R. Artificial vitreous replacements. Biomed Mater Eng. 2003; 13: 59-74.

[27] 27. Ichhpujani P, Jindal A, Jay Katz L. Silicone oil induced glaucoma: a review. Graefe's Arch Clin Exp Ophthalmol. 2009; 247:1585-1593.

[28] 28. La Cour M, Lux A, Heegaard S. Visual loss under silicone oil. Klin Monbl Augenheilkd. 2010; 227: 181-184.

[29] 29. Bhisitkul RB, Gonzalez VH. "Heavy oil" for intraocular tamponade in retinal detachment surgery. Br J Ophthalmol. 2005; 89: 649-650.

[30] 30. Rizzo S, Genovesi-Ebert F, Vento A, et al. Heavy silicone oil(densiron-68) for the treatment of persistent macular holes: densiron-68 endotamponade for persistent macular holes. Graefes Arch Clin Exp Ophthalmol. 2009;247:1471-1476

[31] 31. Maruoka S, Matsuura T, Kawasaki K, et al. Biocompatibility of polyvinylalcohol gel as a vitreous substitute. Curr Eye Res. 2006; 31: 599-606.

[32] 32. Hong Y, Chirila TV, Vijayasekaran S, Dalton PD, Tahija SG, Cuypers MH, et al. Crosslinked poly(1-vinyl-2-pyrrolidinone) as a vitreous substitute. J Biomed Mater Res 1996;30: 441-448.

[33] 33. Hamilton PD, Aliyar HA, Ravi N. Biocompatibility of thiol-containing polyacrylamide polymers suitable for ophthalmic applications. Polym Prep 2004;45: 495-496.

[34] Pritchard CD, Crafoord S, Andréasson S, Arnér KM, O'Shea TM, Langer R, Ghosh FK. Evaluation of viscoelastic poly(ethylene glycol) sols as vitreous substitutes in an experimental vitrectomy model in rabbits. Acta Biomater. 2011;7: 936-943.

[35] Sawhney AS, Pathak CP, Hubbell JA. Bioerodible hydrogels based on photopolymerized poly(ethylene glycol)–co-poly(alpha-hydroxy acid) diacrylate macromers. Macromolecules 1993; 26: 581-587.

[36] Chirila TV, Hong Y, Dalton PD, Constable IJ, Refojo MF. The use of hydrophilic polymers as artificial vitreous. Prog Polym Sci. 1998; 23 (3): 475–508.

[37] Chirila TV, Hong Y. Poly (1-vinyl-2-pyrrolidinone) hydrogels as vitreous substitutes: a rheological study. Polym Int. 1998;46:183–195.

[38] Chaterji S, Kwon IK, Park K. Smart polymeric gels: redefining the limits of biomedical devices. Prog Polym Sci. 2007;32: 1083-122.

[39] Tanaka T, Fillmore D, Sun ST, Nishio I, Swislow G, Shah A. Phase transitions in ionic gels. Phys Rev Lett 1980; 45: 1636-9.

[40] Steijns D, Stilma JS. Vitrectomy: in search of the ideal vitreous replacement. Ned Tijdschr Geneeskd. 2009;153: A 433.

[41] Soman N, Banerjee R. Artificial vitreous replacements. Biomed Mater Eng. 2003; 13: 59-74.

[42] Colthurst MJ, Williams RL, Hiscott PS, Grierson I. Biomaterials used in the posterior segment of the eye. Biomaterials. 2000; 21: 649-665.

[43] Berry MG, Davies DM. Breast augmentation: Part I--A review of the silicone prosthesis. J Plast Reconstr Aesthet Surg. 2010; 63 (11):1761-8.

[44] Stavrou D, Weissman O, Winkler E, Yankelson L, Millet E, Mushin OP, Liran A, Haik J. Silicone-based scar therapy: a review of the literature. Aesthetic Plast Surg. 2010;34 (5):646-51.

[45] Prather CL, Jones DH. Liquid injectable silicone for soft tissue augmentation. Dermatol Ther. 2006; 19 (3):159-68

[46] 46. Gao Q, Mou S, Ge J, et al. A new strategy to replace the natural vitreous by a novel capsular artificial vitreous body with pressure-control valve. Eye. 2008; 22: 461-468.

[47] Gao Q. A novel method and mould for foldable capsular vitreous body, China patent (200810199177.3)(2008).

[48] Chen J, Gao Q, Liu Y, et al. Evaluation of morphology and functions of a foldable capsular vitreous body in rabbit eye. Journal of Biomedical Materials Research: Part B, 2011;97: 396-404.

[49] Gao Q, Chen X, Ge J, et al. Refractive shifts in four selected artificial vitreous substitutes based on Gullstrand-Emsley and Liou-Brennan schematic eyes. Invest Ophthalmol Vis Sci 2009; 50: 3529-3534.

[50] Liu Y, Jiang Z, Gao Q, et al. Technical standards of foldable capsular vitreous body regarding mechanical, optical and biocompatible properties. Artif Organs. 2010; 34: 836-845.

[51] Gampper TJ, Khoury H, Gottlieb W, Morgan RF. Silicone gel implants in breast augmentation and reconstruction. Ann Plast Surg 2007;59: 581–590.

[52] Lin X, Ge J, Gao Q, et al. Evaluation of the flexibility, efficacy, and safety of a foldable capsular vitreous body in the treatment of severe retinal detachment. Invest Ophthalmol Vis Sci. 2011; 52(1):374-381.

[53] Lin X, Wang Z, Gao Q, et al. Preliminary efficacy and safety of a silicone oil-filled foldable capsular vitreous body in the treatment of severe retinal detachment. Retina. 2011, Proof.

[54] Liu Y, Ke Q, Chen J, et al. Dexamethasone sodium phosphate sustained mechanical release in the foldable capsular vitreous body. Invest Ophthalmol Vis Sci. 2010; 51: 1636-1642.

[55] Chen X, Liu Y, Gao Q, et al. Protein kinase Cα downregulation via siRNA-PKCα released from foldable capsular vitreous body in cultured human retinal pigment epithelium cells. Int J Nanomed. 2011; 6: 1303-1311.

6

Endophthalmitis

Phillip S. Coburn and Michelle C. Callegan

University of Oklahoma Health Sciences Center, Dean McGee Eye Institute,
Oklahoma City, Oklahoma,
USA

1. Introduction

Endophthalmitis is an infection of the anterior and posterior segments of the eye resulting from the introduction of microorganisms following a surgical procedure (postoperative), traumatic penetrating injury (posttraumatic), or metastasis from an infection of a distant site in the body (endogenous). Endophthalmitis can develop into panophthalmitis if the infectious agent invades the cornea and sclera. The vast majority of cases of endophthalmitis result from intraocular surgical procedures, in particular cataract surgery (West et al., 2005). Over the past several decades, the number of postoperative endophthalmitis cases has risen steadily, owing to the increase in the number of invasive ocular surgeries performed (West et al., 2005). The etiological agents responsible for endophthalmitis include both Gram-positive and Gram-negative bacteria and fungi. Cases of post-surgical endophthalmitis are usually a result of the introduction of members of the normal microbiota of the eyelid and skin surrounding the eye, the most common cause being coagulase-negative staphylococci (CNS) (West et al., 2005). Cases of posttraumatic endophthalmitis are more frequently caused by environmental bacteria, the most common being *Staphylococcus aureus* and *Bacillus cereus* (Jonas et al., 2000; Meredith, 1999; O'Brien & Choic, 1995; Thompson et al., 1993). Frequent causes of endogenous endophthalmitis (EE) include *S. aureus*, streptococcal species, *B. cereus*, and Gram-negative bacteria including *Klebsiella pneumoniae*, *Escherichia coli*, and fungal agents such as *Candida albicans* (Greenwald et al., 1986; Jackson et al., 2003; Okada et al., 1994; Romero et al., 1999; Shammas, 1977; Shrader et al., 1990).

The clinical hallmarks of endophthalmitis are acute vision loss, severe ocular pain, periorbital swelling, hypopyon, proptosis, and the presence of white cells and flare in the anterior chamber and vitreous (Lemley and Han, 2007). The visual prognosis can vary widely depending on the infectious agent, ranging from mild inflammation and full resolution to devastating blindness and loss of the eye. Therapy for endophthalmitis caused by avirulent skin microbiota typically results in complete resolution and full vision recovery. However, posttraumatic or endogenous endophthalmitis caused by virulent pathogens may not respond to therapeutic intervention and result in partial to complete vision loss, and in some instances, evisceration or enucleation of the infected eye.

This chapter will present a summation of the latest findings of epidemiological studies and discuss current therapeutic modalities. Moreover, the bacteriology and the current state of knowledge regarding the pathogenesis and host/pathogen interactions will be explored.

Given that a number of detailed and authoritative reviews of endophthalmitis in general have been published in the last ten years, and given the paucity of reviews on endogenous bacterial endophthalmitis, this chapter will primarily focus on this route of endophthalmitis.

2. Endogenous endophthalmitis

2.1 Historical perspective

Endogenous or metastatic endophthalmitis results from microorganisms seeding the bloodstream from a distant focus of infection and invading the posterior segment of the eye via a compromised blood retinal barrier (BRB) (Arevalo et al., 2010; Greenwald et al., 1986; Jackson et al., 2003; Okada et al., 1994; Romero et al., 1999; Shammas, 1977; Shrader et al., 1990). While this form of endophthalmitis is rare, the potential for blindness in one or both eyes is high. To date, almost nothing is known about the pathogenesis of endogenous endophthalmitis (EE), even though this disease ranks as one of the most devastating infections of the eye. In the pre-antibiotic era, the majority of cases of endophthalmitis resulted in poor visual outcome. From 1944 to 1966, approximately 73% of endophthalmitis cases resulted in a final visual acuity of hand motion vision or worse. The clinical outcome of endophthalmitis improved somewhat upon the introduction of intravitreal antibiotics and vitrectomy (Neveu and Elliot, 1959; Peyman et al., 1978). Even after the introduction of intravitreal antibiotic therapy and vitrectomy, the visual outcome of EE has not improved significantly in over 50 years (Jackson et al., 2003). Morever, there is a paucity of information on the pathogenic mechanisms of this disease from both the causative agent and host perspectives. The majority of patients have an underlying condition and are immunocompromised (Jackson et al., 2003). The leading predisposing condition of EE is diabetes mellitus type 2, but intravenous drug abuse, immunosuppressive agents, malignancies, and AIDS are also underlying conditions (Arevalo et al., 2010). Symptoms of EE typically include ocular pain, blurring or loss of vision, purulent discharge, and photophobia. EE may present as focal white nodules on the lens capsule, iris, retina, or choroid, or as a ubiquitous inflammation of multiple ocular tissues resulting in purulent exudate throughout the globe. In addition, inflammation can spread to involve the orbital soft tissue (Arevalo et al., 2010).

EE was first identified and described by the German pathologist Rudolf Ludwig Karl Virchow in 1856 (Virchow, 1856). While the causative agent was not identified, it may have been bacterial. In 1894, German ophthalmologist Theodor Axenfeld reported in a treatise on endogenous endophthalmitis that the majority of cases involved only one eye and were a result of the deposition of septic emboli in the uvea (Axenfeld, 1894). However, in one-third of cases, both eyes were affected and infection was selectively localized to the retina. Axenfeld postulated that although bacteria were found in all branches of the carotid and ophthalmic arteries, the predilection for the retina was probably due to the smaller size of the retinal capillaries and „the presence of areas of disease in the capillary walls favoring the lodgment there of micro-organisms" (Tooker, 1938). Collins and Mayou (1925) further speculated that „the retina becomes infiltrated with polymorphonuclear leukocyes, which make their way inward, collecting in large numbers between the retina and the hyaloid membrane and in the neighboring vitreous". Axenfeld noted in his writings that approximately one-third of patients with EE also had endocarditis, and that the vegetations were the likely source of bacteria infecting the eye. In 1916, a case of unilateral EE in a 19 year-old soldier with cerebrospinal meningitis was described (Weakley, 1916). Gram-negative diplococci, presumably *Neisseria meningitidis*, was cultured from both the cerebrospinal fluid and from the anterior chamber of the left eye. The patient was treated with repeated injections of antimeningococcus serum into the spinal column, which resulted in complete resolution of the meningitis. Interestingly, infection and inflammation of the affected eye was also resolved, leading the case author to speculate that the antiserum therapy may have contributed to the rapid clearance of the infection. Regardless of whether the antiserum had any effect on clearing the infection, the patient retained only perception of light visual acuity (Weakley, 1916). In 1938, Tooker described a case of unilateral EE in a patient that was readmitted to the hospital after having undergone ear surgery (Tooker, 1938). The left eye was severely inflamed and visual acuity was perception of light only. Blood cultures were positive for staphylococci and the patient expired from septicemia three days following readmission. An autopsy revealed bronchial pneumonia, vegetative endocarditis, and abscesses in the kidneys, spleen, and liver. Examination of the left eyeball revealed two primary foci in the retina and ciliary body. Tooker concluded that staphylococcal emboli lodged in the retinal and ciliary capillaries, entered the vitreous chamber, and induced a robust inflammatory response. Tooker reported that the patient had been in excellent condition prior to the ear surgery, blood glucose levels were normal, and no other underlying condition was present. It is therefore possible that a systemic inflammatory response induced a breakdown in the blood retinal barrier allowing staphylococci to invade the vitreous humor.

Even after the introduction of antibiotic therapy, visual outcomes following EE remained poor. Walker and Fenwick (1962) reported a case of fulminate bilateral endophthalmitis following streptococcal septicemia. In spite of aggressive treatment with systemic steroids, hydrocortisone ointment, and local and systemic antibiotics, vision in the right eye was perception of light, and in the left was count fingers. More recently, Jackson et al. (2003) reviewed 267 cases of EE and found that the visual prognosis was uniformly poor. These authors offered a number of possible explanations for the poor visual outcome of EE, including misdiagnosis owing to the fact that EE may mimic other ocular conditions, the rapid progression of the disease, and the failure to recognize the overlap between ocular and systemic infection (Jackson et al., 2003). Since the earliest reports of EE, little progress has been achieved in improving the visual prognosis of this disease. This highlights the necessity for studies to characterize the factors that contribute to the pathogenesis of EE, both from the host and the bacterial perspectives.

2.2 Epidemiology and bacteriology

Current epidemiological studies indicate that EE accounts for approximately 2 to 15% of all cases of infectious endophthalmitis (Arevalo et al., 2010; Puliafito et al., 1982). The often poor visual outcome and potential for bilateral blindness make EE one of the most destructive and devastating ocular infections. In recent reviews of cases of bacterial EE, 41% of cases resulted in a final visual acuity of count fingers or better, 26% of infected eyes lost all useful vision, and 29% required enucleation or evisceration (Greenwald et al., 1986; Jackson et al., 2003; Shammas, 1977). The vast majority of infections are unilateral, with disagreement among studies as to whether there is a predilection for the right or left eye (Arevalo et al., 2010; Greenwald et al., 1986; Jackson et al., 2003; Okada et al., 1994). Bilateral infections occur in approximately 25% of patients with EE (Arevalo et al., 2010). As stated earlier, over 50% of EE patients have an underlying medical condition, with diabetes being the most prevalent. Additional populations at risk include immunocompromised patients, patients with prolonged indwelling devices, and intravenous drug abusers. Sources of infection include suppurative liver disease, endocarditis, urinary tract infection, and meningitis (Jackson et al., 2003). Virtually any organism that can infect the bloodstream has the capability to cause EE, but frequent causes include opportunistic and environmental pathogens such as *Staphylococcus aureus, Streptococcus sp., Clostridium septicum,* coagulase-negative *Staphylococcus, Bacillus cereus, Listeria monogocytogenes, Escherichia coli, Klebsiella pneumoniae, Serratia marcescens, Pseudomonas aeruginosa,* and *Neisseria meningitidis* (Arevalo et al., 2010). However, *S. aureus* and *K. pneumoniae* dominate as bacterial causes of Gram-positive and Gram-negative cases of EE, respectively.

S. aureus is a Gram-positive bacterium found as a member of the normal microbiota of skin and mucosa, but can cause a variety of systemic, skin, and deep tissue infections and is a leading cause of contact lens-associated corneal infections (Callegan et al., 1994; Callegan et al., 2002b). The association between *S. aureus* EE and the prolonged use of indwelling prosthetics has been reported in diabetics and patients with other underlying immunocompromise with increasing frequency (Jackson et al., 2003; Major et al., 2010; Ness and Schneider, 2009; Nixdorff et al., 2009; Okada et al., 1994). *S. aureus* causes the majority of the cases of EE in Western countries and Europe (Ho et al., 2011). The emergence of lineages resistant to methicillin in the 1960s has prompted a public health crisis due to the difficulty in treating methicillin-resistant *S. aureus* (MRSA) infections and the increasing trend of infection among individuals with fully competent immune systems. MRSA infections may be community acquired (CA) or healthcare-associated (HA), with CA-MRSA being easier to treat but considerably more virulent. Coinciding with an increase in the prevalence of MRSA strains is an increase in MRSA ocular infections (Blomquist, 2006; Major et al., 2010). Recently, Ho et al. (2011) described a series of 7 patients (8 eyes) from a single institution that were diagnosed with EE caused by MRSA. Treatment of these cases consisted of intravitreal tap and injection of vancomycin and ceftazidime, as well as intravenous vancomycin. While retinal detachment occurred in 6 of 8 eyes, most of the patients experienced improved visual acuity from initial presentation, and only one eye lost all vision and required enucleation. Previous reports found that only 23.5% of cases of MRSA EE resulted in a visual acuity better than 20/200, whereas these authors found that 37.5% of eyes showed a final visual acuity of better than 20/200 (Ho et al., 2011). The authors contend that the higher than usual retinal detachment rate observered in their study might have been due to the higher than normal time between onset of EE and presentation, generally a mean time of 3.5 to 7.1 days versus a mean time of 17 days in their study (Ho et al., 2011).

K. pneumoniae is responsible for the majority of cases of EE due to Gram-negative bacteria and is the leading cause of EE throughout East Asia (Arevalo et al., 2010). Similar to MRSA, *K. pneumoniae* represents a therapeutic challenge due to increasing rates of acquisition of antibiotic resistance determinants. Although *K. pneumoniae* is found in the environment and as a commensal member of the gastrointestinal tract microbiota, it is also a frequent cause of healthcare-associated infections such as pneumonia, bacteremia, and urinary tract infections (Chang et al., 2002; Chuang et al., 2006; Fang et al., 2004; Fung et al., 2002;). *K. pneumoniae* has become the leading cause of pyogenic liver abscess in patients in Taiwan and other countries in the Far East (Chang et al., 2000; Wang et al., 1998), and reports of *K. pneumoniae* EE resulting from septicemia following pyogenic liver abscesses in diabetics are increasing (Chang et al., 2002; Chen et al., 2004; Chuang et al., 2006; Fang et al., 2004; Fung et al., 2002;).

In a case review of 18 patients with EE in Korea, Chung et al. (2011) also reported a close association between diabetes and infection with K. pneumoniae, and these factors were linked to a poor visual prognosis. These findings highlight the necessity for increased scrutiny of diabetic patients that present with ocular symptoms.

2.3 Diagnosis and therapeutic modalities

Early diagnosis and the initiation of treatment are critical to controlling infection and improving the visual prognosis of EE. Diagnosis of EE is difficult to establish based on clinical presentation alone because of the nonspecific nature of the symptomology. Diagnosis is usually based on clinical presentation and additional methods such as fundoscopy, ultrasonography, optical coherence tomography, and magnetic resonance imaging (Jackson et al., 2003). When EE is suspected, cultures of blood, vitreous and aqueous humor, and Gram stains are criticial for confirmation (Arevalo et al., 2010). Symptoms of systemic disease may also be useful in diagnosis, however only 57% of patients with EE manifested systemic signs of infection (Okada et al., 1994). Moreover, EE might be missed in patients with systemic infection until ocular pain and vision loss are experienced. Therapy for diagnosed bacterial EE consists of administration of systemic antibiotics such as third generation cephalosporins, vancomycin, and aminoglycosides (Lemley and Han, 2007). Fourth generation fluoroquinolones are also used at the discretion of the physician (Lemley and Han, 2007). Therapy also consists of intravitreal injection of 1 mg vancomyin per 0.1 ml for Gram-positive and 2.25 mg ceftazidime per 0.1 ml for Gram-negative pathogens and/or the aminoglycoside amikacin (0.4 mg). Jackson et al. (2003) reported in a literature review that vitrectomy is beneficial in cases of severe EE caused by highly virulent organisms and increases the likelihood of a better visual outcome by threefold. Vitrectomy is also indicated for cases of EE complicated by retinal detachment (Arevalo et al., 2010). As stated earlier, however, the visual outcome of EE has not improved in over 50 years. The lack of clinical improvements in EE is likely due to the lack of a reproducible animal model in which to study this disease; a disease model would be beneficial in terms of therapeutic testing and analysis of pathogenesis.

2.4 Pathogenesis

EE is one of the most frequently blinding intraocular infections, however little is known about the interplay of host and bacterial factors that contribute to the development of this disease. Moreover, the pathogenic mechanisms underlying the migration of bacteria toward and into the eye, inflammation, and vision loss have not been addressed. It is also unknown as to why diabetes is a common predisposing condition, although there are a number of possible explanations. Diabetes compromises the eye both immunologically and architecturally, resulting in changes that may weaken the ability of the eye to exclude organisms during systemic infection. One of the most serious and common complications among diabetics, specifically those with type 2 diabetes, is diabetic retinopathy (Aiello et al., 1998; Engler et al., 1991). During the progression of diabetic retinopathy, the vasculature, glia, and neurons of the retina are affected. The initial changes that occur within the retinal vasculature are the death of pericytes and thickening of the basement membrane, which lead to capillary leakage and occlusion. These changes ultimately result in macular edema, formation of new vessels, and neuroretinal degeneration (Asnaghi et al., 2003; Fong et al., 2003; Martin et al., 2004; Neely and Gardner, 1998; Qaum et al., 2001; Takeda et al., 2001).

Increases in vascular endothelial growth factor (VEGF) and the cytokines interleukin (IL)-1β, IL-6, IL-8, and tumor necrosis factor alpha (TNFα) in diabetic retinas contribute to angiogenesis and to breakdown in the BRB, implying an association with inflammation in the disease process (Jo et al., 2010). Intercellular adhesion molecule 1 (ICAM-1) and CD18 are upregulated and contribute to increased leukocyte adhesion to the endothelial wall. This is turn results in endothelial cell injury and death (Funatsu et al., 2005; Miyamoto et al., 1998; Miyamoto et al., 1999; Schroder et al., 1991). Elevated expression of matrix metalloproteases in the retina may also facilitate increases in vascular permeability and degradation of tight junction complexes, leading to BRB dysfunction (Giebel et al., 2005). Retinal pigment epithelia (RPE) and vascular endothelium, barrier cells of the BRB, also undergo changes in hyperglycemic environments *in vitro* and *in vivo*, including increases in VEGF that may contribute to vascular permeability (Amrite et al., 2006; Losso et al., 2010). The deterioration of the BRB during the development of diabetic retinopathy may allow pathogens to more readily invade the interior of the eye and might partially explain the link between diabetes and an increased risk of acquiring EE. Unfortunately, a clinical link between patients with diabetic retinopathy and EE has not been reported, only speculated. Retinal vascular permeability is not the only change occurring in a diabetic individual. Diabetes also compromises the innate immune response and depresses the ability to clear infections in general. Polymorphonuclear leukocytes (PMN) are of critical importance in clearing pathogens from the bloodstream and in the eye during acute bacterial endophthalmitis (Callegan et al., 1999; Ramadan et al., 2006; Ramadan et al., 2008; Wiskur et al., 2008). These important cells are impaired in diabetics. PMN defects in chemotaxis, phagocytosis, and bactericidal activity have been reported in the context of diabetes (Delamaire et al., 1997; Walrand et al., 2004) and PMN from diabetic mice and humans are incapable of phagocytizing and killing both *S. aureus* and *K. pneumoniae* (Lin et al., 2006; Park et al., 2009). These defects in the ability of PMNs to clear bacteria that are destined to cross a compromised blood retinal barrier may also contribute to the development and pathogenesis of EE, but this has not been scientifically analyzed.

Virtually nothing is known about the bacterial factors that contribute to the pathogenesis of EE. *S. aureus* and *K. pneumoniae* possess a repertoire of factors with demonstrable roles in the virulence of these species in a number of animal models of infection, however it is currently unknown if they contribute to the pathogenesis of EE. *S. aureus* expresses a number of adhesins, including the fibronectin binding proteins FnbpA and FnbpB (Green et al., 1995), the fibrinogen-binding proteins ClfA and ClfB (McDevitt et al., 1994), and the collagen binding protein Cna (Patti et al., 1992) that have been shown to mediate attachment to extracellular matrix and plasma proteins, a crucial first step in initiating infections. *S. aureus* synthesizes alpha-toxin, a cytolysin shown to be important in corneal infections (Callegan et al., 1994) and endophthalmitis (Booth et al., 1998; Callegan et al., 2002b). *S. aureus* also secretes a host of other secreted cytolytic toxins including the beta-, gamma- and delta-toxins, and Panton-Valentine leukocidin (Plata et al., 2009) that may contribute to structural damage within the eye, or in the case of Panton-Valentine leukocidin (PVL) have either anti- or pro-inflammatory effects. PVL lyses neutrophils at higher concentrations but is a potent stimulator of the release of proinflammatory cytokines such as IL-8 at lower concentrations (Otto, 2010). Some strains of *S. aureus* are also encapsulated, rendering them resistant to phagocytosis and more virulent in animal models of sepsis (Luong and Lee, 2002; Thakker et al., 1998). Most clinical isolates of *S. aureus* produce either Type 5 or Type 8 capsular polysaccharide (Roghmann et al., 2005). The capsule of *S. aureus* may afford a survival advantage and prevent clearance from the bloodstream as well as the vitreous humor, especially in diabetics with impaired clearance mechanisms.

K. pneumoniae produces at least five major virulence factors that contribute to the pathogenesis of infection and include capsular serotype, hypermucoviscosity phenotype (HMV), lipopolysaccharide (LPS), siderophores, and pili. However, nothing is known about their potential contribution to EE pathogenesis. There are 77 capsular serotypes, however serotype K1 predominates among bacteremia, liver abscess, and EE isolates in Taiwan (Fung et al., 2002). Capsule production is likely to impede clearance of *K. pneumoniae* from the bloodstream and from the eye. The HMV phenotype is enriched among highly virulent, invasive strains of *K. pneumoniae*, especially those causing EE (Fang et al., 2004; Fang et al., 2007; Fung et al., 2002; Karama et al., 2008; Keynan and Rubinstein, 2008; Lee et al., 2006). Strains that express this phenotype possess a thick, viscous capsule-associated mucopolysaccharide web (Wiskur et al., 2008). Two commonly studied genes are associated with HMV: *magA* (mucoviscosity-associated gene A), which encodes a 43 kd outer membrane protein that has not been characterized (Fang et al., 2004), and *rmpA* (regulator of the mucoid phenotype A), a regulatory gene that controls the synthesis of the extracapsular mucopolysaccharide (Nassif et al., 1989). It has been shown that HMV confers resistance to serum killing and phagocytosis, and contributes to virulence in mice (Fang et al., 2004). *magA-* transposon mutants, which lost the HMV phenotype displayed serum sensitivity, became phagocytosis susceptible, and were avirulent in a mouse model (Fang et al., 2004). *magA* was located within a 35-kb locus containing 24 open reading frames (ORFs) with homologies to genes involved in exopolysaccharide biosynthesis or export and glycosylation (Chuang et al., 2006). This locus may represent a novel pathogenicity island responsible for the hypervirulence seen with certain *K. pneumoniae* pathogenic strains (Chuang et al., 2006). HMV+ *K. pneumoniae* are the most common cause of EE in Southeast Asia, with cases of EE caused by HMV+ *K. pneumoniae* on the rise in Western countries (Keynan and Rubinstein, 2008; Lederman and Crum, 2005). Our laboratory has previously shown that the HMV phenotype contributes to the pathogenesis of experimental *K. pneumoniae* endophthalmitis. In this model, an HMV+ strain caused significantly greater inflammation and greater loss of visual function than an HMV- strain following direct injection of bacteria into the vitreous (Wiskur et al., 2008). Further, the HMV+ strain was not readily cleared from the eye in this model (Wiskur et al., 2008). More recently, the *magA* gene was directly linked to the pathogenesis of EE in experimental *K. pneumoniae* endophthalmitis. Hunt et al. compared a wildtype HMV+ *K. pneumoniae* strain with an isogenic mutant defective in the *magA* gene, and found that mice infected with the *magA-* strain showed a significantly improved visual outcome relative to mice infected with the wildtype strain (Hunt et al., 2011). These results clearly demonstrate a role for the HMV phenotype in *K. pneumoniae* endophthalmitis. As this direct injection model circumvents systemic infection, it remains to be seen whether the HMV phenotype is important for crossing the BRB and establishing EBE.

The lipopolysaccharide O side chain has been shown to confer serum resistance to *K. pneumoniae* by preventing the deposition of complement components on the bacterial cell membrane and the ensuing complement-mediated cell lysis (Tomas et al., 1986). It is therefore possible that *K. pneumoniae* LPS from cells migrating near the BRB might elicit increases in permeability in the retinal vasculature that result in leakiness, facilitating entry into the eye. Metrickin et al. (1995), demonstrated that *E. coli* LPS induced a dose-dependent breakdown of the BRB. The siderophores enterobactin and aerobactin could also potentially be involved. While enterobactin is synthesized by nearly all isolates of *K. pneumoniae*, aerobactin is less frequently detected (Podschun et al., 1993). However, only *K. pneumoniae* isolates with capsular serotype K1 or K2 that produced aerobactin were more virulent (LD_{50} $<10^3$ cfu), and transfer of the genes necessary for synthesis of aerobactin into an avirulent strain increased the virulence by 100-fold (Nassif and Sansonetti, 1986). *K. pneumoniae* produce two types of pili or fimbriae, type 1 and type 3, that mediate attachment to epithelial cells. The type 1 fimbrial adhesion gene *fimH* was shown to be enriched among blood isolates (Yu et al., 2006), and the type 3 fimbrial adhesion protein MrkD has been demonstrated to contribute to virulence by binding to epithelial cells of the urogenital, repiratory, and gastrointestinal tracts (Sebghati et al., 1998), and the type 3 fimbrial shaft protein MrkA is required for biofilm formation on intravenous and urinary catheters and human extracellular matrix (Jagnow and Clegg, 2003; Langstraat et al., 2001). It is conceivable that these pili mediate adherence to structures in the eye and aid in the establishment of EE. However, as for all of the above discussed factors, no studies have been conducted evaluating the importance of these virulence traits to EE pathogenesis due to the lack of a well-characterized animal model of this disease.

3. Postoperative endophthalmitis

Postoperative endophthalmitis is the most common type of endophthalmitis and most frequently occurs following cataract surgery, with 90% of cases occuring following this procedure (Lemley and Han, 2007). The rates of postoperative endophthalmitis have been increasing over the past several years, owing to increases in the number of cataract surgeries and other types of intraocular surgeries performed. This raises concerns due to the ever-growing population of the elderly that require cataract surgery. Millions of cataract surgeries are performed each year. Fortunately, the rate of occurrence of post-cataract endophthalmitis remains low, ranging between 0.06% and 0.25% (O'Brien et al., 2007; West et al., 2005). Among the types of cataract surgeries performed, phacoemulsification accounted for approximately 48% of the postoperative endophthalmitis cases, while 38.5% and 6.6% of cases followed extracapsular or intracapsular extraction, respectively (Ng et al., 2005). Postoperative endophthalmitis can occur after other types of surgery such as secondary intraocular lens placement, pars plana vitrectomy, penetrating keratoplasty, and even after corneal suture removal (Lemley and Han, 2007).

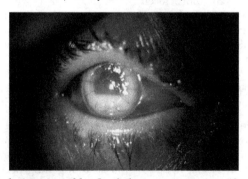

Fig. 1. Acute endophthalmitis caused by *Staphylococcus aureus* in a 43-year-old patient 3 days following a triple surgical procedure (penetrating keratoplasty, cataract extraction, and posterior chamber intraocular lens). Note the hypopion in the anterior chamber. The vitreous was also involved. Reproduced with kind permission from Dr. Rumelt

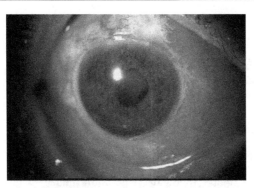

Fig. 2. Bleb-associated endophthalmitis due to *Streptococcus pneumoniae* in the right eye of a 63-year-old patient, 2 weeks after trabeculectomy. Note the whitening of the filtering bleb due to inflammatory infiltrate. There was also inflammation of the anterior and posterior segment. The earliest sign of endophthalmitis is infiltration of the bleb by inflammatory cells, and when the anterior and posterior segments are still normal, this is defined as "blebitis". Reproduced with kind permission from Dr. Rumelt

Preventative measures consist of prophylactic intracameral antibiotics or prophylactic subconjunctival antibiotic injection following cataract surgery (Kelkar et al., 2008). Patients with acute postoperative endophthalmitis generally present between 1 to 2 weeks following surgery. Endophthalmitis has also been reported to occur after intravitreal injection of anti-VEGF agents for the treatment of age-related macular degeneration (AMD). While the rate of endophthalmitis following intravitreal injection of these agents is equivalent to that of postoperative endophthalmitis following cataract surgery, approximately 0.16%, the increasing number of elderly patients requiring this type of therapy is a significant cause for alarm (Gragoudas et al., 2004).

Endophthalmitis must be distinguished from sterile inflammation following surgery. Diagnosis is established by visual acuity measurements, fundoscopy, and ERG, followed by microbiological evaluation of aqueous and vitreous samples (Lemley and Han, 2007). Gram-positive bacteria are the leading cause of postoperative endophthalmitis cases, with coagulase-negative staphylococcal (CNS) isolates being the most common, causing 47–70% of all postoperative endophthalmitis cases (Han et al., 1996). *S. aureus* account for approximately 10%, *Streptococcus* species for 9%, *Enterococcus* species for 2.2%, and Gram-negative bacteria for approximately 6% (Han et al., 1996). Fortunately, postoperative endophthalmitis caused by CNS is relatively mild and is more easily resolved with antibiotic and anti-inflammatory therapy (Josephberg, 2006). The visual prognosis is generally favorable, with 84% of cases resulting in at least 20/100 visual acuity, and 50% of these cases resulted in 20/40 visual acuity (Josephberg, 2006). Less virulent bacteria such as *Propionibacterium acnes* and CNS, and the fungal organism *Candida parapsilosis* are the most common causative agents of chronic endophthalmitis (Lemley and Han, 2007). Patients with this form of endophthalmitis typically present several months following surgery (Lemley and Han, 2007). Postoperative endophthalmitis caused by *S. aureus*, species of streptococci, enterococci, *Bacillus,* and Gram-negative bacteria can cause a more explosive and fulminant infection. The visual outcome of severe infections is uniformly poor, with only 30% of eyes attaining 20/100 visual acuity (Josephberg, 2006). The primary treatment is typically a single intravitreal injection of antibiotics consisting of 1.0 mg vancomycin per 0.1 ml, and 2.25 mg ceftazidime per 0.1 ml or 400 μg amikacin per 0.1 ml. Fourth generation fluoroquinolones can also be employed because of their broad spectrum of activity and usefulness against Gram-negative bacteria. Vitrectomy and corticosteriod therapy are are often advocated as adjunct treatment modalities (Lemley and Han, 2007), however corticosteriod treatment is still considered controversial.

4. Posttraumatic endophthalmitis

Posttraumatic endophthalmitis is a complication of a penetrating injury to the eye and is not as frequent as postoperative endophthalmitis. However, the rate of infection is higher and the visual prognosis is poorer following penetrating injury to the globe than following surgical procedures. The infection rates following traumatic injury to the globe range from 3% to 17% (Meredith, 1999; O'Brien and Choi, 1995; Thompson et al., 1993). The rates increase substantially when a foreign body remains in the globe and range from 11 to 30% (Boldt et al., 1989; Brinton et al., 1984; Thompson et al., 1993). Other risk factors include age greater than 50 and a more than 24 hour delay prior to presentation (Thompson et al., 1993). Those patients who presented for intraocular foregin body removal greater than 24 hours following injury were approximately 4-fold more likely to acquire endophthalmitis (Thompson et al, 1993), highlighting the necessity of seeking immediate medical attention following penetrating injury. Staphylocci and *B. cereus* rank as the number one and two causes, respectively, and together account for 95% of cases (Das et al., 2005; Lemley and Han, 2007).

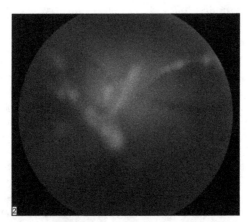

Fig. 3. Fundoscopic exam of a patient with *Staphylococcus aureus* endophthalmitis after a penetrating ocular injury. The findings of endophthalmitis in the vitreous may include not only flare and cells, but also fibrin in various degrees of organization. Organization to fibrotic bands may results in traction retinal detachment due to contraction of such bands. Reproduced with kind permission from Dr. Rumelt

B. cereus is ten times more likely to be the causative agent of posttraumatic than postoperative endophthalmitis, especially in cases involving organic or soil-contaminated intraocular foreign bodies (Das et al., 2005). Other causative agents include CNS, streptococcal species, clostridial species, fungi, and protozoa such as acanthamoeba (Lemley and Han, 2007; Rumelt et al., 2001).

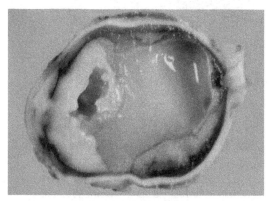

Fig. 4. Gross pathologic specimen of the globe affected by *Pseudomonas aeruginosa* endophthalmitis. The patient lost his vision in the eye and it became a blind, painful eye that underwent enucleation. Note the massive necrosis of the ocular tissues. Reproduced with kind permission from Dr. Rumelt

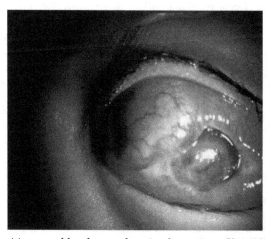

Fig. 5A. Endophthalmitis caused by the gas-forming bacterium *Clostridium bifermentans*. The endophthalmitis was caused following ocular penetrating injury be a soiled-contaminated foreign body. Note the brownish discoloration of the conjunctiva and a subconjunctival gas bubble. The patient was treated with intravenous and intravitreal panicillin and clyndamycin, but lost his vision despite the treatment. Reproduced with kind permission from Elsevier, Inc., in Rehany U, Dorenboim Y, Lefler E, Schirer E. Ophthalmology. 1994;101:839-42.

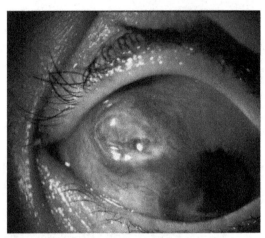

Fig. 5B. The same patient as in 5A a few days later. Note that the conjunctiva has become necrotic, the color became purple, and the gas bubble ruptured. Reproduced with kind permission from Elsevier, Inc., in Rehany U, Dorenboim Y, Lefler E, Schirer E. Ophthalmology. 1994;101:839-42.

When penetrating injury occurs, the foreign body should be removed as soon as possible, especially when the material is organic or soil contaminated due to the potential for *B. cereus* contamination (Lemley and Han, 2007). In some cases, for example where the foreign body is inert glass and is located in a sensitive position such as the retina, it may not be desirable to remove the object. Even relatively minor injuries to the eye can result in severe endophthalmitis with devastating outcomes. Cases have been described following penetrating injury to the eye due to orthodontic headgear (Blum-Hareuveni et al., 2006). Diagnosis of posttraumatic endophthalmitis is established by visual acuity tests, slit-lamp examination, and ophthalmoscopy, as well as computed tomography and ultrasound (Lemley and Han, 2007). For posttraumatic endopthalmitis, treatment consists of administration of intravitreal 1 mg vancomycin per 0.1 ml, 2.25 mg ceftazidime per 0.1 ml or 400 µg amikacin per 0.1 ml (Lemley and Han, 2007). Even with early therapy, the outcomes are often poor due to the potential virulence of the infecting bacterium and the explosive inflammatory response.

5. Experimental endophthalmitis and the roles of bacterial and host factors

A rabbit model of experimental endophthalmitis has been used to assess the contribution of both bacterial and host factors to the development of endophthalmitis. This model mimics the infection course after introduction of bacteria directly into the posterior segment of the eye that would occur following a surgical procedure or penetrating injury, but does not allow for the analysis of host immunological status and bacterial factors that contribute to the development of EE. This model system allows intravitreal injection across the pars plana of low inocula that allow the bacterium under study to adapt to the intraocular environment of the eye and replicate (Booth et al., 1995; Booth et al., 1997; Callegan et al., 1999a; Jett et al., 1992; Sanders et al., 2010; Sanders et al., 2011). Depending on the infecting organisms, infection symptoms in the rabbit model develop over a period ranging from 6 hours to 3 days, and a number of infection parameters can be repeatedly monitored and quantitative data obtained. Parameters that can be monitored include ocular inflammation, fibrin deposition, electrophysiologic measurement of retinal function, and bacterial growth and distribution. Infiltration of inflammatory cells can be quantified by slit lamp biomicroscopy in which progressive inflammation is scored in different anatomical locations within the eye (Callegan et al., 1999a). Inflammation and fibrin deposition can be qualitatively assessed by analysis of thin-section histopathology. Retinal damage as a result of the production of toxin by the bacterium under study or by bystander damage due to PMN activity in the eye can be measured by electroretinography (ERG). Using the rabbit model, Callegan et al. (1999a) found that supernatants from from *B. cereus* and *S. aureus* caused retinal damage and were highly inflammogenic, suggesting that secreted toxins are of primary importance to the pathogenesis of endophthalmitis. Callegan and colleagues did not find individual roles for the *B. cereus* membrane damaging toxins hemolysin BL, phosphatidylinositol-specific phopholipase C, and phosphatidylcholine-specific phospholipase C in this model, however, other toxins controlled by the global regulator *plcR* were found to contribute to pathogenesis of experimental *B. cereus* endophthalmitis (Callegan et al., 1999b; Callegan et al., 2002a; Callegan et al., 2003). The *S. aureus* alpha- and beta-toxins, but not the gamma-toxin, were shown to make an important contribution to endophthalmitis (Booth et al., 1998; Callegan et al., 2002b). Isogenic mutants deficient in each of the toxin-encoding genes were compared in this model. Injection of rabbit eyes with the gamma-toxin deficient mutant had no impact on retinal function when compared with the wildtype strain. However, the alpha- and beta-toxin deficient mutants were attenuated when compared with the wildtype. After 2 days, rabbit eyes infected with the alpha- or beta-toxin deficient mutant showed 40% and 60% retinal function retained, respectively, as compared with 20% retained in rabbits infected with the wildtype strain. Moreover, a cumulative effect was observed as a result of inactivation of all three toxin loci on retention of retinal function (Callegan et al., 2002b). This model has also been used as a sensitive measure of the contribution of enterococcal virulence factors to pathogenesis. Jett et al. (1992) demonstrated that the course and severity of disease was significantly determined by the *E. faecalis* biocomponent cytolysin. The cytolysin destroyed the neural tissue of the retina and its architecture over a period of 24 – 72 hours. The toxicity to retinal tissue was not attenuated by either antibiotic and/or anti-inflammatory therapy when infection involved a cytolytic strain, although an isogenic, non-cytolytic infection completely resolved when both of these treatments were provided 24 h postinfection. These studies showed not only the contribution of the cytolysin to the pathogenesis of enterococcal endophthalmitis, but also the importance of inflammatory sequelae. Engelbert et al. (2004) demonstrated that the *E. faecalis* gelatinase and serine protease in concert contributed to pathogenesis in this model as double mutants in these genes were significantly attenuated when compared to the single mutants. Callegan et al. (1999a) also utilized this model to implicate the contribution of bacterial cell wall components in inciting an inflammatory response during endophthalmitis. Injection of metabolically inactive bacteria or cell wall sacculi elicited significant intraocular inflammation. The rabbit model has also been used to implicate the *Streptococcus pneumoniae* capsule in the pathogenesis of endopthalmitis (Sanders et al., 2011). Infection with an isogenic unencapsulated *S. pneumoniae* mutant strain resulted in significantly lower slit lamp examination scores, significantly greater retinal function, and significantly less neutrophil infiltration into the eye compared with the wildtype parental strain in this model. Moreover, they demonstrated the efficacy of immunizing with the *S. pneumoniae* pneumolysin in protecting the eye from retinal damage during *S. pneumoniae* endophthalmitis (Sanders et al., 2010). In summary, the rabbit model of experimental endophthalmitis has proven invaluable in assessing the role of bacterial virulence factors and identifiying potentially new therapeutic targets.

More recently, a mouse model of experimentally induced endophthalmitis has been employed to explore various aspects of disease development, course, and outcome. As with the rabbit model, infection parameters can be qualitatively and quantitatively measured including bacterial growth, ocular inflammation, and retinal function. Ocular inflammation can be qualitatively assessed via thin-section histopathology as well as quantified by slit-lamp biomicrosopy and indirect measurements of PMN influx by a myeloperoxidase ELISA (Ramadan et al., 2006). As stated earlier, Wiskur et al. (2008) implicated the HMV phenotype in the persistence of *K. pneumoniae* in the eye by comparing the bacterial growth of an HMV+ to that of an HMV- strain after intravitreal injection of 100 CFU. The HMV- strain did not grow to the same level as the HMV+ strain and were cleared with 27 hours. HMV+ infected eyes underwent phthisis within 24 hours. This study provided evidence that the HMV phenotype makes an important contribution to *K. pneumoniae* endophthalmitis pathogenesis. As discussed above, Hunt et al. (2011) confirmed these findings using a *magA-*mutant of *K. pneumoniae* in the mouse endophthalmitis model. *S. aureus* cell wall teichoic acids have also been shown to contribute to the pathogenesis of endophthalmitis and that inhibitors of cell wall teichoic acid synthesis might serve as candidates for therapy of *S. aureus* endophthalmitis in this model (Suzuki et al., 2011).

An important aspect of the murine model of experimental endophthalmitis is that factors of the host immune system can be assessed by comparison of the infection course in genetic knockout mouse strains with that in wildtype strains of the same genetic background. Ramadan and colleagues (2006) showed that as early as 4 hours post-injection with *B. cereus*, significant decline in retinal function and PMN infiltration were observed, which coincided with an increase in the proinflammatory cytokine TNF-α. In TNF-α knockout mice, *B. cereus* replicated more rapidly, retinal function declined more sharply, and fewer PMN infiltrated the eye. These findings illustrate the power of this model in allowing the repeated measurement of multiple infection parameters and showed that damage to the retina occurred earlier than was previously thought. Furthermore, the necessity of TNF-α in PMN recruitment and control of *B. cereus* replication was established. Engelbert and Gilmore (2005) used C3 and FasL knockout out mice to dissect components of the innate immune and ocular immune privilege systems in controlling *S. aureus* endophthalmitis. The infection course in C3 knockout eyes followed a similar course to their wildtype counterparts, suggesting that complement does not play a significant role in ocular defense against *S. aureus* infection. On the other hand, the membrane-bound Fas ligand (FasL), which functions to maintain the immune privilege status of the eye by inducing apoptosis in infiltrating inflammatory cells, was found to be criticial in bacterial clearance. Mice deficient in FasL were unable to control *S. aureus* infection after injection of an inoculum that is cleared in wildtype mice (Engelbert and Gilmore, 2005). The host heat shock protein alphaB-crystallin was shown to be upregulated in the retina and prevent apoptosis and retinal damage during murine *S. aureus* endopthalmitis (Whiston et al., 2008). These authors found that mice deficient in the production of this molecular chaperone displayed increased retinal apoptosis and damage, and that *S. aureus* produced a protease capable of cleaving this protective protein. Finally, Kumar et al. (2010) suggested that the host toll-like receptor (TLR) 2 is involved in controlling infection by *S. aureus* in this model by showing that pretreatment of mice with intravitreal injections of the TLR2 ligand Pam3Cys reduced bacterial load when compared with mock-injected animals. In summary, the murine model of experimental endopthalmitis has proven to be invaluable in analyzing both host and bacterial factors that contribute to this disease. The growing number of available genetic knockouts in components of the innate and adaptive immune systems and the relative ease of use will continue to make the murine model key to understanding the complex interplay between host and bacterial factors during the initiation, course, and resolution of endophthalmitis.

6. Conclusions

Endophthalmitis remains a relatively rare infection, but the potential for vision loss and/or blindness is significant. The potential for poor prognosis, which depends on the causative organism and the immune status of the patient, remains high despite antibiotic and surgical intervention. Research on the contribution of bacterial virulence factors has implicated both secreted toxins and proteases, capsules, and the intraocular host response to bacterial cell wall components in the pathogenesis of experimental *B. cereus, S. aureus, E. faecalis, S. pneumoniae,* and *K. pneumoniae* endophthalmitis. Moreover, components of the host inflammatory response and mediators of ocular immune privilege have been shown to play critical roles in controlling experimental *B. cereus* and *S. aureus* endophthalmitis. Virtually nothing is known about the contribution of bacterial or host virulence factors to the development of EE. The fact that visual prognosis of EE and other types of bacterial endophthalmitis caused by pathogenic organisms remains uniformly poor highlights the need for continuing research on the interactions between the offending pathogen, the internal structures of the eye, underlying disease state and the immune response.

7. Acknowledgments

Portions of the work presented in this review were supported by the National Institutes of Health Grant R01EY012985 (to MCC), a Lew R. Wasserman Award from Research to Prevent Blindness (to MCC), a National Institutes of Health CORE Grant P30EY012190 (to Robert E. Anderson, OUHSC), and an unrestricted grant to the Dean A. McGee Eye Institute from Research to Prevent Blindness.

8. References

Aiello, L., Gardner, T., King, G., Blankenship, G., Cavallerano, J., Ferris, F., Klein, R. (1998). Diabetic retinopathy. *Diabetes Care*, Vol.21, pp. 143-156.

Amrite, A., Ayalasomayajula, S., Cheruvu, N., Kompella, U. (2006). Single periocular injection of celecoxib-PLGA microparticles inhibits diabetes-induced elevations in retinal PGE2, VEGF, and vascular leakage. *Invest. Ophthalmol. Vis. Sci.*, Vol.47, pp. 1149-1160.

Arevalo, J., Jap, A., Chee, S., Zeballos, D. (2010). Endogenous endophthalmitis in the developing world. *Int. Ophthalmol. Clin.*, Vol.50, pp. 173-187.

Asnaghi, V., Gerhardinger, C., Hoehn, T., Adeboje, A., Lorenzi, M. (2003). A role for the polyol pathway in the early neuroretinal apoptosis and glial changes induced by diabetes in the rat. *Diabetes*, Vol.52, pp. 506-511.

Axenfeld, T. (1894). *Arch. F. Ophth.*, pp. 103.

Blomquist, P. (2006). Methicillin-resistant *Staphylococcus aureus* infections of the eye and orbit (an American Ophthalmological Society thesis). *Trans. Am. Ophthalmol. Soc.*, Vol.104, pp. 322-345.

Blum-Hareuveni, T., Rehany, U., Rumelt, S. (2006). Devastating endophthalmitis following penetrating ocular injury during night sleep from orthodontic headgear: case report and literature review. *Graefes Arch. Clin. Exp. Ophthalmol.*, Vol.244, pp. 253-258.

Boldt, H., Pulido, J., Blodi, C., Folk, J., Weingeist, T. (1989). Rural endophthalmitis. *Ophthalmology*, Vol.96, pp. 1722-1726.

Booth, M., Atkuri, R., Nanda, S., Iandolo, J., Gilmore, M. (1995). Accessory gene regulator controls *Staphylococcus aureus* virulence in endophthalmitis. *Invest. Ophthalmol. Vis. Sci.*, Vol.36, pp. 1828-1836.

Booth, M., Cheung, A., Hatter, K., Jett, B., Callegan, M., Gilmore, M. (1997). Staphylococcal accessory regulator (*sar*) in conjunction with *agr* contributes to *Staphylococcus aureus* virulence in endophthalmitis. *Infect. Immun.*, Vol.65, pp. 1550-1556.

Booth, M., Hatter, K., Miller, D., Davis, J., Kowalski, R., Parke, D., Chodosh, J., Jett, B., Callegan, M., Penland, R., Gilmore, M. (1998). Molecular epidemiology of *Staphylococcus aureus* and *Enterococcus faecalis* in endophthalmitis. *Infect. Immun.*, Vol.66, pp. 356-360.

Brinton, G., Topping, T., Hyndiuk, R., Aaberg, T., Reeser, F., Abrams, G. (1984). Posttraumatic endophthalmitis. *Arch. Ophthalmol.*, Vol.102, pp. 547-550.

Callegan, M., Booth, M., Jett, B., Gilmore, M. (1999a). Pathogenesis of gram-positive bacterial endophthalmitis. Infect. Immun., Vol.67, pp. 3348-3356.

Callegan, M., Cochran, D., Kane, S., Gilmore, M., Gominet, M., Lereclus, D. (2002a). Contribution of membrane-damaging toxins to *Bacillus* endophthalmitis pathogenesis. *Infect.Immun.*, Vol.70, pp. 5381–5389.

Callegan, M., Engelbert, M., Parke, D., Jett, B., Gilmore, M. (2002b). Bacterial endophthalmitis: epidemiology, therapeutics, and bacterium-host interactions. *Clin. Microbiol. Rev.*, Vol.15, pp. 111-124.

Callegan, M., Engel, L., Hill, J., O'Callaghan, R. (1994). Corneal virulence of *Staphylococcus aureus*: roles of alpha-toxin and protein A in pathogenesis. *Infect. Immun.*, Vol.62, pp. 2478-2482.

Callegan, M., Jett, B., Hancock, L., Gilmore, M. (1999b). Role of hemolysin BL in the pathogenesis of extraintestinal *Bacillus cereus* infection assessed in an endophthalmitis model. *Infect. Immun.*, Vol. 67, pp. 3357-3366.

Callegan, M., Kane, S., Cochran, D., Gilmore, M., Gominet, M., Lereclus, D. (2003). Relationship of *plcR*-regulated factors to *Bacillus* endophthalmitis virulence. *Infect. Immun.*, Vol.71, pp. 3116–3124.

Chang, S., Fang, C., Hsueh, P., Chen, Y., Luh, K. (2000). *Klebsiella pneumoniae* isolates causing liver abscess in Taiwan. *Diagn. Microbiol. Infect. Dis.*, Vol.37, pp. 279-284.

Chen, Y., Kuo, H., Wu, P., Kuo, M., Tsai, H., Liu, C., Chen, C. (2004). A 10-year comparison of endogenous endophthalmitis outcomes: an east Asian experience with *Klebsiella pneumoniae* infection. *Retina*, Vol.24, pp. 383-390.

Chuang, Y., Fang, C., Lai, S., Chang, S., Wang, J. (2006). Genetic determinants of capsular serotype K1 of *Klebsiella pneumoniae* causing primary pyogenic liver abscess. *J. Infect. Dis.*, Vol.193, pp. 645-654.

Chung, K., Kim, Y., Song, Y., Kim, C., Han, S., Chin, B., Gu, N., Jeong, S., Baek, J., Choi, J., Kim, H,, Kim, J. (2011). Clinical review of endogenous endophthalmitis in Korea: a 14-year review of culture positive cases of two large hospitals. *Yonsei Med. J.*, Vol.52, pp. 630-634.

Collins, E., and Mayou, M. (1925). In: *Pathology and Bacteriology of the Eye*, P. Blakiston's Son & Co., Philadelphia.

Das, T., Kunimoto, D., Sharma, S., Jalali, S., Majji, A., Nagaraja, R., Gopinathan, U., Athmanathan, S. (2005). Relationship between clinical presentation and visual outcome in postoperative and posttraumatic endophthalmitis in south central India. *Indian J. Ophthalmol.*, Vol.53, pp. 5-16.

Delamaire, M., Maugendre, D., Moreno, M., Le Goff, M., Allannic, H., Genetet, B. (1997). Impaired leucocyte functions in diabetic patients. *Diabet. Med.*, Vol.14, pp. 29-34.

Engelbert, M., Gilmore, M. (2005). Fas ligand but not complement is critical for control of experimental *Staphylococcus aureus* endophthalmitis. *Invest. Ophthalmol. Vis. Sci.*, Vol.46, pp. 2479-2486.

Engelbert, M., Mylonakis, E., Ausubel, F., Calderwood, S., Gilmore, M. (2004). Contribution of gelatinase, serine protease, and fsr to the pathogenesis of *Enterococcus faecalis* endophthalmitis. *Infect. Immun.*, Vol.72, pp. 3628-3633.

Engler, C., Krogsaa, B., Lund-Andersen, H. (1991). Blood-retina barrier permeability and its relation to the progression of diabetic retinopathy in type 1 diabetics. An 8-year follow-up study. *Graefes Arch. Clin. Exp. Ophthalmol.*, Vol.229, pp. 442-446.

Fang, C., Chuang, Y., Shun, C., Chang, S., Wang, J. (2004). A novel virulence gene in *Klebsiella pneumoniae* strains causing primary liver abscess and septic metastatic complications. *J. Exp. Med.*, Vol.199, pp. 697-705.

Fang, C., Lai, S., Yi, W., Hsueh, P., Liu, K., Chang, S. (2007). *Klebsiella pneumoniae* genotype K1: an emerging pathogen that causes septic ocular or central nervous system complications from pyogenic liver abscess. *Clin. Infect. Dis.*, Vol.45, pp. 284-293.

Fong, D., Aiello, L., Gardner, T., King, G., Blankenship, G., Cavallerano, J., Ferris, F., Klein, R. (2003). American Diabetes Association: Diabetic retinopathy. *Diabetes Care*, Vol.26, pp. 226-229.

Funatsu, H., Yamashita, H., Sakata, K., Noma, H., Mimura, T., Suzuki, M., Eguchi, S., Hori, S. (2005). Vitreous levels of vascular endothelial growth factor and intercellular adhesion molecule 1 are related to diabetic macular edema. *Ophthalmology*, Vol.112, pp. 806-16.

Fung, C., Chang, F., Lee, S., Hu, B., Kuo, B., Liu, C., Ho, M., Siu, L. (2002). A global emerging disease of *Klebsiella pneumoniae* liver abscess: is serotype K1 an important factor for complicated endophthalmitis? *Gut*, Vol.50, pp. 420-424.

Giebel, S., Menicucci, G., McGuire, P., Das, A. (2005). Matrix metalloproteinases in early diabetic retinopathy and their role in alteration of the blood-retinal barrier. *Lab. Invest.*, Vol.85, pp. 597-607.

Gragoudas, E., Adamis, A., Cunningham, E., Feinsod, M., Guyer, D. (2004). Pegaptanib for neovascular age-related macular degeneration. *N. Engl. J. Med.*, Vol.351, pp. 2805-2816.

Greene, C., McDevitt, D., François, P., Vaudaux, P., Lew, D., Foster, T. (1995). Adhesion properties of mutants of *Staphylococcus aureus* defective in fibronectin binding proteins and studies on the expression of the *fnb* genes. *Mol. Microbiol.*, Vol.17, pp. 1143-1152.

Greenwald, M., Wohl, L., Sell, C. (1986). Metastatic bacterial endophthalmitis: a contemporary reappraisal. *Surv Ophthalmol.*, Vol.31, pp. 81-101.

Han, D., Wisniewski, S., Wilson, L., Barza, M., Vine, A., Doft, B., Kelsey, S. (1996). Spectrum and susceptibilities of microbiologic isolates in the Endophthalmitis Vitrectomy Study. *Am. J. Ophthalmol.*, Vol.122, pp. 1-17. Erratum in: *Am. J. Ophthalmol.*, Vol.122, pp. 920.

Ho, V., Ho, L., Ranchod, T., Drenser, K., Williams, G., Garretson, B. (2011). Endogenous methicillin-resistant *Staphylococcus aureus* endophthalmitis. *Retina*, Vol.31, pp. 596-601.

Hunt, J., Wang, J., Callegan, M. (2011). Contribution of mucoviscosity associated gene A (*magA*) to virulence in experimental *Klebsiella pneumoniae* endophthalmitis. *Invest. Opthalmol. Vis. Sci.*, Vol. 52, pp. 6860-6866.

Jackson, T., Eykyn, S., Graham, E., Stanford, M. (2003). Endogenous bacterial endophthalmitis: a 17-year prospective series and review of 267 reported cases. *Surv Ophthalmol.*, Vol.48, pp. 403-423.

Jagnow, J., Clegg, S. (2003). *Klebsiella pneumoniae* MrkD-mediated biofilm formation on extracellular matrix- and collagen-coated surfaces. *Microbiology*, Vol.149, pp. 2397-2405.

Jett, B., Jensen, H., Nordquist, R., Gilmore, M. (1992). Contribution of the pAD1-encoded cytolysin to the severity of experimental *Enterococcus faecalis* endophthalmitis. *Infect. Immun.*, Vol.60, pp. 2445-2452.

Jo, D., Kim, J., Kim, J. (2010). How to overcome retinal neuropathy: the fight against angiogenesis-related blindness. *Arch. Pharm. Res.*, Vol.33, pp. 1557-65.

Jonas, J., Knorr, H., Budde, W. (2000). Prognostic factors in ocular injuries caused by intraocular or retrobulbar foreign bodies. *Ophthalmology*, Vol.107, pp. 823–828.

Josephberg, R. (2006). Endophthalmitis: the latest in current management. *Retina*, Vol.26, pp. S47-S50.

Karama, E., Willermain, F., Janssens, X., Claus, M., Van den Wijngaert, S., Wang, J., Verougstraete, C., Caspers, L. (2008). Endogenous endophthalmitis complicating *Klebsiella pneumoniae* liver abscess in Europe: case report. *Int. Ophthalmol.*, Vol.28, pp. 111-113.

Kelkar, A., Kelkar, J., Amuaku, W., Kelkar, U., Shaikh, A. (2008). How to prevent endophthalmitis in cataract surgeries? *Indian J. Ophthalmol.*, Vol.56, pp. 403–407.

Keynan, Y., Rubinstein, E. (2008). Endogenous endophthalmitis caused by hypermucoviscous *Klebsiella pneumoniae*: an emerging disease in Southeast Asia and beyond. *Curr. Infect. Dis. Rep.*, Vol.10, pp. 343-345.

Kumar, A., Singh, C., Glybina, I., Mahmoud, T., Yu, F. (2010). Toll-like receptor 2 ligand-induced protection against bacterial endophthalmitis. *J. Infect. Dis.*, Vol.201, pp. 255-263.

Langstraat, J., Bohse, M., Clegg, S. (2001). Type 3 fimbrial shaft (MrkA) of *Klebsiella pneumoniae*, but not the fimbrial adhesin (MrkD), facilitates biofilm formation. *Infect. Immun.*, Vol.69, pp. 5805-5812.

Lederman, E., Crum, N. (2005). Pyogenic liver abscess with a focus on *Klebsiella pneumoniae* as a primary pathogen: an emerging disease with unique clinical characteristics. *Am. J. Gastroenterol.*, Vol.100, pp. 322-331.

Lee, H., Chuang, Y., Yu, W., Lee, N., Chang, C., Ko, N., Wang, L., Ko, W. (2006). Clinical implications of hypermucoviscosity phenotype in *Klebsiella pneumoniae* isolates: association with invasive syndrome in patients with community-acquired bacteraemia. *J. Intern. Med.*, Vol.259, pp. 606-614.

Lemley, C., Han, D. (2007). Endophthalmitis: a review of current evaluation and management. *Retina*, Vol.27, pp. 662-680.

Lin, J., Siu, L., Fung, C., Tsou, H., Wang, J., Chen, C., Wang, S., Chang, F. (2006). Impaired phagocytosis of capsular serotypes K1 or K2 *Klebsiella pneumoniae* in type 2 diabetes mellitus patients with poor glycemic control. *J. Clin. Endocrinol. Metab.*, Vol.91, pp. 3084-3087.

Losso, J., Truax, R., Richard, G. (2010). Trans-resveratrol inhibits hyperglycemia-induced inflammation and connexin downregulation in retinal pigment epithelial cells. *J. Agric. Food Chem.* Vol.58, pp. 8246-8252.

Luong, T., Lee, C. (2002). Overproduction of type 8 capsular polysaccharide augments *Staphylococcus aureus* virulence. *Infect. Immun.*, Vol.70, pp. 3389-3395.

Major, J., Engelbert, M., Flynn, H., Miller, D., Smiddy, W., Davis, J. (2010). *Staphylococcus aureus* endophthalmitis: antibiotic susceptibilities, methicillin resistance, and clinical outcomes. *Am. J. Ophthalmol.*, Vol.149, pp. 278-283.

Martin, P., Roon, P., Van Ells, T., Ganapathy, V., Smith, S. (2004). Death of retinal neurons in streptozotocin induced diabetic mice. *Invest. Ophthalmol. Vis. Sci.*, Vol.45, pp. 3330-3336.

McDevitt, D., François, P., Vaudaux, P., Foster, T. (1994). Molecular characterization of the fibrinogen receptor (clumping factor) of *Staphylococcus aureus*. *Mol. Microbiol.*, Vol.11, pp. 237-248.

Meredith, T. (1999). Posttraumatic endophthalmitis. *Arch. Ophthalmol.*, Vol.117, pp. 520-521.

Metrickin, D., Wilson, C., Berkowitz, B., Lam, M., Wood, G., Peshock, R. (1995). Measurement of blood-retinal barrier breakdown in endotoxin-induced endophthalmitis. *Invest. Ophthalmol. Vis. Sci.*, Vol. 36, pp. 1361-1370.

Miyamoto, K., Hiroshiba, N., Tsujikawa, A., Ogura, Y. (1998). In vivo demonstration of increased leukocyte entrapment in retinal microcirculation of diabetic rats. *Invest. Opthalmol. Vis. Sci.*, Vol.39, pp. 2190-2194.

Miyamoto, K., Khosrof, S., Bursell, S-E., et al. (1999). Prevention of leukostasis and vascular leakage in streptozotocin-induced diabetic retinopathy via intercellular adhesion molecule-1 inhibition. *Proc. Natl. Acad. Sci. USA.*, Vol.96, pp. 10836-10841.

Nassif, X., Honoré, N., Vasselon, T., Cole, S., Sansonetti, P. (1989). Positive control of colanic acid synthesis in *Escherichia coli* by *rmpA* and *rmpB*, two virulence-plasmid genes of *Klebsiella pneumoniae*. *Mol. Microbiol.*, Vol.3, pp. 1349-1359.

Nassif, X., Sansonetti, P. (1986). Correlation of the virulence of *Klebsiella pneumoniae* K1 and K2 with the presence of a plasmid encoding aerobactin. *Infect. Immun.*, Vol.54, pp. 603-608.

Neely, K., Gardner T. (1998). Ocular neovascularization: clarifying complex interactions. *Am. J. Pathol.*, Vol.153, pp. 665-670.

Ness, T., Schneider, C. (2009). Endogenous endophthalmitis caused by methicillin-resistant *Staphylococcus aureus* (MRSA). *Retina*, Vol.29, pp. 831-834.

Neveu, M., Elliot, A. (1959). Prophylaxis and treatment of endophthalmitis. *Am. J. Ophthalmol.*, Vol.48, pp. 368-373.

Ng, J., Morlet, N., Pearman, J., Constable, I., McAllister, I., Kennedy, C., Isaacs, T., Semmens, J., Team EPSWA. (2005). Management and outcomes of postoperative endophthalmitis since the endophthalmitis vitrectomy study: the Endophthalmitis Population Study of Western Australia (EPSWA)'s fifth report. *Ophthamology*, Vol.112, pp. 1199–1206.

Nixdorff, N., Tang, J., Mourad, R., Skalweit, M. (2009). SAME is different: a case report and literature review of *Staphylococcus aureus* metastatic endophthalmitis. *South Med. J.*, Vol.102, pp. 952-956.

O'Brien, T., Arshinoff, S., Mah, F. (2007). Perspectives on antibiotics for postoperative endophthalmitis prophylaxis: potential role of moxifloxacin. *J. Cataract Refract. Surg.*, Vol.33, pp. 1790-1800.

O'Brien, T., Choi, S. (1995). Trauma-related ocular infections. *Int. Ophthalmol. Clin. N. Am.*, Vol.8, pp. 667–679.

Okada, A., Johnson, R., Liles, W., D'Amico, D., Baker, A. (1994). Endogenous bacterial endophthalmitis. Report of a ten-year retrospective study. *Ophthalmology*, Vol.101, pp. 832-838.

Otto, M. (2010). Basis of virulence in community-associated methicillin-resistant Staphylococcus aureus. *Annu. Rev. Microbiol.*, Vol.64, pp. 143-16.

Park, S., Rich, J., Hanses, F., Lee, J. (2009). Defects in innate immunity predispose C57BL/6J-Leprdb/Leprdb mice to infection by *Staphylococcus aureus. Infect. Immun.*, Vol.77, pp. 1008-1014.

Patti, J., Jonsson, H., Guss, B., Switalski, L., Wiberg, K., Lindberg, M., Höök, M. (1992). Molecular characterization and expression of a gene encoding a *Staphylococcus aureus* collagen adhesion. *J. Biol. Chem.*, Vol.267, pp. 4766–4772.

Peyman, G., Vastine, D., Raichard, M. (1978). Postoperative endophthalmitis: experimental aspects and their clinical application. *Ophthalmology*, Vol.85, pp. 374-385.

Plata, K., Rosato, A., Wegrzyn, G. (2009). *Staphylococcus aureus* as an infectious agent: overview of biochemistry and molecular genetics of its pathogenicity. *Acta. Biochim. Pol.*, Vol.56, pp. 597-612.

Podschun, R., Sievers, D., Fischer, A., Ullmann, U. (1993). Serotypes, hemagglutinins, siderophore synthesis, and serum resistance of *Klebsiella* isolates causing human urinary tract infections. *J. Infect. Dis.*, Vol.168, pp. 1415-1421.

Puliafito, C., Baker, A., Haaf, J., Foster, C. (1982). Infectious endophthalmitis. Review of 36 cases. *Ophthalmology.*, Vol.89, pp. 921-929.

Qaum, T., Xu, Q., Joussen, A., Clemens, M., Qin, W., Miyamoto, K., Hassessian, H., Wiegand, S., Rudge, J., Yancopoulos, G., Adamis, A. (2001). VEGF-initiated blood-retinal barrier breakdown in early diabetes. *Invest. Ophthalmol. Vis. Sci.*, Vol.42, pp. 2408-2413.

Ramadan, R., Moyer, A., Callegan, M. (2008). A role for tumor necrosis factor-alpha in experimental *Bacillus cereus* endophthalmitis pathogenesis. *Invest. Ophthalmol. Vis. Sci.*, Vol.49, pp. 4482-4489.

Ramadan, R., Ramirez, R., Novosad, B., Callegan, M. (2006). Acute inflammation and loss of retinal architecture and function during experimental *Bacillus* endophthalmitis. *Curr. Eye Res.*, Vol.31, pp. 955-965.

Roghmann, M., Taylor, K., Gupte, A., Zhan, M., Johnson, J., Cross, A., Edelman, R., Fattom, A. (2005). Epidemiology of capsular and surface polysaccharide in *Staphylococcus aureus* infections complicated by bacteraemia. *J. Hosp. Infect.*, Vol.59, pp. 27-32.

Romero, C., Rai, M., Lowder, C., Adal, K. (1999). Endogenous endophthalmitis: case report and brief review. *Am Fam Physician*, Vol.60, pp. 510-514.

Rumelt, S., Cohen, I., Lefler, E., Rehany, U. (2001). Corneal co-infection with *Scedosporium apiospermum* and *Acanthamoeba* after sewage-contaminated ocular injury. *Cornea*, Vol.20, pp. 112-116.

Sanders, M., Norcross, E., Moore, Q., Fratkin, J., Thompson, H., Marquart, M. (2010). Immunization with pneumolysin protects against both retinal and global damage caused by *Streptococcus pneumoniae* endophthalmitis. *J. Ocul. Pharmacol. Ther.*, Vol.26, pp. 571-577.

Sanders, M., Norcross, E., Robertson, Z., Moore, Q., Fratkin, J., Marquart, M. (2011). The *Streptococcus pneumoniae* capsule is required for full virulence in pneumococcal endophthalmitis. *Invest.Ophthalmol. Vis. Sci.*, Vol.52, pp. 865-872.

Schroder, S., Palinski, W., Schmid-Schonbein, G. (1991). Activated monocytes and granulocytes, capillary nonperfusion, and neovascularization in diabetic retinopathy. *Am. J. Pathol.*, Vol.139, pp. 81-100.

Sebghati, T., Korhonen, T., Hornick, D., Clegg, S. (1998). Characterization of the type 3 fimbrial adhesins of *Klebsiella* strains. *Infect. Immun.*, Vol.66, pp. 2887-2894.

Shammas, H. (1977). Endogenous *E. coli* endophthalmitis. *Surv Ophthalmol.*, Vol.21, pp. 429-435.

Shrader, S., Band, J., Lauter, C., Murphy, P. (1990). The clinical spectrum of endophthalmitis: incidence, predisposing factors, and features influencing outcome. *J Infect Dis.*, Vol.162, pp. 115-120.

Suzuki, T., Campbell, J., Swoboda, J., Walker, S., Gilmore, M. (2011). Role of wall teichoic acids in *Staphylococcus aureus* endophthalmitis. *Invest. Ophthalmol. Vis. Sci.*, Vol.52, pp. 3187-3192.

Takeda, M., Mori, F., Yoshida, A., Takamiya, A., Nakagomi, S., Sato, E., Kiyama, H. (2001). Constitutive nitric oxide synthase is associated with retinal vascular permeability in early diabetic rats. *Diabetologia*, Vol.44, pp. 1043-1050.

Thakker, M., Park, J., Carey, V., Lee, J. (1998). *Staphylococcus aureus* serotype 5 capsular polysaccharide is antiphagocytic and enhances bacterial virulence in a murine bacteremia model. *Infect. Immun.* Vol.66, pp. 5183-5189.

Thompson, S., Parver, L., Enger, C., Meiler, W., Liggett, P. (1993). Infectious endophthalmitis after penetrating injuries with retained intraocular foreign bodies. *Ophthalmology*, Vol.100, pp. 1468–1474.

Tomás, J., Benedí, V., Ciurana, B., Jofre, J. (1986). Role of capsule and O antigen in resistance of *Klebsiella pneumoniae* to serum bactericidal activity. *Infect. Immun.*, Vol.54, pp. 85-89.

Tooker, C. (1938). Metastatic septic endophthalmitis with ring abscess of the cornea-case report, clinical history, and pathologic anatomy. *Trans. Am. Ophthalmol. Soc.*, Vol.36, pp. 77-88.

Virchow, R. (1856). Uber capillare embolie. *Virchow Arch. Pathol. Anato.*, Vol.9, pp. 307-308.

Walker, C., Fenwick, P. (1962). Bilateral fulminating endophthalmitis with streptocococcal septicaemia. *Br. J. Ophthalmol.*, Vol.46, pp. 281-284.

Walrand, S., Guillet, C., Boirie, Y., Vasson, M. (2004). *In vivo* evidences that insulin regulates human polymorphonuclear neutrophil functions. *J. Leukoc. Biol.*, Vol.76, pp. 1104-1110.

Wang, J., Liu, Y., Lee, S., Yen, M., Chen, Y., Wang, J., Wann, S., Lin, H. (1998). Primary liver abscess due to *Klebsiella pneumoniae* in Taiwan. *Clin. Infect. Dis.*, Vol.26, pp. 1434-1438.

Weakley, A. (1916). Metastatic endophthalmitis in a case of cerebro-spinal meningitis. *Br. Med. J.*, Vol.1, pp. 47-48.

West, E., Behrens, A., McDonnell, P., Tielsch, J., Schein, O. (2005). The incidence of endophthalmitis after cataract surgery among the US Medicare population increased between 1994 and 2001. *Ophthalmology, Vol.*112, pp. 1388-1394.

Whiston, E., Sugi, N., Kamradt, M., Sack, C., Heimer, S., Engelbert, M., Wawrousek, E., Gilmore, M., Ksander, B., Gregory, M. (2008). alphaB-crystallin protects retinal tissue during *Staphylococcus aureus*-induced endophthalmitis. *Infect. Immun.*, Vol.76, pp. 1781-1790.

Wiskur, B., Hunt, J., Callegan, M. (2008). Hypermucoviscosity as a virulence factor in experimental *Klebsiella pneumoniae* endophthalmitis. *Invest. Ophthalmol. Vis. Sci.*, Vol.49, pp. 4931-4938.

Yu, W., Ko, W., Cheng, K., Lee, H., Ke, D., Lee, C., Fung, C., Chuang, Y. (2006). Association between *rmpA* and *magA* genes and clinical syndromes caused by *Klebsiella pneumoniae* in Taiwan. *Clin. Infect. Dis.*, Vol.42, pp. 1351-1358.

7

Regulation of Angiogenesis in Choroidal Neovascularization of Age Related Macular Degeneration by Endogenous Angioinhibitors

Venugopal Gunda[1] and Yakkanti A. Sudhakar[1,2]
[1]Cell Signaling, Retinal and Tumor Angiogenesis Laboratory,
Department of Genetics, Boys Town National Research Hospital, Omaha, NE,
[2]Department of Biochemistry and Molecular Biology,
University of Nebraska Medical Center, Omaha, NE,
USA

1. Introduction

The sense of vision has utmost significance and the loss of vision leads to the impairment of active human behavior as evident in pathological disorders that affect vision. Among different pathological visual disorders, Age Related Macular Degeneration (AMD/ARMD) is of serious concern as a leading cause of blindness, observed with aging globally. The clinical manifestation of AMD includes retinal damage with the degeneration of macula, leading to the partial or complete loss of acuity in vision. One form of pathologic AMD named, "wet form of AMD", involves the growth of new blood vessels from the choroid which lies underneath the retina, leading to the pathological blood vessel growth termed as Choroidal Neovascularization (CNV), with subsequent damage to the retina. Thus, choroidal neovascularization reflects a pathological angiogenic condition, where the loss of regulation over angiogenesis leads to the retinal damage. It also indicates that, the regulation of pathological angiogenesis can be an efficient strategy in preventing CNV of AMD. Though, some genetic disposition and aging factors are identified as peculiar etiological factors causing AMD; recent studies have shown that different cellular mechanisms regulating angiogenesis are common in different angiogenic scenarios including CNV. Further, the role of different endogenous angiogenesis inhibitors/angioinhibitors conferring the tissues with angiogenic regulation has been deciphered, which can be applied for regulation of CNV in AMD through inhibition of angiogenic signaling mechanisms. The present chapter provides an overview of the role of factors leading to choroidal neovascularization, the mechanisms underlying such angiogenesis and also the scope for endogenous angioinhibitors in regulation of CNV of AMD.

1.1 Retina and choroid

Retina is the inner most layer of the eye, which possesses anatomically ten distinct layers that are broadly categorized into two layers. The inner neural layer comprising of extensive nervous tissue towards the vitreous chamber and the outer retinal pigmented epithelium (RPE) adhering to the choroid. Some of the functions of the RPE include the phagocytosis of outer retinal segmental discs, maintenance of chorio-capillaries, fluid and electrolyte balance in subretinal space. Choroid is the highly vascular and pigmented tissue of the eye lying between the retina and the sclera. It consists of lamina suprachoroidea adhering to sclera, followed by lamina vesculosa, chorio-capillaries, stroma and Bruch membrane adhering to the RPE. Choroid is rich in vasculature and the extracellular matrix (ECM) components, including collagen and elastin fibers. It provides nutrient, metabolite and gaseous exchange to the retina by diffusion through chorio-capillaries.

1.2 Choroidal neovascularization in age related macular degeneration

The histological proximity between retinal pigmented epithelium and choroid confers not only physiological but also pathological effect on RPE. The mechanical barrier that separates the RPE from choroid is the Bruch membrane, which in turn consists of basement membrane secreted by RPE, inner collagenous layer, elastic layer, outer collagenous zone and the basement membrane of chorio-capillaries acting as a mechanical barrier for the underlying chorio-capillaries, but facilitating diffusion of metabolites and gaseous exchange for RPE. In cases of CNV the Bruch membrane is distorted with initial deposition of lipid and protienaceous component called 'drusen' followed by the growth and penetration of blood capillaries from choroid into Bruch membrane, finally leading to the leakage of fluid into sub-retinal spaces and retinal or retinal pigmented epithelial damage (Green, 1999; Green and Enger, 1993; Jager et al., 2008).

1.3 Factors for choroidal neovascularization in age related macular degeneration

Pathological neovascularization in CNV of AMD is considered to be contributed by both the angiogenesis and vasculogenesis, which are the processes of *de-novo* blood vessel formation (Chan-Ling et al., 2011; Jager et al., 2008). Angiogenesis is the process of formation of new blood vessels from the pre-existing ones, which involves the role of different cell types and remodeling of ECM. The inception of different cell types involved in the angiogenesis, such as, the endothelial cells (ECs) of RPE and choroid involved in CNV, mural cells and inflammatory cells occurs through vasculogenesis, by the differentiation of endothelial progenitor cells (EPCs). The EPCs found in the normal circulation are recruited into angiogenic sites, where they differentiate into different cell types leading to angiogenesis (Chan-Ling et al., 2011; Jager et al., 2008). However, the salient feature of neovascularization involves the common sequential events of angiogenesis including the proliferation of ECs, degradation of ECM or vascular basement membrane (VBM) by ECs through secretion of proteases, migration and differentiation of ECs into tip and stalk cells, lumen development, ECM reorganization and finally vessel anastomosing into functional capillaries (Carmeliet and Jain, 2000). These sequential steps of angiogenesis are considered to be common for CNV, which are initiated by the release of angiogenic factors by the RPE and other cell types differentiated from EPCs or infiltrating through the leaky capillaries in response to aging evoked stress (Alon et al., 1995; Grossniklaus et al., 2002). The initiating cellular and physiological factors that lead to the secretion of angiogenic factors by ECs and other cell types have been identified in different studies, which can be systematically framed for synergistic interpretation of etiological factors leading to CNV.

The normal function of phagocytosis and degradation of phagocytosed membranes is impaired with aging in RPE, leading to the accumulation of lipofuscin in these cells, with senescence (Marshall, 1987; Young and Bok, 1969). Ischemia and hypoxia evident in the ocular tissues of CNV are identified as factors promoting free radical generation in RPE and also the release of cellular lipids and proteinaceous deposits into the Bruch membrane (Spaide et al., 2003). Thus, impairing Bruch membrane's barrier function and in turn leading to the secretion of different angiogenic factors like vascular endothelial growth factor (VEGF), transforming growth factor-β (TGF- β), basic fibroblast growth factor (bFGF), insulin-like growth factor-1 and platelet derived growth factor (PDGF) by the RPE and the macrophages and stromal cells that are recruited by the differentiation of EPCs (Alon et al., 1995; Grossniklaus et al., 2002; Lu and Adamis, 2006; Penn et al., 2008; Young and Bok, 1969). Damage to the Bruch membrane is considered to enhance the diffusion of the growth factors, which elicit angiogenic signaling in the ECs (Lu and Adamis, 2006; Marshall, 1987; Penn et al., 2008).

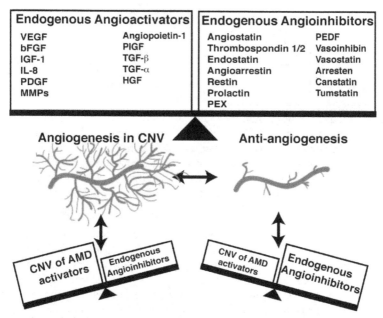

Fig. 1. **The angiogenic balance between endogenous angioactivators and angioinhibitors regulate vascular homeostasis.** Angiogenesis under physiological and pathological conditions is associated with up-regulation of endogenous angioactivators and/or down-regulation of endogenous angioinhibitors. Up-regulation of angioinhibitors and/or down-regulation of angioactivators may be associated with impaired neovascularization capacity in the choroidal neovascularization in age related macular degeneration (CNV of AMD). VEGF, vascular endothelial growth factor; bFGF, basic fibroblast growth factor; IGF-I, insulin-like growth factor-I; IL-8, interleukin-8; PDGF, platelet-derived growth factor; PlGF, placental growth factor; TGF-α and β, transforming growth factor-α and β; HGF, Hepatocyte growth factor

Endogenous Angioactivators	Potent Receptors	Angiogenic action
Vascular endothelial growth factor (VEGF) & Placental growth factor (PIGF)	VEGFRs (Flt-1, Flk-1, KDR, Flt-4), Neuropilins, HSPG, integrins	Increases EC permeability, proliferation, migration, NO, uPA/PAI-1 & MMP production Inhibiting EC apoptosis, Promotes ECM degradation Monocyte migration
Transforming growth factor-β (TGF-α, –β)	Transforming growth factor receptors	Increased vessel stability and organization, promote secretion of ECM components
basic Fibroblast growth factor (bFGF)	FGFRs, HSPG, integrins	Promotes EC proliferation, migration, tube formation, ECM degradation, vessel maturation
Insulin-like growth factor-1 (IGF-1)	Insulin-like growth factor receptors	Promotes EC migration, proliferation, tube formation
Platelet derived growth factor (PDGF)	PDGF-α, –β, GPCRs, integrins	Increases EC permeability, proliferation, migration
Angiopoietin-1	Tie-2, integrins	EC sprouting, Vessel stabilization
Hepatocyte growth factor (HGF)	Hepatocyte growth factor receptor	Promotes tubulogenesis along with other factors
Interleukin-8 (IL-8)	C-X-C chemokine receptor type (CXCR-1,2)	Activates neovascularization increasing invasiveness of different cell types
Matrix metalloproteinases (MMPs)		Degradation of ECM components promoting EC migration and vessel organization, release of ECM or cell surface bound/sequestred angiogenic fcators

Table 1. Endogenous activators, their receptors and angiogenic activities (EC: endothelial cell, ECM: extracellular matrix, FGFRs: Fibroblast growth factor receptors, Flk-1: Fetal liver kinase-1, Flt-1, 4: fms-related tyrosine kinase, GPCRs: G-protein coupled receptors, HSPG: Heparan sulfate proteoglycan, KDR: kinase insert domain receptor, MMP: matrix metallo proteinase, NO: nitric oxide, Pak: p21 protein activated kinase, PDGF: platelet derived growth factor, Tie: tyrosine kinase with immunoglobulin-like and EGF-like domains, VEGFRs: vascular endothelial growth factor receptors)

The integrins and other ECM binding receptors present on ECs are essential in maintaining the ECM promoted survival and migration in angiogenesis (Avraamides et al., 2008; Mettouchi and Meneguzzi, 2006). The synergistic activation of integrins and other ECM binding receptors on ECs by the growth factors and cytokines leads to the activation of different signaling cascades mediated by the kinases, secondary messengers, transcription factors such as, nuclear factor kappa β (NF-κβ), hypoxia inducible factor-1α (HIF-1α), and other enzymes such as, inducible nitric oxide synthase (iNOS), cyclooxygenase-2 (COX-2) and metalloproteinases (MMPs) (Avraamides et al., 2008; Boosani et al., 2007; Egeblad and Werb, 2002; Mettouchi and Meneguzzi, 2006; Oklu et al., 2010). The transcription factors that are stabilized, up-regulated or expressed under hypoxia also lead to activation of different signaling cascades that promote effective survival and proliferation of ECs. The secretion of proteases such as matrix metallo-proteinases (MMPs) including collagenases and elastases, which degrade the collagen and elastin of vascular basement membrane (VBM) promote the migration of ECs. The urokinase is another proteinase, which binds to its receptors (urikanse binding receptor, uPAR) and activates signaling cascades leading to the secretion of MMPs, which promote migration of ECs and angiogenesis. The organization and differentiation of migrating ECs into tip and stalk cells is further enumerated to be regulated by Wingless type (Wnt)/Frizzled-Notch signaling that provides an insight about formation of functional capillaries in neovascular vessels (Dejana, 2010; Zerlin et al., 2008).

The inflammatory cells that are recruited through the expression of cytokines such as monocyte chemo-attractant protein-1 (Ccl2/MCP-1), Chemokine (C-X-C motif) liagnd 1 (CXCL1), macrophage inflammatory protein-1/-2 (MIP-1, MIP-2) are also considered to play role in CNV progression (Hendricks, 2006). Further, the intriguing stimulative role of Bruch membrane in promoting AMD is also being deciphered by identifying the complement components 3a and 5a (C3a and C5a), which lead to the up-regulation of VEGF-A (Nozaki et al., 2006). Thus, the orchestration of various signaling events at different stages of angiogenesis leads to the neovascularization. The angiogenic ECs lining the neovascular vessels arising due to the above factors in CNV are found to possess fenestrations and also organize into defective capillaries leading to the leakage of macromolecules as well as vascular cells into the Bruch membrane and sub-retinal spaces leading to the degeneration of macula of retina (Dvorak et al., 1995; Roberts and Palade, 1995).

2. Endogenous angioinhibitors

In addition to the angiogenic factors, which activate angiogenesis, tissues and ECM also possess angioinhibitors, which have the potency to inhibit the angiogenesis and thus, regulating the pathological angiogenesis by inhibiting the signaling mechanisms activated by angiogenic factors (Boosani et al., 2010; Sudhakar and Kalluri, 2010, Zhang and Ma, 2007). Nearly, 40 endogenous angioinhibitors have been characterized and some of them are found in the ocular tissues or secreted into vasculature and released into ocular tissues, where they exhibit angio-inhibition and finally regulation of CNV (Boosani et al., 2011; Sudhakar and Kalluri, 2010). The significance of imbalance in the levels of endogenous angioinhibitors and angioactivators in regulation of vascular homeostasis can be summarized as in Figure 1. This significance was also ascertained by the evaluations showing the correlation between the decrease in specific angioinhibitors and the progression of CNV (Bhutto et al., 2008).

2.1 Mechanisms of regulation of CNV by endogenous angioinhibitors

2.1.1 Vasoinhibins

The vasoinhibins (14-18 kDa) are antiangiogenic peptides found in the pituitary, retina and extrapituitary tissues. They constitute the amino terminal regions of three different precursors; prolactin, growth hormone and placental lactogen. Though their precursors do not exhibit angioinhibitory activities; vasoinhibins found in the tissues or those expressed using recombinant methods exhibit antiangiogenic properties (Clapp et al., 2008). The therapeutic potential of vasoinhibins in regulating angiogenesis in CNV and tumor growth was evaluated and studies indicate that adenovirus mediated expression of vasoinhibins inhibits CNV, *in-vivo* and also angiogenesis (Zhou et al., 2010). Mechanisms of regulation of EC survival, proliferation and migration by the vasoinhibins have been deciphered in different studies; nevertheless, the receptors through which the mechanisms are mediated still remain enigmatic. Vasoinhibins regulate the EC migration and survival through inhibition of VEGF and bFGF stimulated MAPK activation (D'Angelo et al., 1995).

Endogenous Angioinhibitor	Parent molecule	Receptors	Mode of action/ Inhibition pathways
Vasoinhibins	Prolactin, growth hormone	Not known	Sos/Ras/MAPK or eNOS /Raf/MAPK, Ca2+/ eNOS/protein phosphatase 2, Ras/Tiam-1/Rac1/Pak1, Bcl-XL, NF-kβ, caspases
PEDF	PEDF	Not known	Possible apoptosis
Arresten	Collagen IV, α1 NC1	α1β1 integrin, HSPG	Raf/MEK/ERK1/2/p38-MAPK, HIF-1α, MMPs
Canstatin	Collagen IV, α2 NC1	αVβ3, αVβ5 integrins, Fas	procaspse-8 and -9, Akt/ FAK/mToR, eIF-4EBP-1, Ribosomal S6-kinase
Tumstatin	Collagen IV, α3NC1	CD47/IAP, αVβ3, α6β1 integrins	FAK/Akt/PI3K/mTOR/ eIF-4EBP1/NFκB, COX-2 signaling
Endostatin	Collagen XVIII-NC1	αVβ1/α5β1 integrins, HSP, glypican, caveolin-1	Ras/Raf/KDR/Flk-1 / ERK/p38-MAPK/p125 FAK/HIF1α/Ephrin/TNFα/NFκB, Wnt signaling
Angiostatin	Plasminogen	ATP synthases, αVβ3 integrin, angiomotin	αVβ3 integrin mediated apoptotis, ATP synthase
Thrombospondins	TSP	CD36, IAP, CD47, HSPG, α3β1 , other integrins	Src-family kinases/ Caspase-3/p38 MAPK, TGF-β signaling
Endorepellin	Perlecan	α2β1 integrins, lipid rafts, caveolin	cAMP-PKA/FAK/p38-MAPK/Hsp27, SHP-1, Ca2+ signaling

Table 2. Endogenous angioinhibitors, their precursors, cell surface receptors and mode of action AMD/ARMD: Age related macular degeneration, Akt: protein kinase B, Bcl-XL: B-cell lymphoma-extra large, bFGF: basic fibroblast growth factor, Ccl2/MCP-1: chemoattractant protein-1, CD(CD47, CD36): cluster of differentiation, CNV: choroidal neovascularization, COX-2: cyclooxygenase-2, eIF-4EBP-1: eukaryotic translation initiation factor-4E binding protein-1, eNOS: endothelial nitric oxide synthase, ECs: endothelial cells, ECM: extracellular matrix, EPCs: endothelail progenitor cells, ERK1/2: extracellular signal-regulated kinase1/2, FAK: focal adhesion kinase, Flk-1: fetal liver kinase-1, HIF-1α: hypoxia inducible factor-1α, Hsp: heat shock protein, HSPG: Heparan sulfate proteoglycan, IAP: integrin associated protein, KDR: kinase insert domain receptor, MAPK: Mitogen activated protein kinase, MEK: MAPK-ERK kinase, MMPs: matrix metallo proteinases, mToR: mammalian target of rapamycin, NF-kβ: nuclear factor kappa β, Pak: p21 protein activated kinase, PDGF: platelet derived growth factor, PEDF: Pigment epithelium derived factor, PEX: noncatalytic Carboxy-terminal hemopexin-like domain of MMP, PI3K: phosphatidyl inositol 3-kinase, Rac: Ras-related C3 botulinin toxin susbtrate 1, Raf: Ras activated factor, Ras: Rat sarcoma, RPE: retinal pigmented epithelium, SHP: Src homology region 2 domain-conatining phopshatase, Sos: Son of sevenless, Src: Schmidt-Ruppin A-2 sarcoma viral oncogene homolog, Tiam: T-lymphoma invasion and metastasis-inducing protein, TGF-β: transforming growth factor β, TNFα: tumor necrosis factorα, TSP: thrombospondin, VBM: vascular basement membrane, VEGF: vascular endothelial growth factor, Wnt: wingless-type

VEGF activated Sos/Ras/MAPK or eNOS/Raf/MAPK-mediated proliferative signaling and Ca2+/eNOS/protein phosphatase-2 mediated vascular permeability and vasodilatation were shown to be inhibited by the vasoinhibins (Gonzalez et al., 2004; Ziche and Morbidelli, 2000). In addition vasoinhibins also inhibit the migration of EC stimulated by IL-1β through Ras/Tiam-1/Rac-1/Pak1 and promote apoptosis through conversion of Bcl-XL to proapoptoctic Bcl-Xs and NF-kβ mediated activation of initiator and effector caspases (Martini et al., 2000; Tabruyn et al., 2003).

2.1.2 Pigment Epithelium Derived Factor (PEDF)

Pigment epithelium derived factor (PEDF) is a 50 kDa, secreted, serpin family glycoprotein, first identified from the cultured fetal RPE conditioned media (Tombran-Tink et al., 1991). PEDF accumulates in the vitreous humor and is also expressed in different adult tissues (Tombran-Tink et al., 1991). Addition of PEDF to the cultured HUVECs increased the number of TUNEL positive cells suggesting apoptotic mode of action of PEDF and thus, possibly preventing EC response to ischemia *in-vivo* (Ho et al., 2007). The levels of PEDF were found to be decreased in Bruch membrane with progression of AMD and concomitant increase in VEGF levels were also identified with decrease in PEDF levels (Bhutto et al., 2008). Different methods of PEDF upregulation have been applied to investigate the effect of PEDF on CNV. Intravitreous injections of adenovirus expressing the PEDF and ultrasound-microbubble technique of noninvasive gene transfer of PEDF gene in rats exhibited significant decrease in the CNV (Gehlbach et al., 2003; Zhou et al., 2009). However, studies also demonstrate that PEDF at lower doses (90μg/ml) has negative effect on CNV whereas; higher doses (2-4 fold) can augment CNV; thus, indicating a strategic approach to be developed during clinical trials for CNV treatment with PEDF (Apte et al., 2004).

2.1.3 Angiostatin

Angiostatins are 38-45 kDa kringle domains derived by the protease activity of parent molecule plasminogen, which itself has significant role in activation of fibrinogen and blood clotting (Hayashi et al., 2008). Some of the angiostatin peptide derivates exhibit anti-angiogenic properties including inhibition of EC proliferation, tube formation and migration. The application of angiostatins in regulating CNV of AMD was evaluated by the expression of the angiostatins *in-vivo*, using viral vectors (Lai et al., 2001). Angiostatins bind to ATP synthases on the surface of ECs leading to their apoptotic death (Burwick et al., 2005; Tarui et al., 2001). Further αVβ3 integrin and angiomotin are also shown to bind angiostatin and induce apoptosis (Burwick et al., 2005; Tarui et al., 2001).

2.1.4 Thrombospondins

Thrombospondins (TSPs) are secreted ECM glycoproteins playing key role in the cellular and ECM interactions (Bornstein, 2001; Lawler, 2000). The NH2-terminal peptides derived from the TSPs, by the action of different proteases are identified to possess angioinhibitory properties. TSP-1 and TSP-2 are trimeric globular domain subunits (145 kDa) categorized into subgroup-A and subgroup-B consists of TSP's 3-5, which are pentameric subunits (110 kDa) (Bornstein, 2009). TSP-1 was the first identified ECM derived endogenous angioinhibitor from many normal tissues and produced by a variety of cells including platelets, megakaryocytes, epithelial, endothelial and stromal cells (Bornstein, 2009). TSP-1 is secreted by the retinal-pigmented epithelium (RPE) and regulates angiogenesis in normal eye (Miyajima-Uchida et al., 2000). Immunolocalization studies showed decrease in the levels of TSP in the chorio-capillaries and the Bruch membrane of AMD samples (Bhutto et al., 2008). Wispostatin-1 (WISP-1) repeat derived peptide from TSP-1 was shown to inhibit the CNV in LASER induced CNV mice models (Cano Mdel et al., 2009). TSP-1 induces apoptosis in ECs through CD36 and integrin associated protein (IAP)/Src-family protein kinases/Caspase-3/p38 MAPK signaling (Dawson et al., 1997). In addition TSP-1 can also bind to different integrins, including CD47 and heparin sulfated proteoglycans (Kaur et al., 2011). Thus the significance of TSPs in regulation of CNV have been evaluated through detection of endogenous levels in pathological tissues and also by evaluating the effects of TSPs both *in vitro* and *in vivo*.

2.1.5 Arresten

Arresten [α1(IV)NC1], is the 26 kDa collagen type IV, α1 chain derived non-collagenous domain, which functions via binding to α1β1 integrin and heparan sulfate proteolgycans, regulating bFGF and VEGF stimulated activation of ECs (Boosani and Sudhakar, 2006; Colorado et al., 2000; Sudhakar et al., 2005). It inhibits the survival of mouse lung endothelial cells through inhibition of FAK phopshorylation in AKT independent manner (Sudhakar et al., 2005). FAK inhibition by arresten via α1β1 integrin leads to inhibition of downstream Raf/MEK/ERK1/2/p38 MAPK signaling and HIF-1α expression **(Figure 2)**. Inhibition of HIF-1α by arresten is critical in preventing hypoxic survival of ECs through VEGF regulation (Sudhakar et al., 2005). Arresten inhibited VEGF-mediated angiogenesis by promoting apoptosis, caspase-3/PARP activation and negatively impacting FAK/p38-MAPK phosphorylation, Bcl-2 and Bcl-x$_L$ expressions leading to mouse retinal endothelial cell (MREC) death (Boosani et al., 2009). In addition angioinhibitory activity of arresten was found to inhibit bFGF induced proliferation of MREC *in-vitro* in a dose dependent manner. It also inhibited the bFGF-induced migration of MREC mediated by MMP-2 activity but not the expression levels of MMP-2 (Boosani et al., 2010). Thus, arresten was shown to effect the proliferation and migration of choroidal endothelial cells and regulate CNV of AMD. The endothelial specific inhibitory actions of arresten may be of benefit in the treatment of a variety of eye diseases with a neovascular component.

2.1.6 Canstatin

It is the 24 kDa collagen type IV, α2 derived non-collagenous domain [α2(IV)NC1], which binds to the αVβ3 and αVβ5 integrins and inhibits EC proliferation, migration and tube formation by enhancing apoptosis in these cells (Magnon et al., 2005; Magnon et al., 2007; Petitclerc et al., 2000; Roth et al., 2005). The antiangiogenic efficacy of canstatin in regulating the neovascularization of cornea was also evaluated using the recombinant canstatin in alkali burn induced neovascularization study (Lima et al., 2006; Wang et al., 2011). Cantstain was shown to induce apoptosis through the induction of Fas-ligand, activation of procaspse-8 and -9 cleavage, reduction in membrane potential, inhibition of Akt, FAK, mToR, eIF-4E/4E-BP1 and ribosomal S6-kinase phosphorylations, in cultured HUVECs **(Figure 2)** (Panka and Mier, 2003).

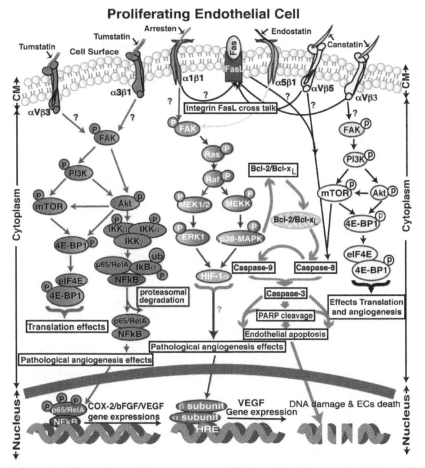

Fig. 2. **Schematic illustration of distinct angioinhibitory signaling mediated by different
extracellular matrix (ECM) reloaded molecules.** Tumstatin, arresten, canstatin and
endostatin interact with $\alpha V\beta3/\alpha3\beta1$, $\alpha1\beta1$, $\alpha V\beta3/\alpha V\beta5$ and $\alpha5\beta1$ integrins respectively, to
inhibit the phosphorylation of focal adhesion kinase (FAK). Tumstatin: It binds to $\alpha V\beta3$ and
$\alpha3\beta1$ integrins and inhibits the pathway that includes phosphorylation of FAK, PI3-K, Akt,
mTOR, 4E-BP1 and eIF4E to decrease endothelial cell protein synthesis and proliferation. In
addition tumstatin also inhibits NFκB mediated signaling in hypoxic conditions leading to
the inhibition of COX-2, VEGF and bFGF expressions, resulting in inhibition of hypoxic
tumor angiogenesis. Arresten: It binds to $\alpha1\beta1$ integrin and inhibit phosphorylation FAK,
causes inhibition of Ras, Raf, extra cellular signal related kinase 1 (ERK1) and p38 MAPK
pathways that leads to inhibition of HIF-1α and VEGF expression resulting in inhibition of
endothelial cell migration, proliferation and tube formation. In addition arresten initiates
two apoptotic pathways, involving activation of caspase-9 and -8, leading to activation of
caspase-3 and PARP cleavage. (a) Arresten activates caspase-3 directly through inhibition of
FAK/p38-MAPK/Bcl-2/Bcl-x$_L$ and activation of caspase-9; (b) Integrin $\alpha1\beta1$ cross talk with
Fas-L through mitochondrial pathway and leads to activation of caspase-8 and-3 in

proliferating endothelial cells. Canstatin: It binds to αVβ3/αVβ5 integrins and inhibits two apoptotic pathways, involving activation of caspase-8 and casoase-9, leading to activation of caspase-3. Canstatin activates procaspase-9 not only through inhibition of the FAK/PI3K/AKT pathways but also by integrins cross talking mitochondrial pathway through Fas-L dependent caspase-8 activation leads to endothelial cell apoptosis. CM represents cell membrane. Endostatin: It binds to α5β1 integrin and inhibit phosphorylation FAK, causes inhibition of Ras, Raf, extra cellular signal related kinase-1 (ERK1) and p38 MAPK pathways that leads to inhibition of endothelial cell migration and tube formation.

2.1.7 Tumstatin

Tumstatin [α3(IV)NC1], is a 28 kDa collagen type IV, α3 chain derived non-collagenous domain with anti-angiogenic and proapoptotic activities. It binds to the CD47/IAP, αVβ3, α3β1 and α6β1 integrins and inhibits the signaling cascade mediated by FAK, Akt, PI3K/mTOR/eIF-4E/4E-BP1 and NFκB/COX-2 (Boosani et al., 2007; Hamano et al., 2003; Maeshima et al., 2002; Monboisse et al., 1994; Sudhakar et al., 2003). Inhibition of eIF-4E/4E-BP1 by tumstatin leads to the regulation of cap dependent translational level of genes, whereas inhibition of transcriptional factor signaling such as NFκB leads to regulation of genes such as COX-2 at transcriptional level (Figure 2) (Boosani et al., 2007). Thus, tumstatin exhibits gene regulation in endothelail cell-specific and integrin-dependent manner. Angioinhibitory effect of tumstatin has been evaluated in regulation of CNV in mice (Boosani et al., 2011). Recombinant tumstatin regulated tube formation by mouse corneal endothelial cells (MCECs) *in-vitro* and adenoviral mediated expression of tumstatin *in-vivo* in mice has shown reduction in CNV (Boosani et al., 2011; Gunda et al., 2011).

2.1.8 Endostatin

Endostatin is the partial 20-kDa fragment of collagen type XVIII, carboxy terminal non-collagenous domain, derived from the parent collagen by proteolytic cleavage activities of elastase and cathepsin-L (Felbor et al., 2000). Endostatin is found in normal circulation enabling it to be utilized as an effective angioinhibitor without toxic effects (Fukai et al., 2002). Lower levels of endostatin have been recorded in CNV samples compared to the healthy donor eyes and within the tissues of progressive AMD (Bhutto et al., 2008; Fukai et al., 2002). Deletion of endostatin or collagen type XVIII massively up-regulates LASER induced CNV; where as administration of physiological concentrations of endostatin was able to inhibit such CNV in these mice (Marneros et al., 2007). Endostatin also down regulates the expression of VEGF in experimental CNV rat models (Takahashi et al., 2003). These observations along with the evidence of inhibition of CNV with intravenous injection of adenoviral vectors that express secretable endostatin, confirm the significance of endostatin in regulation of CNV (Mori et al., 2001; Wickstrom et al., 2003).

Endostatin elicits the anti-proliferative and anti-migratory effects by binding to different EC surface molecules and regulating the signaling cascades (Faye et al., 2009). Recombinant endostatin binds to αV integrin as shown in human endothelial cells (Rehn et al., 2001). Further studies have also shown localization of endostatin in the lipid rafts and association with caveolae (Wickstrom et al., 2002; Wickstrom et al., 2003). Surface plasmon resonance assays characterized the binding of endostatin to both αVβ1 integrins and the heparin sulfates and also localization to the lipid rafts (Ricard-Blum et al., 2004). *In-vitro* assays using ECs also showed the co-localization of endostatin with α5β1 integrin, actin stress fibers, membrane anchor protein and caveolin-1, which enumerates the interaction of endostatin with caveolae, inhibiting EC migration through the disassembly of actin stress fibers/focal adhesions, activation of Src and impaired fibronectin deposition by ECs in response to bFGF (Wickstrom et al., 2002; Wickstrom et al., 2003; Sudhakar et al., 2003). Binding of endostatin with integrins also down-regulates the activity of RhoA-GTPase and inhibits signaling pathways mediated by small kinases of the Ras and Raf families (Ricard-Blum et al., 2004). In addition, binding to the KDR/Flk-1, endostatin inhibits the VEGF-induced tyrosine phosphorylation of KDR/Flk-1 and activation of ERK, p38 MAPK, and p125FAK in HUVECs (Kim et al., 2002; Sudhakar et al., 2003). Further signaling cascades regulated by the endostatin are being identified, which are mediated by activator protein 1 (Id), HIF1α, ephrin, tumor necrosis factor-α (TNFα), nuclear factor-κB (NFκB), coagulation cascades, adhesion molecules and Wnt, which indicate the potential role of endostatin as an endogenous angioinhibitor (Nyberg et al., 2005) **(Figure 2)**.

2.2 Scope for endogenous angioinhibitors in CNV treatment

Current modalities of treatment for the CNV in AMD include the regulation of angiogenesis as angiogenesis being one of the pathological factors of neovascularization. The therapies such as LASER photocoagulation, photodynamic therapy and anti-VEGF therapies using Macugen or Lucentis, that are currently being applied to regulate the CNV have their own constraints such as development of lesions, loss of acuity in vision and frequent administration, respectively (Gallemore and Boyer, 2006). Alternative strategies for the treatment of CNV in AMD are therefore being developed in which the specific targeting on angiogenesis can be possible. Endogenous angioinhibitors are considered as one of the area to be explored in this arena to include them in regimens of complementary treatments for the regulation of CNV (Chappelow and Kaiser, 2008; Do, 2009). The signaling cascades regulated by some of endogenous angioinhibitors have been identified **(Table 2 and Figure 2)**, which enabled the application of those inhibitors in CNV.

3. Conclusions

The cellular, extracellular milieu and genetic factors responsible for the neovascularization arising in AMD are being deciphered with emphasis on identifying those factors that play a key role in the inception and progression of CNV. In this scenario, different etiological factors have been identified which regulate angiogenesis, effecting both extracellular milieu and intracellular angiogenic signaling pathways. Identification of the signaling cascades leading to the pathological angiogenesis in CNV has further lead to the possibility of regulating CNV, by focusing on signaling pathways as one of the targets. Application of endogenous angioinhibitors has proven as a promising strategy in this scenario of inhibiting angiogeneic pathways that are identified in CNV. The inhibitors such as vasoinhibins, PEDF, angiostatin, endostatin, tumstatin, canstatin and arresten that have been so far evaluated for regulation of CNV have not only shown promising evidence of CNV regulation, but also provided new strategies for inhibiting CNV through differential mode of actions. Such variation exhibited by different endogenous angioinhibitors can be beneficial in targeting CNV using different combinations of these inhibitors. It can be realized that these naturally occurring inhibitors can pose low immune reactions and thus, an efficient way of regulating diseases. Further, clinical studies using individual and combinations of endogenous angioinhibitors, included in different regimens along with current therapies of CNV would elaborate the application of endogenous angioinhibitors for regulating CNV of AMD.

4. Acknowledgements

This study was supported by Flight Attendant Medical Research Institute Young Clinical Scientist Award Grant FAMRI-062558, NIH/NCI Grant RO1CA143128, Dobleman Head and Neck Cancer Institute Grant DHNCI-61905 and startup research funds of Cell Signaling, Retinal and Tumor Angiogenesis Laboratory at Boys Town National Research Hospital to YAS.

5. References

Alon, T., Hemo, I., Itin, A., Pe'er, J., Stone, J., and Keshet, E. (1995). Vascular endothelial growth factor acts as a survival factor for newly formed retinal vessels and has implications for retinopathy of prematurity. Nat Med 1, 1024-1028.

Apte, R. S., Barreiro, R. A., Duh, E., Volpert, O., and Ferguson, T. A. (2004). Stimulation of neovascularization by the anti-angiogenic factor PEDF. Invest Ophthalmol Vis Sci 45, 4491-4497.

Avraamides, C. J., Garmy-Susini, B., and Varner, J. A. (2008). Integrins in angiogenesis and lymphangiogenesis. Nat Rev Cancer 8, 604-617.

Bhutto, I. A., Uno, K., Merges, C., Zhang, L., McLeod, D. S., and Lutty, G. A. (2008). Reduction of endogenous angiogenesis inhibitors in Bruch's membrane of the submacular region in eyes with age-related macular degeneration. Arch Ophthalmol 126, 670-678.

Boosani, C. S., Gunda, V., Wang, S., Sheibani, N., and Sudhakar, A. Y. (2011). Tumstatin inhibits Choroidal Neovascularisation by Inhibiting MMP-2 activation in-vitro and in-vivo. Mol Vision. (Publication ahead of print).

Boosani, C. S., Mannam, A. P., Cosgrove, D., Silva, R., Hodivala-Dilke, K. M., Keshamouni, V. G., and Sudhakar, A. (2007). Regulation of COX-2 mediated signaling by alpha3 type IV noncollagenous domain in tumor angiogenesis. Blood 110, 1168-1177.

Boosani, C.S., Nalabothula, N., Munugalvadla, V., Cosgrove, D., Keshamouni, V. G., Sheibani, N., and Sudhakar, A. (2009). FAK and p38-MAP kinase-dependent activation of apoptosis and caspase-3 in retinal endothelial cells by $\alpha1(IV)NC1$. Invest. Ophthalmol. Vis. Sci. 50, 4567-4575.

Boosani, C. S., Nalabothula, N., Sheibani, N., and Sudhakar, A. (2010). Inhibitory effects of arresten on bFGF-induced proliferation, migration, and matrix metalloproteinase-2 activation in mouse retinal endothelial cells. Curr Eye Res 35, 45-55.

Boosani, C. S., and Sudhakar, A. (2006). Cloning, purification, and characterization of a non-collagenous anti-angiogenic protein domain from human alpha1 type IV collagen expressed in Sf9 cells. Protein Expr Purif 49, 211-218.

Bornstein, P. (2001). Thrombospondins as matricellular modulators of cell function. J Clin Invest 107, 929-934.

Bornstein, P. (2009). Thrombospondins function as regulators of angiogenesis. J Cell Commun Signal 3, 189-200.

Burwick, N. R., Wahl, M. L., Fang, J., Zhong, Z., Moser, T. L., Li, B., Capaldi, R. A., Kenan, D. J., and Pizzo, S. V. (2005). An Inhibitor of the F1 subunit of ATP synthase (IF1) modulates the activity of angiostatin on the endothelial cell surface. J Biol Chem 280, 1740-1745.

Cano Mdel, V., Karagiannis, E. D., Soliman, M., Bakir, B., Zhuang, W., Popel, A. S., and Gehlbach, P. L. (2009). A peptide derived from type 1 thrombospondin repeat-containing protein WISP-1 inhibits corneal and choroidal neovascularization. Invest Ophthalmol Vis Sci 50, 3840-3845.

Carmeliet, P., and Jain, R. K. (2000). Angiogenesis in cancer and other diseases. Nature 407, 249-257.

Chan-Ling, T., Dahlstrom, J. E., Koina, M. E., McColm, J. R., Sterling, R. A., Bean, E. G., Adamson, S., Hughes, S., and Baxter, L. C. (2011). Evidence of hematopoietic differentiation, vasculogenesis and angiogenesis in the formation of human choroidal blood vessels. Exp Eye Res 92, 361-376.

Chappelow, A. V., and Kaiser, P. K. (2008). Neovascular age-related macular degeneration: potential therapies. Drugs 68, 1029-1036.

Clapp, C., Thebault, S., Arnold, E., Garcia, C., Rivera, J. C., and de la Escalera, G. M. (2008). Vasoinhibins: novel inhibitors of ocular angiogenesis. Am J Physiol Endocrinol Metab 295, E772-778.

Colorado, P. C., Torre, A., Kamphaus, G., Maeshima, Y., Hopfer, H., Takahashi, K., Volk, R., Zamborsky, E. D., Herman, S., Sarkar, P. K., Ericksen, M. B., Dhanabal, M., Simons, M., Post, M., Kufe, D. W., Weichselbaum, R. R., Sukhatme, V. P., and Kalluri, R. (2000). Anti-angiogenic cues from vascular basement membrane collagen. Cancer Res 60, 2520-2526.

D'Angelo, G., Struman, I., Martial, J., and Weiner, R. I. (1995). Activation of mitogen-activated protein kinases by vascular endothelial growth factor and basic fibroblast growth factor in capillary endothelial cells is inhibited by the antiangiogenic factor 16-kDa N-terminal fragment of prolactin. Proc Natl Acad Sci U S A 92, 6374-6378.

Dawson, D. W., Pearce, S. F., Zhong, R., Silverstein, R. L., Frazier, W. A., and Bouck, N. P. (1997). CD36 mediates the In vitro inhibitory effects of thrombospondin-1 on endothelial cells. J Cell Biol 138, 707-717.

Dejana, E. (2010). The role of wnt signaling in physiological and pathological angiogenesis. Circ Res 107, 943-952.

Do, D. V. (2009). Antiangiogenic approaches to age-related macular degeneration in the future. Ophthalmology 116, S24-26.

Dvorak, H. F., Brown, L. F., Detmar, M., and Dvorak, A. M. (1995). Vascular permeability factor/vascular endothelial growth factor, microvascular hyperpermeability, and angiogenesis. Am J Pathol 146, 1029-1039.

Egeblad, M., and Werb, Z. (2002). New functions for the matrix metalloproteinases in cancer progression. Nat Rev Cancer 2, 161-174.

Faye, C., Moreau, C., Chautard, E., Jetne, R., Fukai, N., Ruggiero, F., Humphries, M. J., Olsen, B. R., and Ricard-Blum, S. (2009). Molecular interplay between endostatin, integrins, and heparan sulfate. J Biol Chem *284*, 22029-22040.

Felbor, U., Dreier, L., Bryant, R. A., Ploegh, H. L., Olsen, B. R., and Mothes, W. (2000). Secreted cathepsin L generates endostatin from collagen XVIII. EMBO J *19*, 1187-1194.

Fukai, N., Eklund, L., Marneros, A. G., Oh, S. P., Keene, D. R., Tamarkin, L., Niemela, M., Ilves, M., Li, E., Pihlajaniemi, T., and Olsen, B. R. (2002). Lack of collagen XVIII/endostatin results in eye abnormalities. EMBO J *21*, 1535-1544.

Gallemore, P. R., and Boyer, D. S. (2006). PDT or Anti-VEGF for AMD treatment. Review of Ophthalmology online.

Gehlbach, P., Demetriades, A. M., Yamamoto, S., Deering, T., Duh, E. J., Yang, H. S., Cingolani, C., Lai, H., Wei, L., and Campochiaro, P. A. (2003). Periocular injection of an adenoviral vector encoding pigment epithelium-derived factor inhibits choroidal neovascularization. Gene Ther *10*, 637-646.

Gonzalez, C., Corbacho, A. M., Eiserich, J. P., Garcia, C., Lopez-Barrera, F., Morales-Tlalpan, V., Barajas-Espinosa, A., Diaz-Munoz, M., Rubio, R., Lin, S. H., Martinez de la Escalera, G., and Clapp, C. (2004). 16K-prolactin inhibits activation of endothelial nitric oxide synthase, intracellular calcium mobilization, and endothelium-dependent vasorelaxation. Endocrinology *145*, 5714-5722.

Green, W. R. (1999). Histopathology of age-related macular degeneration. Mol Vis *5*, 27.

Green, W. R., and Enger, C. (1993). Age-related macular degeneration histopathologic studies. The 1992 Lorenz E. Zimmerman Lecture. Ophthalmology *100*, 1519-1535.

Grossniklaus, H. E., Ling, J. X., Wallace, T. M., Dithmar, S., Lawson, D. H., Cohen, C., Elner, V. M., Elner, S. G., and Sternberg, P., Jr. (2002). Macrophage and retinal pigment epithelium expression of angiogenic cytokines in choroidal neovascularization. Mol Vis *8*, 119-126.

Gunda, V., Wang, S., Sheibani, N., and Sudhakar, A. (2011). Inhibitory effect of tumstatin on corneal neovascularization both in-vitro and in-vivo. J Clinic Experment Ophthalmol (publication ahead of time).

Hamano, Y., Zeisberg, M., Sugimoto, H., Lively, J. C., Maeshima, Y., Yang, C., Hynes, R. O., Werb, Z., Sudhakar, A., and Kalluri, R. (2003). Physiological levels of tumstatin, a fragment of collagen IV alpha3 chain, are generated by MMP-9 proteolysis and suppress angiogenesis via alphaV beta3 integrin. Cancer Cell *3*, 589-601.

Hayashi, M., Tamura, Y., Dohmae, N., Kojima, S., and Shimonaka, M. (2008). Plasminogen N-terminal activation peptide modulates the activity of angiostatin-related peptides on endothelial cell proliferation and migration. Biochem Biophys Res Commun *369*, 635-640.

Hendricks, R. L. (2006). Interaction of angiogenic and immune mechanisms in the eye. Semin Ophthalmol *21*, 37-40.

Ho, T. C., Chen, S. L., Yang, Y. C., Liao, C. L., Cheng, H. C., and Tsao, Y. P. (2007). PEDF induces p53-mediated apoptosis through PPAR gamma signaling in human umbilical vein endothelial cells. Cardiovasc Res *76*, 213-223.

Jager, R. D., Mieler, W. F., and Miller, J. W. (2008). Age-related macular degeneration. N
Engl J Med *358*, 2606-2617.

Kaur, S., Kuznetsova, S. A., Pendrak, M. L., Sipes, J. M., Romeo, M. J., Li, Z., Zhang, L., and
Roberts, D. D. (2011). Heparan sulfate modification of the transmembrane receptor
CD47 is necessary for inhibition of T cell receptor signaling by thrombospondin-1. J
Biol Chem *286*, 14991-15002.

Kim, Y. M., Hwang, S., Pyun, B. J., Kim, T. Y., Lee, S. T., Gho, Y. S., and Kwon, Y. G. (2002).
Endostatin blocks vascular endothelial growth factor-mediated signaling via direct
interaction with KDR/Flk-1. J Biol Chem *277*, 27872-27879.

Lai, C. C., Wu, W. C., Chen, S. L., Xiao, X., Tsai, T. C., Huan, S. J., Chen, T. L., Tsai, R. J., and
Tsao, Y. P. (2001). Suppression of choroidal neovascularization by adeno-associated
virus vector expressing angiostatin. Invest Ophthalmol Vis Sci *42*, 2401-2407.

Lawler, J. (2000). The functions of thrombospondin-1 and-2. Curr Opin Cell Biol *12*, 634-640.

Lima, E. S. R., Kachi, S., Akiyama, H., Shen, J., Aslam, S., Yuan Gong, Y., Khu, N. H., Hatara,
M. C., Boutaud, A., Peterson, R., and Campochiaro, P. A. (2006). Recombinant non-
collagenous domain of alpha2(IV) collagen causes involution of choroidal
neovascularization by inducing apoptosis. J Cell Physiol *208*, 161-166.

Lu, M., and Adamis, A. P. (2006). Molecular biology of choroidal neovascularization.
Ophthalmol Clin North Am *19*, 323-334.

Maeshima, Y., Colorado, P. C., Torre, A., Holthaus, K. A., Grunkemeyer, J. A., Ericksen, M.
B., Hopfer, H., Xiao, Y., Stillman, I. E., and Kalluri, R. (2000). Distinct antitumor
properties of a type IV collagen domain derived from basement membrane. J Biol
Chem *275*, 21340-21348.

Maeshima, Y., Sudhakar, A., Lively, J. C., Ueki, K., Kharbanda, S., Kahn, C. R., Sonenberg,
N., Hynes, R. O., and Kalluri, R. (2002). Tumstatin, an endothelial cell-specific
inhibitor of protein synthesis. Science *295*, 140-143.

Magnon, C., Galaup, A., Mullan, B., Rouffiac, V., Bouquet, C., Bidart, J. M., Griscelli, F.,
Opolon, P., and Perricaudet, M. (2005). Canstatin acts on endothelial and tumor
cells via mitochondrial damage initiated through interaction with alphavbeta3 and
alphavbeta5 integrins. Cancer Res *65*, 4353-4361.

Magnon, C., Opolon, P., Ricard, M., Connault, E., Ardouin, P., Galaup, A., Metivier, D.,
Bidart, J. M., Germain, S., Perricaudet, M., and Schlumberger, M. (2007). Radiation
and inhibition of angiogenesis by canstatin synergize to induce HIF-1alpha-
mediated tumor apoptotic switch. J Clin Invest *117*, 1844-1855.

Marneros, A. G., She, H., Zambarakji, H., Hashizume, H., Connolly, E. J., Kim, I.,
Gragoudas, E. S., Miller, J. W., and Olsen, B. R. (2007). Endogenous endostatin
inhibits choroidal neovascularization. FASEB J *21*, 3809-3818.

Marshall, J. (1987). The ageing retina: physiology or pathology. Eye (Lond) *1 (Pt 2)*, 282-295.

Martini, J. F., Piot, C., Humeau, L. M., Struman, I., Martial, J. A., and Weiner, R. I. (2000). The
antiangiogenic factor 16K PRL induces programmed cell death in endothelial cells
by caspase activation. Mol Endocrinol *14*, 1536-1549.

Mettouchi, A., and Meneguzzi, G. (2006). Distinct roles of beta1 integrins during
angiogenesis. Eur J Cell Biol *85*, 243-247.

Miyajima-Uchida, H., Hayashi, H., Beppu, R., Kuroki, M., Fukami, M., Arakawa, F., Tomita, Y., and Oshima, K. (2000). Production and accumulation of thrombospondin-1 in human retinal pigment epithelial cells. Invest Ophthalmol Vis Sci 41, 561-567.

Monboisse, J. C., Garnotel, R., Bellon, G., Ohno, N., Perreau, C., Borel, J. P., and Kefalides, N. A. (1994). The alpha 3 chain of type IV collagen prevents activation of human polymorphonuclear leukocytes. J Biol Chem 269, 25475-25482.

Mori, K., Ando, A., Gehlbach, P., Nesbitt, D., Takahashi, K., Goldsteen, D., Penn, M., Chen, C. T., Melia, M., Phipps, S., Moffat, D., Brazzell, K., Liau, G., Dixon, K. H., and Campochiaro, P. A. (2001). Inhibition of choroidal neovascularization by intravenous injection of adenoviral vectors expressing secretable endostatin. Am J Pathol 159, 313-320.

Nozaki, M., Raisler, B. J., Sakurai, E., Sarma, J. V., Barnum, S. R., Lambris, J. D., Chen, Y., Zhang, K., Ambati, B. K., Baffi, J. Z., and Ambati, J. (2006). Drusen complement components C3a and C5a promote choroidal neovascularization. Proc Natl Acad Sci U S A 103, 2328-2333.

Nyberg, P., Xie, L., and Kalluri, R. (2005). Endogenous inhibitors of angiogenesis. Cancer Res 65, 3967-3979.

Oklu, R., Walker, T. G., Wicky, S., and Hesketh, R. (2010). Angiogenesis and current antiangiogenic strategies for the treatment of cancer. J Vasc Interv Radiol 21, 1791-1805; quiz 1806.

Panka, D. J., and Mier, J. W. (2003). Canstatin inhibits Akt activation and induces Fas-dependent apoptosis in endothelial cells. J Biol Chem 278, 37632-37636.

Penn, J. S., Madan, A., Caldwell, R. B., Bartoli, M., Caldwell, R. W., and Hartnett, M. E. (2008). Vascular endothelial growth factor in eye disease. Prog Retin Eye Res 27, 331-371.

Petitclerc, E., Boutaud, A., Prestayko, A., Xu, J., Sado, Y., Ninomiya, Y., Sarras, M. P., Jr., Hudson, B. G., and Brooks, P. C. (2000). New Functions for Non-collagenous Domains of Human Collagen Type IV. Novel integrin ligands inhibiting angiogenesis and tumor growth in vivo. J Biol Chem 275, 8051-8061.

Rehn, M., Veikkola, T., Kukk-Valdre, E., Nakamura, H., Ilmonen, M., Lombardo, C., Pihlajaniemi, T., Alitalo, K., and Vuori, K. (2001). Interaction of endostatin with integrins implicated in angiogenesis. Proc Natl Acad Sci U S A 98, 1024-1029.

Ricard-Blum, S., Feraud, O., Lortat-Jacob, H., Rencurosi, A., Fukai, N., Dkhissi, F., Vittet, D., Imberty, A., Olsen, B. R., and van der Rest, M. (2004). Characterization of endostatin binding to heparin and heparan sulfate by surface plasmon resonance and molecular modeling: role of divalent cations. J Biol Chem 279, 2927-2936.

Roberts, W. G., and Palade, G. E. (1995). Increased microvascular permeability and endothelial fenestration induced by vascular endothelial growth factor. J Cell Sci 108 (Pt 6), 2369-2379.

Roth, J. M., Akalu, A., Zelmanovich, A., Policarpio, D., Ng, B., MacDonald, S., Formenti, S., Liebes, L., and Brooks, P. C. (2005). Recombinant alpha2(IV)NC1 domain inhibits tumor cell-extracellular matrix interactions, induces cellular senescence, and inhibits tumor growth in vivo. Am J Pathol 166, 901-911.

Spaide, R. F., Armstrong, D., and Browne, R. (2003). Continuing medical education review: choroidal neovascularization in age-related macular degeneration--what is the cause? Retina 23, 595-614.

Sudhakar, A., and Boosani, C. S. (2008). Inhibition of tumor angiogenesis by tumstatin: insights into signaling mechanisms and implications in cancer regression. Pharm Res 25, 2731-2739.

Sudhakar, A., and Kalluri, R. (2010). Molecular mechanisms of angiostatis. Encyclopedia of the eye 3 M-P, 52-59.

Sudhakar, A., Nyberg, P., Keshamouni, V. G., Mannam, A. P., Li, J., Sugimoto, H., Cosgrove, D., and Kalluri, R. (2005). Human alpha1 type IV collagen NC1 domain exhibits distinct antiangiogenic activity mediated by alpha1beta1 integrin. J Clin Invest 115, 2801-2810.

Sudhakar, A., Sugimoto, H., Yang, C., Lively, J., Zeisberg, M., and Kalluri, R. (2003). Human tumstatin and human endostatin exhibit distinct antiangiogenic activities mediated by alpha vbeta 3 and alpha 5beta 1 integrins. Proc Natl Acad Sci U S A 100, 4766-4771.

Tabruyn, S. P., Sorlet, C. M., Rentier-Delrue, F., Bours, V., Weiner, R. I., Martial, J. A., and Struman, I. (2003). The antiangiogenic factor 16K human prolactin induces caspase-dependent apoptosis by a mechanism that requires activation of nuclear factor-kappaB. Mol Endocrinol 17, 1815-1823.

Takahashi, K., Saishin, Y., Silva, R. L., Oshima, Y., Oshima, S., Melia, M., Paszkiet, B., Zerby, D., Kadan, M. J., Liau, G., Kaleko, M., Connelly, S., Luo, T., and Campochiaro, P. A. (2003). Intraocular expression of endostatin reduces VEGF-induced retinal vascular permeability, neovascularization, and retinal detachment. FASEB J 17, 896-898.

Tarui, T., Miles, L. A., and Takada, Y. (2001). Specific interaction of angiostatin with integrin alpha(v)beta(3) in endothelial cells. J Biol Chem 276, 39562-39568.

Tombran-Tink, J., Chader, G. G., and Johnson, L. V. (1991). PEDF: a pigment epithelium-derived factor with potent neuronal differentiative activity. Exp Eye Res 53, 411-414.

Wang, Y., Yin, H., Chen, P., and Xie, L. (2011). Inhibitory Effect of Canstatin in Alkali Burn-Induced Corneal Neovascularization. Ophthalmic Res 46, 66-72.

Wickstrom, S. A., Alitalo, K., and Keski-Oja, J. (2002). Endostatin associates with integrin alpha5beta1 and caveolin-1, and activates Src via a tyrosyl phosphatase-dependent pathway in human endothelial cells. Cancer Res 62, 5580-5589.

Wickstrom, S. A., Alitalo, K., and Keski-Oja, J. (2003). Endostatin associates with lipid rafts and induces reorganization of the actin cytoskeleton via down-regulation of RhoA activity. J Biol Chem 278, 37895-37901.

Young, R. W., and Bok, D. (1969). Participation of the retinal pigment epithelium in the rod outer segment renewal process. J Cell Biol 42, 392-403.

Zerlin, M., Julius, M. A., and Kitajewski, J. (2008). Wnt/Frizzled signaling in angiogenesis. Angiogenesis 11, 63-69.

Zhang, S. X., and Ma, J. X. (2007). Ocular neovascularization: Implication of endogenous angiogenic inhibitors and potential therapy. Prog Retin Eye Res 26, 1-37.

Zhou, S. Y., Xie, Z. L., Xiao, O., Yang, X. R., Heng, B. C., and Sato, Y. (2010). Inhibition of mouse alkali burn induced-corneal neovascularization by recombinant adenovirus encoding human vasohibin-1. Mol Vis *16*, 1389-1398.

Zhou, X. Y., Liao, Q., Pu, Y. M., Tang, Y. Q., Gong, X., Li, J., Xu, Y., and Wang, Z. G. (2009). Ultrasound-mediated microbubble delivery of pigment epithelium-derived factor gene into retina inhibits choroidal neovascularization. Chin Med J (Engl) *122*, 2711-2717.

Ziche, M., and Morbidelli, L. (2000). Nitric oxide and angiogenesis. J Neurooncol *50*, 139-148.

8

NRF2 and Age-Dependent RPE Degeneration

Yan Chen, Zhenyang Zhao,
Paul Sternberg and Jiyang Cai
Vanderbilt Eye Institute,
Vanderbilt University Medical Center, Nashville, TN,
USA

1. Introduction

Retinal pigment epithelium (RPE) is a single layer of epithelial cells lined between the neurosensory retina and choriocapillaris. It is part of the blood-retinal barrier and is a central component of the visual phototransduction pathway. RPE cells regenerate 11-cis-retinal by RPE65 isomerase and its related enzymes and chaperones (Moiseyev et al., 2006; Xue et al., 2004). They are professional phagocytes and are responsible for the clearance of daily shed photoreceptor outer segments (POS) (Young, 1967; Young & Bok, 1969). The multi-step process of phagocytosis includes receptor-mediated binding of POS to the RPE (Finnemann et al., 1997), internalization (Feng et al., 2002; Finnemann & Silverstein, 2001), transport to lysosome and degradation. The importance of RPE phagocytosis has been clearly illustrated by the Royal College of Surgeons (RCS) rats, which carry a mutation in *Mertk* gene (D'Cruz et al., 2000). MERTK is a membrane-associated receptor tyrosine kinase and is activated upon binding of POS to the RPE (Feng et al. 2002). In RCS rats, loss-of-function mutation of *Mertk* causes defects in phagocytosis and consequently these animals develop inherited retinal dystrophy and photoreceptor apoptosis (Tso et al., 1994). In addition to their roles in the visual cycle, RPE cells provide vital support for the structure and function of the outer retina. They transport ions, water and nutrients between choroidal blood supply and the retina, and synthesize melanin which absorbs light and shields the retina. RPE-produced growth factors, such as vascular endothelial growth factor (VEGF), are indispensable for the choroidal vasculature (Saint-Geniez et al., 2009).

Degeneration of the RPE with aging is an initiating event in age-related macular degeneration (AMD), a major cause of blindness in elderly people. Approximately 11% of persons between ages 65 and 74 have AMD, with prevalence rates rising to 30% in individuals at age 75 or older (Lee et al., 2003). Vision loss in AMD occurs through photoreceptor loss in the macula, the central area of the retina, and results either from a gradual "geographic atrophy" of the RPE (dry or atrophic disease) or from leakage and/or bleeding from choroidal neovascularization (CNV) (wet or neovascular disease). During CNV, blood vessels break through Bruch's membrane, leading to rapid loss of central vision in many cases. In recent years anti-VEGF agents have achieved unprecedented success in preserving visual acuity in patients with CNV (Brown et al., 2006; Rosenfeld et al., 2006; Galbinur et al., 2009). Detailed clinical aspects of wet AMD and anti-VEGF therapy are covered by other chapters of this book.

The genetic and biochemical mechanisms of RPE degeneration in dry AMD, however, remain largely unknown. Several hypothetical models have been proposed, including accumulation of lipofuscin and its bisretinoid fluorophore (Sparrow et al., 2003; Zhou et al., 2006), iron overload (Dunaief, 2006; Hahn et al., 2004), autoimmune response (Hollyfield et al., 2008) and exposure to double strand RNA (Ambati, 2011; Kaneko et al., 2011). All of them have suggested clinical associations with AMD and their causal relationships to the disease have been demonstrated by respective animal models (Ramkumar et al., 2010). Oxidative stress is a common mechanism underlying these diversified pathological processes. Photooxidation of the bisretinoids can produce singlet oxygen and release methylglyoxal to form advanced glycation end product (Wu et al., 2010). Iron overload increased isoprostane, a marker of lipid peroxidation, in the RPE/choroid (Hadziahmetovic et al., 2008). Mice immunized with serum albumin conjugated with carboxyethylpyrrole, an oxidation product of docosahexaenoic acid, developed signs of RPE degeneration and deposition of complement proteins in the Bruch's membrane (Hollyfield et al., 2008). Oxidative stress can downregulate DICER1, a RNA processing enzyme whose deficiency was shown to cause Alu RNA-induced cytotoxicity and RPE apoptosis (Kaneko et al., 2011).

Results from earlier clinical and laboratory studies also support the contributing roles of oxidative stress to AMD. Smoking is the strongest environmental risk factor of AMD (Cano et al., 2010; Smith et al., 2001) and has been clearly associated with oxidative stress (DeBlack, 2003; Mitchell et al., 2002; Pryor et al., 1983; Smith et al., 2001). A number of interventional studies showed that antioxidant supplementation had protective effects against development of AMD or limiting its progression. Experimental animals fed with diets supplemented with antioxidants demonstrated an increased resistance to retinal degeneration (Ham et al., 1984; Organisciak et al., 1985; Tso et al., 1984). Results from the Age-Related Eye Disease Study (AREDS) showed that supplemental antioxidants (vitamin C, vitamin E and beta carotene) and zinc can decrease the risk of progression from intermediate AMD to advanced AMD by 25% (AREDS 2000 & 2001). Taken together, the findings from the research of the past two decades suggest that AMD is a multifactorial disease, with oxidative stress viewed as a common mechanism involved in the gene-environmental interaction of its etiololgy.

Oxidative stress is due to an imbalance between the generation of reactive oxygen species and their clearance by antioxidant systems. The RPE has powerful endogenous antioxidant capacity to overcome the high level of oxidative stress, which is caused by both focal light exposure and high metabolic rate of the retina. In addition to utilizing direct radical scavengers such as β-carotene, ascorbic acid and α-tocopherol, RPE cells have an elaborate enzymatic antioxidant system that can prevent and repair oxidative injury. Nuclear factor erythroid 2-related factor 2 (NRF2) is a master regulator of cellular antioxidant and detoxification responses (Kensler et al., 2007). We and others have shown previously that elevating the transcriptional activity of NRF2 can protect against oxidative injury to the RPE; while mice that are deficient of NRF2 developed pathological features similar to human AMD (Zhao et al., 2011; Cano et al., 2010). Oral zinc supplementation, which was used in the AREDS to slow AMD progression, can activate NRF2-dependent antioxidant system in the RPE (Ha et al., 2006). More recently, a newer class of NRF2 inducers, which are based on synthetic triterpenoid 2-cyano-3,12-dioxooleana-1,9-dien-28-oic acid (CDDO) and its derivatives, have achieved potent protection in various models of retinal damage (Pitha-Rowe et al. 2009). In this chapter we will review past and recent literature reports, based on cell culture, animal models and human clinical studies, to address how NRF2 regulates RPE function both *in vitro* and *in vivo*.

2. NRF2-dependent antioxidant defense

NRF2 is a transcription factor that controls the expression of phase 2 detoxification genes. It heterodimerizes with members of the Maf family of transcription factors and binds to the *cis*-acting antioxidant response element in the promoter regions of various phase 2 genes (Katsuoka et al., 2005; Motohashi et al., 2004). The latter encode a group of enzymes, such as glutamate-cysteine ligase, glutathione S-transferase, glutathione peroxidase, heme oxygenase, NAD(P)H:quinone reductase and glutamate-cysteine exchanger, which are essential for detoxification of xenobiotics and endogenous reactive intermediates (Kensler et al., 2007; Wakabayashi et al. 2010). NRF2-deficient mice showed increased sensitivity to a variety of pharmacological and environmental toxicants (Kensler et al., 2007; Rangasamy et al., 2004). The protective effects of NRF2 inducers have been tested in a number of models of human diseases, including cancer, neurodegeneration, cardiovascular disease, and liver and lung injury (Kensler et al., 2007; Wakabayashi et al., 2010).

Activation of NRF2 is subjected to multiple levels of regulation. Under basal conditions, NRF2 is sequestered by its inhibitor protein, Keap1, and is targeted for Cullin 3/Rbx1-mediated ubiquitination and degradation (Cullinan et al., 2004; Furukawa & Xiong, 2005; Kobayashi et al., 2004). Upon conditions of oxidative stress or exposure to electrophilic compounds, NRF2 protein can be liberated from Keap1 and will translocate into nucleus to mediate gene trasncription. As illustrated in Fig. 1, there are six Neh (NRF2 ECH homology) domains that are responsible for most of the functions of NRF2. The Neh domains show amino acid sequence homology conserved between different species including human, rodents and chicken (McMahon et al., 2004; Zhang et al., 2007).

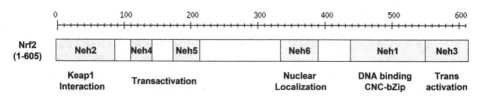

Fig. 1. Illustration of the Neh domains of the NRF2 protein. Human NRF2 is a polypeptide of 605 amino acids and contains 6 Neh domains. The relative positions of each domain and their putative functions are listed. Neh1 contains the signature cap-n-collar motif which is a highly conserved basic leucine zipper domain for DNA binding. The nuclear localization and export signals are present in both Neh6 and Neh1.

3. NRF2-mediated protection in cultured RPE cells

Compounds that promote the nuclear translocation of Nrf2 and elevate its transcriptional activity can protect against oxidative injury in cultured RPE cells. In 2001, Talalay and colleagues first reported that sulforaphane could prevent RPE cell death caused by treatments with menadione, t-butyl hydroperoxide, 4-hydroxynonenal and peroxynitrite (Gao et al., 2001). Since then numerous other studies reported the protective effects of a wide range of structurally-different NRF2 inducers including isothiocyanates (sulforaphane) (Gao & Talalay, 2004), polyphenols (curcumin, resveratrol and flavonoids) (Alex et al., 2010; Johnson et al., 2009; Mandal et al., 2009), 1,2,dithiole-3-thiones (oltipraz) (Nelson et al., 2002), zinc (Ha et al., 2006) or triterpenoids (Pitha-Rowe et al., 2009). Many of them are naturally occurring compounds present in fruits and vegetables, making them ideal for dietary supplementation. Some of the compounds have either gone through human clinical trials or are currently used for other applications. For instances, zinc was used in the AREDS supplementation either alone or with antioxidant vitamins. Oltipraz, a dithiole derivate, is used in treating schistosomiasis and cancer chemoprevention (Jacobson et al., 1997). A common mechanism underlying the antioxidant and detoxification functions of NRF2 is to increase cellular glutathione (GSH) synthesis.

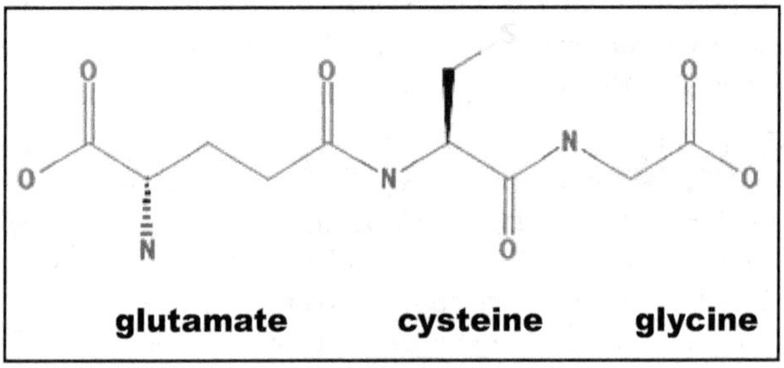

glutamate   cysteine   glycine

Fig. 2. Structure of glutathione. The γ-glutamylcysteine is formed by a peptide bond between the carboxylate group of glutamate and animo group of cysteine. The sulfhydryl group of cysteine is responsible for the antioxidant function of the tripeptide.

GSH is a tripeptide consisted of glutamate, cysteine and glycine. It contains a unique peptide bond between the amine group of cysteine and the carboxyl group of the glutamate side chain so that it is much more resistant to degradation by peptidase (Fig. 2). The sulfhydryl group of cysteine of GSH can be used by glutathione S-transferase to conjugate electrophilic centers on a wide variety of substrates (Pool-Zobel et al., 2005). GSH is also used by glutathione peroxidase to reduce lipid hydroperoxides and hydrogen peroxide to alcohols and water, respectively. The glutamate cysteine ligase (GCL) is the rate-limiting enzyme of GSH synthesis. It generates γ-glutamylcysteine from glutamate and cysteine. NRF2 inducers can elevate the mRNA levels of the catalytic and modulatory subunits of GCL. Cystine uptake by the RPE is mediated by a sodium independent, cystine/glutamate exchanger (Bridges et al., 2001; Ishii et al., 1992). The transporter is consisted of two subunits, xCT as the light chain and 4F2hc as the heavy chain (Wagner et al., 2001). NRF2 controls the expression of xCT gene (Sato et al., 1999). In xCT knock out mice, the plasma cystine concentration almost doubled, resulted from decreased tissue uptake (Sasaki et al., 2002). The $xCT^{-/-}$ mice showed more several renal injury caused by ischemia-reperfusion (Shibasaki et al., 2009). Thus, NRF2 inducers can increase both the rate of GSH synthesis and cellular concentration of its amino acid precursor.

Monitoring the RPE glutathione content is a reliable assay for initial screening of model compounds designed to activate NRF2. For instance, RPE cells pretreated with oltipraz showed increased total and mitochondrial GSH. At 50 μM, oltipraz increased total cellular GSH by 18% and mitochondrial GSH by 50%, and achieved significant protection against tert-butylhydroperoxide-induced RPE cell death (Nelson et al., 2002). Similar results were obtained from cells pretreated with dimethylfumarate (DMF) for 24 hours (Nelson et al., 1999). However, when the time course of the DMF was evaluated, a transient decrease in GSH levels was found that preceded the increase noted at later time points. Compared to vehicle-treated control cells, cells pretreated with DMF for 3 hours showed a significant reduction in viability when further challenged by peroxide (Nelson et al, 1999). Thus, the initial decrease of GSH after DMF treatment rendered the RPE cells more sensitive to oxidative injury, although it can subsequently lead to a feedback increase of GSH synthesis and a more robust antioxidant response (Nelson et al., 1999). Many of the NRF2 inducers are thiol-reacting compounds and may cause a similar initial depletion of cellular GSH. Therefore, although the *in vitro* culture system does not present the complexity of the retinal microenvironment and cell-cell interaction *in vivo*, it is a valuable tool for assessing both the pharmacological properties of new NRF2 inducers and their potential toxicities. For treatment of a chronic disease like AMD, the RPE cells are already stressed by oxidative burden and may not tolerate transient GSH depletion after repeated administration of agents that react with cellular thiols with low selectivity.

4. Ocular pathology of *Nrf2* knockout mice

Nrf2 knockout mice have normal embryonic development (Chan et al., 1996) and their basal level of antioxidant status in many tissues is not different from age-matched wild type mice. However, the *Nrf2* null mice show increased sensitivity to a variety of pharmacological and environmental toxicants (Cano et al., 2010; Kensler et al., 2007; Osburn & Kensler, 2008). Depending upon the stimuli, injuries occur in different organs and tissues. The phenotypes vary, but commonly involve oxidative and inflammatory stress. For ocular pathology, neonatal *Nrf2* knockout mice develop more severe retinal vaso-obliteration at early phase after hyperoxia exposure (Uno et al., 2010). NRF2 also modulates the innate immune response in the retina and iris-ciliary body in a mouse model of uveitis induced by intraperitoneal injection of lipopolysaccaride (Nagai et al., 2009).

Aging and smoking are the major demographic and environmental risk factor of AMD, respectively. Cano and colleagues (2010) reported that NRF2-deficient mice were more susceptible to smoking-induced retinal injury. At 8 months, *Nrf2* null mice showed a mild degree of ultrastructural change in the RPE. Comparing to age-matched wild type mice, RPE of the knockout mice exposed to cigarette smoking for 6 months (starting at 2 months) displayed markedly increased staining of 8-hydroxydeoxyguanosine, an indicator of accumulated oxidative DNA damage (Cano et al., 2010). On electron microscopy, *Nrf2-/-* smoking mice displayed abnormal RPE basal infoldings and vacuoles, without apparent changes of the choroidal endothelium or sub-RPE deposit formation (Cano et al., 2010). Thickening and deposits in the outer collagenous layer of Bruch's membrane were often observed in smoking mice. The data suggest that NRF2-mediated protection to the RPE is important against chronic environmental toxicities associated with AMD.

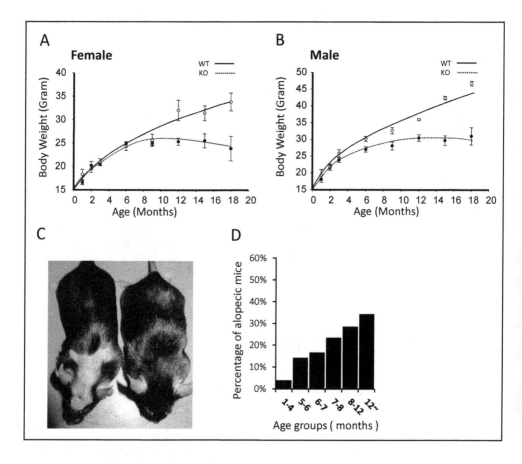

Fig. 3. Accelerated aging in *Nrf2-/-* mice. (A) and (B) Growth curves of male and female *Nrf2-/-* mice and their age-matched littermates. Knockout animals showed a lower body weight after the first year. (C) and (D) Hair loss in *Nrf2-/-* mice. A representative picture of a 12-month-old alopecic *Nrf2-/-* mice is shown in (C). Hair loss was often first observed between 5 to 6 months of age (D).

We recently reported that *Nrf2-/-* mice developed age-related RPE and choroidal degeneration resembling cardinal features of human AMD (Zhao et al., 2011). The *Nrf2-/-* mice have accelerated aging. Some of the animals exhibited extensive hair loss (alopecia), which began as early as 4 months and peaked at 8 months (Fig. 3). Interestingly, more female *Nrf2-/-* mice suffered from hair loss than male ones; this could possibly be attributed to the higher susceptibility of female mice to autoimmune diseases as reported by Takahashi and colleagues (Yoh et al., 2001). After 12 months, the *Nrf2-/-* mice started to show lower body weight than the age-matched wild type littermates (Fig. 3). The life expectancy of *Nrf2-/-* mice is about 20 months which is only 60% of wild type mice with the same genetic background (Pearson et al., 2008).

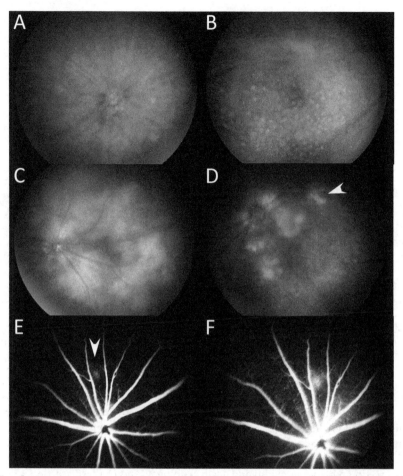

Fig. 4. Fundus examinations of *Nrf2-/-* mice. (A) Normal fundus image taken from a 12-month-old wild type mouse. (B) Drusen like deposits developed in the peripheral retina of an 8-month-old *Nrf2-/-* mouse. (C) Yellowish patchy lesions found in a 14-month-old *Nrf2-/-* mouse. (D-F) A 16-month-old knockout mouse developed extensive RPE lesions (D), one of which showed hyperfluorescence in both early (E) and late (F) phase of fluorescein angiography. Arrowheads in D and E indicate the same lesion.

Drusen-like deposits were noted in around 70% of eyes from *Nrf2-/-* mice, as examined by funduscopy between 8 to 11 months (Fig. 4B). With aging, these small, dome-shaped whitish spots in the fundus tended to become confluent yellowish lesions, gradually increasing in area (Fig. 4C). Atrophic RPE lesions were frequently seen in *Nrf2-/-* mice after the first year (Fig 4C and 4D). Some of these lesions would eventually develop into sites of CNV, which were identified by both fundus fluorescein angiography (Fig 4E and 4F) and histopathology (Zhao et al., 2011). Moderate but statistically significant decreases in both a- and b-wave amplitudes on ERG were observed between the *Nrf2-/-* and wild-type mice at 12 months of age (Zhao et al., 2011), indicating compromised visual function in knockout mice.

The fundus phenotype in aged *Nrf2-/-* mice was further confirmed by histology (Fig. 5 and Zhao et al., 2011), which showed drusen formation, extensive RPE atrophy with numerous vacuoles, increased autofluorescence inside the RPE layer and CNV. Thickening of the Bruch's membrane with age and basal laminar and basal linear deposit were found exclusively in *Nrf2-/-* mice by electron microscopy (Zhao et al., 2011). Immunostaining of eye sections revealed increased deposition of proteins that are related to innate immunity (i.e., C3d, vitronectin and serum amyloid P) and marker of oxidative injury (nitrotyrosine) between the RPE and Bruch's membrane in *Nrf2-/-* mice (Zhao et al., 2011). The same proteins have been found in drusen and Bruch's membrane of human AMD eyes (Crabb et al., 2002; Mullins et al., 2000).

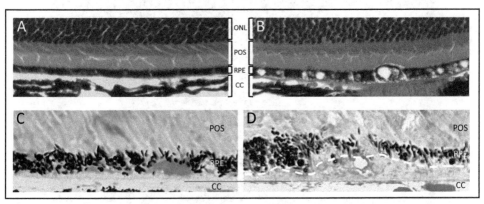

Fig. 5. Histology examination of retina of *Nrf2-/-* mice. (A) A 14-month-old wild type mouse showed normal structure of the outer retina. (B) Representative image of RPE degeneration with big vacuoles, taken from a 14-month-old *Nrf2-/-* mouse. (C-D) Semi-thin sections from a 12-month-old wild-type mouse (C) and an age-matched *Nrf2-/-* mouse (D). Bruch's membranes of the two were aligned at the same level (red line). Note that the RPE layer was elevated due to heterogeneous deposits (under the dotted line) in the sub-RPE space. (A and B: Paraffin section with hematoxylin and eosin staining. C and D: Plastic section with toluidine blue staining. ONL: outer nuclear layer; POS: photoreceptor outer segment; CC: choriocapillaris)

The accelerated degeneration after middle age and the typical pathology of the RPE/choroid indicate that the *Nrf2-/-* model shares many features of human AMD. At advanced age, the retinal pathology progressed from atrophic form to neovascularization and about 15% of the *Nrf2-/-* mice developed spontaneous CNV (Zhao et al., 2011). Photoreceptor degeneration was moderate and was probably secondary to RPE dysfunction. Rodents do not have macula and, therefore, cannot be used to generate ideal models of AMD. On the other hand, mechanistic studies exploring the molecular and biochemical mechanisms of age-related RPE degeneration and CNV can greatly benefit from animal models that at least partially reproduce representative lesions commonly seen in human AMD eyes. Animal models, such as the *Nrf2-/-* mice, will display the dynamic process of the disease and offer windows of intervention that can either slow down or accelerate the progression. Similar experiments will be difficult if not impossible to perform with human eyes mainly at late stages of AMD.

5. Pharmacological interventions that activate NRF2 *in vivo*

A number of *in vivo* studies have investigated the protective roles of NRF2 inducers in models of retinal injury and inflammation. A study by Yodoi and colleagues (Tanito et al., 2005) showed that sulforaphane, a prototypic NRF2 inducer, could upregulate thioredoxin in both the RPE and neural retina, and was effective in protecting photoreceptors from photo-oxidative damage. Compared to vehicle-treated controls, mice received sulforaphane showed fewer apoptotic cells in the outer nuclear layer and RPE, and had moderate but statistically significant improvement of both a- and b-wave amplitudes. At four days after light exposure, the ONL was significantly thicker in sulforaphane-treated mice (Tanito et al., 2005). Sulforaphane also delayed photoreceptor cell death in *tubby* mouse, a model of Usher syndrome (Kong et al., 2007). Homozygous *tubby* mice develop progressive photoreceptor degeneration shortly after birth. Sulforaphane-treated *tub/tub* mice showed significantly increased ONL thickness and b-wave amplitude at P28 and P34, as compared to vehicle-treated animals (Kong et al., 2007).

For human clinical studies, AREDS reported (2001) that supplementation with zinc alone, or antioxidants plus zinc, decreased the risk of progression towards advanced AMD by 20%. We showed that zinc could activate NRF2 both in cultured RPE cells and in RPE of NRF2 reporter mice (Chen et al., data not shown). In an ancillary study of AREDS, we analyzed the effects of long-term zinc supplementation on plasma thiol metabolites and their redox status (Moriarty-Craige et al., 2007). There was a significant decrease in plasma cystine concentration in the zinc-supplemented group. The systemic effects may be due to increased tissue uptake of cystine, as NRF2 regulates the transporter protein xCT (Sasaki et al., 2002). These results prove the concept that long term dietary supplementation of an NRF2 inducer is a feasible approach for treating early stage AMD patients.

A new class of synthetic triterpenoids derivatives of oleanolic acid have been tested both in cultured RPE cells and *in vivo*. These agents exerted highly potent activity at concentration as low as 10 nM. They reacted with a broad range of accessible protein thiols and activate NRF2 about 10 times more potently (by the ARE reporter assay) than previously used compounds (Pitha-Rowe et al., 2009). The *in vivo* protection against light-induced retinal toxicity has been demonstrated. Mice receiving 200 mg/kg CDDO-trifluoroethylamide (-TFEA) showed significantly increased ONL thickness after light-induced retinal degeneration (Pitha-Rowe et al., 2009). CDDO-imidazolide decreased mouse leukocyte adherence to retinal vasculature after lipopolysaccharide treatment, and reduced expression of inflammatory mediators including ICAM-1, IL-6, COX-2, TNF-α and MCP-1 (Nagai et al., 2009; Cano et al., 2010). CDDO-methyl ester inhibited neutrophil infiltration in vitreous and internal limiting membrane after retinal ischemia-reperfusion induced by high intraocular pressure, and inhibited degeneration of retinal capillary (Wei et al., 2011). The CDDO compounds are currently under clinical trials for chronic kidney disease and type 2 diabetes. Their potential applications in treating dry AMD can be explored in human studies in the near future.

6. Signaling pathways that regulate NRF2 activation

The interaction between Keap1 and NRF2 is considered as a major determinant of the stability and function of NRF2 (Dinkova-Kostova et al., 2002; Hong et al., 2005). Electrophilic compounds, such as sulforaphane, can directly react with various cysteine residues of Keap1 and consequently cause dissociation and activation of NRF2 (Eggler et al., 2005). Keap1-

deficient hepatocytes had increased NRF2 activity and were more resistant to acetaminophen (Okawa et al., 2006). In addition to thiol modification and redox regulation, it is well established that there are cross-talk between the protein kinase pathways and NRF2-dependent antioxidant system (Sherratt et al., 2004).

Several phosphorylation sites of NRF2 protein have been mapped out and associated to its activity (Fig. 6). Phosphorylation of NRF2 at Serine 40 by protein kinase C promotes its dissociation from Keap1 and translocation into the nucleus (Bloom and Jaiswal, 2003; Huang et al., 2002). Phosphorylation at Tyrosine 568 by a Src subfamily kinase Fyn controls the export and inactivation of NRF2 at the late phase of induction (Jain and Jaiswal, 2006; Salazar et al., 2006). Other Src subfamily kinases, Src, Yes and Fgr, can also function as negative regulators of NRF2 by phosphorylating the protein at Tyr568 (Niture et al., 2011). A recent study by Rada et al (2011) demonstrated that a serine cluster in the Neh6 domain (Ser335, 338, 342, 347, 351, and 355) (Fig. 1) of NRF2 can be phosphorylated by glycogen synthase kinase-3β (GSK-3β). The phosphorylation enhanced the association between Nrf2 and SCF/β-TrCP, which is an adaptor protein for ubiquitin ligase and targets NRF2 for cullin-1/Rbx1-mediated degradation (Rada et al., 2011). Thus, phosphorylation of NRF2 by GSK-3β will facilitate it proteosomal degradation and inhibit its transactivation function. GSK-3β may also act upstream of Src family kinases (Jain and Jaiswal, 2006; Kaspar and Jaiswal, 2011). It remains elusive whether those two mechanisms work independently or additively. Mitogen-activated protein kinases (MAPKs) have been shown to phosphorylate NRF2 at Ser215, 408, 558, 577 and Tyr559; however, impacts on NRF2 location and activity were marginal after phosphorylation at those residues (Sun et al., 2009).

Results from the functional studies consistently showed that inhibition of the PI3K/Akt pathway decreased NRF2 activation induced by a variety of stimuli in different cell lines, while expression of a constitutive active mutant of Akt increased NRF2 activity, indicating that PI3K/Akt signalling is a positive regulator of NRF2 (Chen et al., 2009; Jain and Jaiswal, 2006; Kang et al., 2000; Lee et al., 2001; Wang et al., 2008). PI3K/Akt controls NRF2 via multiple indirect mechanisms. They can facilitate translocation of NRF2 into the nucleus via rearrangement of cytoskeletal actin (Kang et al., 2002). They are upstream kinases of GSK-3β. Akt phosphorylates GSK-3β at Ser9 and inhibits its kinase activity, which in turn will potentiate NRF2 activation because GSK-3β is its negative regulator (Jain and Jaiswal, 2006; Niture et al., 2011; Rada et al., 2011; Salazar et al., 2006).

There are other kinases that can be positive regulators of NRF2. PKR-like endoplasmic reticulum kinase phosphorylates and activates NRF2 under conditions of ER stress (Cullinan and Diehl, 2004; Cullinan et al., 2003). Casein kinase 2 phosphorylates endogenous NRF2 and regulates its activity and degradation (Pi et al., 2007). MAPK family proteins, extracellular signal-regulated protein kinases (ERKs) and the c-Jun N-terminal kinases (JNK), also play positive roles in NRF2-signaling pathway (Shen et al., 2004; Yu et al., 2000a; Zipper and Mulcahy, 2003). However, the positive regulation by ERKs and JNK may not through direct phosphorylation of NRF2 (Shen et al., 2004; Zipper and Mulcahy, 2003). Instead, they may upregulate NRF2 activity by phosphorylating and activating Nrf2 binding partner, such as the nuclear transcriptional coactivator CBP (Shen et al., 2004; Yu et al., 2000a). The p38 kinase may either stimulate or inhibit NRF2 activity, depending on the different type of cells and the pharmacological agents used for the studies (Yu et al., 2000b; Zipper and Mulcahy, 2000).

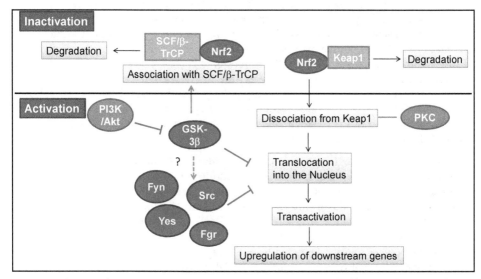

Fig. 6. Regulation of NRF2 activity by protein phosphorylation. There are positive and negative regulators of upstream kinases that function at various steps of the signalling pathway. Phosphorylation can leads to either its activation or degradation/inactivation.

Because of the multiple putative phosphorylation sites of NRF2, and its dual regulation by cellular redox status and protein phosphorylation, it is difficult to clearly define its upstream signalling network both at basal level and in response to oxidative stress. Identification of authentic phosphorylation sites and development of antibodies specific for phosphorylated NRF2 can greatly advance our knowledge in this area. More importantly, most of the works on signal transduction of NRF2 have been performed in transformed cancer cells, which harbour genetic and biochemical variations and function quite differently from the RPE. Future mechanistic studies of NRF2 will be needed to address cell type-specific signalling mechanisms involved in RPE aging and degeneration.

7. Potential mechanisms linking NRF2 to AMD

A unique pathology of AMD is that RPE degeneration occurs before severe loss of photoreceptors, a retinal phenotype also seen in NRF2-deficient mice. In contrast, in model systems of retinal toxicities, animals exposed to excessive levels of oxidative stress often showed much more severe retinal degeneration than the RPE damage. Compared to epithelial cells, neurons are less efficiently protected by the endogenous antioxidant system. The outer segments of rods and cones have very low GSH (Winkler 2008). As shown in both the SOD1- and SOD2-deficient mice, severe loss of neurons occurred before or at the same time of RPE degeneration (Imamura et al. 2006; Justilien et al., 2007). In $Vldlr^{-/-}$ mice, antioxidant supplementation protected retinal degeneration and improved the retinal electrophysiology (Dorrell et al., 2009). The fact that $Nrf2^{-/-}$ mice showed preferential loss of RPE suggests that NRF2 can have functions other than antioxidant protection.

It is noteworthy that the retinal ultrastructure of aged Nrf2-/- mice showed signs of dysregulated autophagy (Zhao et al., 2011). Autophagy is a major self-renewal process which is essential for organelle turnover and removal of aggregated proteins that cannot be processed by proteasome (Klionsky 2007). During autophagy, unwanted proteins and organelles are sorted to double-membrane autophagosomes, which are further delivered to and fused with lysosomes to degrade the sequestered cargos. The accumulation of various intermediate forms of autophagic vacuoles and multivesicular bodies in the RPE and Bruch's membrane was evident on EM images of aged Nrf2-/- mice (Zhao et al. 2011). This can be caused by either increased autophagic flux or decreased final degradation by lysosome. Similar findings of dysregulated autophagy were reported in another study using human AMD eyes (Wang et al., 2009).

Autophagy is of particular importance in non-dividing cells like neurons and RPE which, unlike proliferating cells, are incapable of diluting the waste products by mitosis. Dysregulated autophagy is considered as pathogenic in various neurodegenerative diseases; and the underlying mechanisms are disease-specific. In Alzheimer's disease, mutations in presenilin-1 impairs lysosomal targeting of v-ATPase V0a1, which is essential for lysosome acidification and protease activation (Lee et al., 2010). In Parkinson's disease, mutated α-synuclein cannot be efficiently degraded by autophagy (Cuervo et al., 2004). In Huntington's disease, mutant huntingtin may impair the initial cargo assembly of autophagic vesicles (Martinez-Vicente et al., 2010). It has been hypothesized that dysregulated autophagy is also involved in AMD (Wang et al., 2009; Kaarniranta 2010).

NRF2 can be an important regulator of RPE autophagy via multiple mechanisms. In normal RPE cells, autophagy is responsible for the removal of ubiquitinated and/or aggregated proteins. Cargos inside autophagosomes will be delivered to lysosome for degradation and recycled for catabolism. NRF2 is likely involved in autophagosome formation. Several previous studies reported that p62, which is a receptor protein of ubiquitinated proteins and essential for the initial assembly of autophagosome, is transcriptionally regulated by NRF2 (Komatsu et al., 2010). Whether NRF2 controls other specific molecular components of the autophagy pathway remains to be characterized by future studies. Accelerated accumulation of lipofuscin was observed in Nrf2-/- RPE (Zhao et al., 2011). Reactive metabolites from bisretinoids inhibit lysosome-mediated autophagic degradation. NRF2-dependent detoxification can be protective in both formation and elimination of lipofuscin-related metabolic waste products. Thus, compromised NRF2 signalling can impact both the early and late stages of RPE autophagy.

NRF2 may also be involved in the innate immune response that amplifies the initial RPE lesions in AMD. As shown in the uveitis model, NRF2-deficient retina had higher number of infiltrated leukocytes and increased production of pro-inflammatory cytokines (Cano et al., 2010). Thioredoxin 1, a downstream protein of NRF2, can interact with complement factor H and regulate its activation (Inomata et al., 2008). Autophagy can be a possible mechanistic link between oxidative stress and inflammation (Levine et al., 2011). Elevated cellular stress will cause increased damage to proteins and organelles and overwhelm the degradation capacity of RPE autophagy. Consequently, the undigested wastes could be exported into Bruch's membrane via exocytosis and deposited in the sub-RPE space (Wang et al., 2009). The exported proteins, possibly in oxidatively modified forms, may further promote drusen formation and cause local inflammation mediated by complement proteins and macrophages. Loss of endothelial fenestration was observed in choriocapillaris of aged *Nrf2-/-* mice (Zhao et al., 2011). In human AMD eyes, choroidal vascular degeneration occurs in areas of geographic atrophy (McLeod et al., 2009; Mullins et al. 2011). Decreased transport function of choroidal vessels can facilitate the accumulation of damaged proteins in the sub-RPE space and Bruch's membrane.

Single nucleotide polymorphisms (SNPs) in the coding region of *NRF2* gene have been detected in human cancerous tissues (Shibata et al. 2008). Functional polymorphisms in the promoter region of *NRF2* have been reported (Marzec et al., 2007). However, according to the GWAS data (Chen et al., 2010), NRF2 is not a major risk allele of AMD and SNPs of *NRF2* are unlikely to be a major genetic factor. A recent study showed that age-dependent decline of NRF2 function could be caused by upstream regulatory mechanisms, such as GSK-3β, that control its localization and activity (Tomobe et al., 2011). Defining these mechanisms will open up new revenues of intervention to prevent oxidative injury and RPE loss during dry AMD. Unlike the inherited genetic variations, the biochemical changes associated with RPE aging are likely treatable.

8. Conclusion

NRF2 is a protein that has been extensively studied in cancer and other chronic human diseases. Accumulating evidence suggests that NRF2-mediated signalling pathways have central roles in protecting the RPE cells from aging and age-related degeneration. The *Nrf2-/-* mice represent a new model for translational and mechanistic studies of AMD. Agents that activate Nrf2 are potential candidates for treating AMD and other retinal diseases involving oxidative and inflammatory stress.

9. Acknowledgment

This work was supported by International Retinal Research Foundation, NIH grants EY019706, EY07892, EY018715, P30 EY08126, and Research to Prevent Blindness, Inc.

10. References

AREDS (2000). The Age-Related Eye Disease Study: a clinical trial of zinc and antioxidants--AREDS Report No. 2. *Journal of Nutrition* Vol.130, No.5S (Suppl), (May 2000), pp. 1516S-1519S, ISSN 0022-3166

AREDS (2001).A randomized, placebo-controlled, clinical trial of high-dose supplementation with vitamins C and E, beta carotene, and zinc for age-related macular degeneration and vision loss: AREDS report no. 8. *Archives of Ophthalmology* Vol.119, No.10, (October 2001), pp. 1417-1436, ISSN 0003-9950

Alex, A.F., Spitznas, M., Tittel, A.P., Kurts, C., & Eter, N. (2010). Inhibitory effect of epigallocatechin gallate (EGCG), resveratrol, and curcumin on proliferation of human retinal pigment epithelial cells in vitro. *Current Eye Resesearch* Vol.35, No.11, (November 2010), pp. 1021-1033, ISSN 1460-2202

Ambati, J. (2011). Age-related macular degeneration and the other double helix. The Cogan Lecture. *Investigative Ophthalmology & Visual Science* Vol.52, No.5, (April 2011), pp. 2165-2169, ISSN 0146-0404

Bloom, D.A., & Jaiswal, A.K. (2003). Phosphorylation of Nrf2 at Ser40 by protein kinase C in response to antioxidants leads to the release of Nrf2 from INrf2, but is not required for Nrf2 stabilization/accumulation in the nucleus and transcriptional activation of antioxidant response element-mediated NAD(P)H:quinone oxidoreductase-1 gene expression. *Journal of Biological Chemistry* Vol.278, No.45, (November 2003), pp. 44675-44682, ISSN 0021-9258

Bridges, C.C., Kekuda, R., Wang, H., Prasad, P.D., Mehta, P., Huang, W., Smith, S.B., & Ganapathy, V. (2001). Structure, function, and regulation of human cystine/glutamate transporter in retinal pigment epithelial cells. *Investigative Ophthalmology & Visual Science* Vol.42, No.1, (January 2001), pp. 47-54, ISSN 0146-0404

Brown, D.M., Kaiser, P.K., Michels, M., Soubrane, G., Heier, J.S., Kim, R.Y., Sy, J.P., & Schneider, S. (2006). Ranibizumab versus verteporfin for neovascular age-related macular degeneration. *New England Journal of Medicine* Vol.355, No.14, (October 2006), pp. 1432-1444, ISSN 0028-4793

Cano, M., Thimmalappula, R., Fujihara, M., Nagai, N., Sporn, M., Wang, A.L., Neufeld, A.H., Biswal, S., & Handa, J.T. (2010). Cigarette smoking, oxidative stress, the anti-oxidant response through Nrf2 signaling, and Age-related Macular Degeneration. *Vision Reseseach* Vol.50, No.7, (March 2010), pp. 652-664, ISSN 0042-6989

Chan, K., Lu, R., Change, J.C. & Kan, Y.W. (1996) NRF2, a member of the NFE2 family of transcription factors, is not essential for murin erythropoiesis, growth, and development. *Proceedings of the National Academy of Sciences of the United States of America* Vol.93, No.24, (November 1996), pp. 13943-13948, ISSN 1091-6490

Chen, J. B., Wang, L., Chen, Y., Sternberg, P., & Cai, J. (2009). Phosphatidylinositol 3 Kinase Pathway and 4-Hydroxy-2-Nonenal-Induced Oxidative Injury in the RPE. *Investigative Ophthalmology & Visual Science* Vol.50, No.2, (February 2009), pp. 936-942, ISSN 0146-0404

Chen, W., Stambolian, D., Edwards, A.O., Branham, K.E., Othman, M., et al. (2010) Genetic variants near TIMP3 and high-density lipoprotein-associated loci influence susceptibility to age-related macular degeneration. *Proceedings of the National Academy of Sciences of the United States of America* Vol.107, No.16, (April 2010), pp. 7401-7406, ISSN 1091-6490

Crabb, J.W., Miyagi, M., Gu, X., Shadrach, K., West, K.A., Sakaguchi, H., Kamei, M., Hasan, A., Yan, L., Rayborn, M.E., et al. (2002). Drusen proteome analysis: an approach to the etiology of age-related macular degeneration. *Proceedings of the National Academy of Sciences of the United States of America* Vol.99, No.23, (November 2002), pp. 14682-14687, ISSN 1091-6490

Cullinan, S.B., & Diehl, J.A. (2004). PERK-dependent activation of Nrf2 contributes to redox homeostasis and cell survival following endoplasmic reticulum stress. *Journal of Biological Chemistry* Vol.279, No.19, (May 2004), pp. 20108-20117, ISSN 0021-9258

Cullinan, S.B., Gordan, J.D., Jin, J., Harper, J.W., & Diehl, J.A. (2004). The Keap1-BTB protein is an adaptor that bridges Nrf2 to a Cul3-based E3 ligase: oxidative stress sensing by a Cul3-Keap1 ligase. *Molecular and Cell Biology* Vol.24, No.19, (October 2004), pp. 8477-8486, ISSN 0270-7306

Cullinan, S. B., Zhang, D., Hannink, M., Arvisais, E., Kaufman, R. J., & Diehl, J. A. (2003). Nrf2 is a direct PERK substrate and effector of PERK-dependent cell survival.

Molecular and Cellular Biology Vol.23, No.20, (October 2003), pp. 7198-7209, ISSN 0270-7306

Cuervo, A.M., Stefanis, L., Fredenburg, R., Lansbury, P.T. & Sulzer, D. (2004) Impaired degradation of mutant α-synuclein by chaperone-mediated autophagy. *Science* Vol.305, No.5688, (August 2004), pp. 1292-1295, ISSN 0036-8075

D'Cruz, P.M., Yasumura, D., Weir, J., Matthes, M.T., Abderrahim, H., LaVail, M.M., & Vollrath, D. (2000). Mutation of the receptor tyrosine kinase gene Mertk in the retinal dystrophic RCS rat. *Human Molecular Genetics* Vol.9, No.4, (March 2000), pp. 645-651, ISSN 0964-6906

DeBlack, S.S. (2003). Cigarette smoking as a risk factor for cataract and age-related macular degeneration: a review of the literature. *Optometry* Vol.74, No.2, (February 2003), pp. 99-110, ISSN 1558-1527

Dinkova-Kostova, A.T., Holtzclaw, W.D., Cole, R.N., Itoh, K., Wakabayashi, N., Katoh, Y., Yamamoto, M., & Talalay, P. (2002). Direct evidence that sulfhydryl groups of Keap1 are the sensors regulating induction of phase 2 enzymes that protect against carcinogens and oxidants. *Proceedings of the National Academy of Sciences of the United States of America* Vol.99, No.18, (September 2002), pp. 11908-11913, ISSN 1091-6490

Dorrell, M.I., Aguilar, E., Jacobson, R., Yanes, O., Gariano, R., Heckenlively, J., Banin, E., Ramirez, G.A., Gasmi, M., Bird, A., Siuzdak G. & Friedlander, M. Antioxidant or neurotrophic factor treatment preserves function in a mouse model of neovascularization-associated oxidative stress. *Journal of Clinical Investigation* Vo.119, No.3, (March 2009), pp. 611-623, ISSN 0021-9738

Dunaief, J.L. (2006). Iron induced oxidative damage as a potential factor in age-related macular degeneration: the Cogan Lecture. *Investigative Ophthalmology & Visual Science* Vol.47, No.11, (November 2006), pp. 4660-4664, ISSN 0146-0404

Eggler, A.L., Liu, G., Pezzuto, J.M., van Breemen, R.B., & Mesecar, A.D. (2005). Modifying specific cysteines of the electrophile-sensing human Keap1 protein is insufficient to disrupt binding to the Nrf2 domain Neh2. *Proceedings of the National Academy of Sciences of the United States of America* Vol.102, No.29, (July 2005), pp. 10070-10075, ISSN 1091-6490

Feng, W., Yasumura, D., Matthes, M.T., LaVail, M.M., and Vollrath, D. (2002). Mertk triggers uptake of photoreceptor outer segments during phagocytosis by cultured retinal pigment epithelial cells. *Journal of Biological Chemistry* Vol.277, No.19, (May 2002), pp. 17016-17022, ISSN 0021-9258

Finnemann, S.C., Bonilha, V.L., Marmorstein, A.D., & Rodriguez-Boulan, E. (1997). Phagocytosis of rod outer segments by retinal pigment epithelial cells requires alpha(v)beta5 integrin for binding but not for internalization. *Proceedings of the National Academy of Sciences of the United States of America* Vol.94, No.24, (November 1997), pp. 12932-12937, ISSN 1091-6490

Finnemann, S.C., & Silverstein, R.L. (2001). Differential roles of CD36 and alphavbeta5 integrin in photoreceptor phagocytosis by the retinal pigment epithelium. *Journal of Experimental Medicine* Vol.194, No.9, (November 2001), pp. 1289-1298, ISSN 0022-1007

Furukawa, M., & Xiong, Y. (2005). BTB protein Keap1 targets antioxidant transcription factor Nrf2 for ubiquitination by the Cullin 3-Roc1 ligase. *Molecular and Cell Biology* Vol.25, No.1, (January 2005), pp. 162-171, ISSN 0270-7306

Galbinur, T., Averbukh, E., Banin, E., Hemo, I., & Chowers, I. (2009). Intravitreal bevacizumab therapy for neovascular age-related macular degeneration associated with poor initial visual acuity. *British Journal of Ophthalmology* Vol.93, No.10, (October 2009), pp. 1351-1352, ISSN 0007-1161

Gao, X., Dinkova-Kostova, A.T., & Talalay, P. (2001). Powerful and prolonged protection of human retinal pigment epithelial cells, keratinocytes, and mouse leukemia cells against oxidative damage: the indirect antioxidant effects of sulforaphane. *Proceedings of the National Academy of Sciences of the United States of America* Vol.98, No.26, (December 2001), pp. 15221-15226, ISSN 0027-8424

Gao, X., & Talalay, P. (2004). Induction of phase 2 genes by sulforaphane protects retinal pigment epithelial cells against photooxidative damage. *Proceedings of the National Academy of Sciences of the United States of America* Vol.101, No.28, (July 2004), pp. 10446-10451, ISSN 0027-8424

Ha, K.N., Chen, Y., Cai, J., & Sternberg, P., Jr. (2006). Increased glutathione synthesis through an ARE-Nrf2-dependent pathway by zinc in the RPE: implication for protection against oxidative stress. *Investigative Ophthalmology & Visual Science* Vol.47, No.6, (June 2006), pp. 2709-2715, ISSN 0146-0404

Hadziahmetovic, M., Dentchev, T., Song, Y., Haddad, N., He, X., Hahn, P., Pratico, D., Wen, R., Harris, Z.L., Lambris, J.D., et al. (2008). Ceruloplasmin/hephaestin knockout mice model morphologic and molecular features of AMD. *Investigative Ophthalmology & Visual Science* Vol.49, No.6, (June 2008), pp. 2728-2736, ISSN 0146-0404

Hahn, P., Qian, Y., Dentchev, T., Chen, L., Beard, J., Harris, Z.L., & Dunaief, J.L. (2004). Disruption of ceruloplasmin and hephaestin in mice causes retinal iron overload and retinal degeneration with features of age-related macular degeneration. *Proceedings of the National Academy of Sciences of the United States of America* Vol.101, No.38, (September 2004), pp. 13850-13855, ISSN 0027-8424

Ham, W.T., Jr., Mueller, H.A., Ruffolo, J.J., Jr., Millen, J.E., Cleary, S.F., Guerry, R.K., and Guerry, D., 3rd (1984). Basic mechanisms underlying the production of photochemical lesions in the mammalian retina. *Current Eye Research* Vol.3, No.1, (January 1984), pp. 165-174, ISSN 0271-3683

Hollyfield, J.G., Bonilha, V.L., Rayborn, M.E., Yang, X., Shadrach, K.G., Lu, L., Ufret, R.L., Salomon, R.G., and Perez, V.L. (2008). Oxidative damage-induced inflammation initiates age-related macular degeneration. *Nature Medicine* Vol.14, No.2, (February 2008), pp. 194-198, ISSN 1078-8956

Hong, F., Sekhar, K.R., Freeman, M.L., & Liebler, D.C. (2005). Specific patterns of electrophile adduction trigger Keap1 ubiquitination and Nrf2 activation. *Journal of Biological Chemistry* Vol.280, No.36, (September 2005), pp. 31768-31775, ISSN 0021-9258

Huang, H.C., Nguyen, T., & Pickett, C.B. (2002). Phosphorylation of Nrf2 at Ser-40 by protein kinase C regulates antioxidant response element-mediated transcription. *Journal of Biological Chemistry* Vol.277, No.45, (November 2002), pp. 42769-42774, ISSN 0021-9258

Imamura, Y., Noda, S.,Hashizume, K., Shinoda, K., Yamaguchi, M., Uchlyama, S., Shimizu, T., Mizushima, Y., Shirasawa, T. & Tsubota, K. Drusen, choroidal neovascularization, and retinal pigment epithelium dysfunction in SOD1-deficient mice: a model of age-related macular degeneration. *Proceedings of the National Academy of Sciences of the United States of America* Vol.103, No.30, (July 2006), pp. 11282-11287, ISSN 0027-8424

Imomata, Y., Tanibara, H., Tanito, M., Okyama, H., Hoshino, Y., Kinumi, T., Kawaji, T., Kondo, N., Yodoi, J & Nakamura H. Suppression of choroidal neovascularization by thioredoxin-1 via interaction with complement factor H. *Investigative Ophthalmology & Visual Science* Vol.49, No.11, (November 2008), pp. 5118-5125, ISSN 0146-0404

Ishii, T., Sato, H., Miura, K., Sagara, J., & Bannai, S. (1992). Induction of cystine transport activity by stress. *Annals of the New York Academy of Sciences* Vol.663, (November 1992), pp. 497-498, ISSN 0077-8923

Jacobson, L.P., Zhang, B.C., Zhu, Y.R., Wang, J.B., Wu, Y., Zhang, Q.N., Yu, L.Y., Qian, G.S., Kuang, S.Y., Li, Y.F., et al. (1997). Oltipraz chemoprevention trial in Qidong, People's Republic of China: study design and clinical outcomes. *Cancer Epidemiology, Biomarkers & Prevention* Vol.6, No.4, (April 1997), pp. 257-265, ISSN 1055-9965

Jain, A. K., & Jaiswal, A.K. (2006). Phosphorylation of tyrosine 568 controls nuclear export of Nrf2. *Journal of Biological Chemistry* Vol.281, No.17, (April 2006), pp. 12132-12142, ISSN 0021-9258

Johnson, J., Maher, P., and Hanneken, A. (2009). The flavonoid, eriodictyol, induces long-term protection in ARPE-19 cells through its effects on Nrf2 activation and phase 2 gene expression. *Investigative Ophthalmology & Visual Science* Vol.50, No.5, (May 2009), pp. 2398-2406, ISSN 0146-0404

Justilien, V., Pang, J.J., Renganathan, K., Zhan, X., Crabb, J.W., Kim, S.R., Sparrow, J.R., Hauswirth, W.W. & Lewin, A.S. SOD2 knockdown mouse model of early AMD. *Investigative Ophthalmology & Visual Science* Vol.48, No.10, (October 2007), pp. 4407-4420, ISSN 0146-0404

Kaarniranta, K. (2010) Autophagy-hot topic in AMD. *Acta Ophthalmologica* Vol.88, No.4, (June 2010), pp. 387-388, ISSN 1755-3768

Kaneko, H., Dridi, S., Tarallo, V., Gelfand, B.D., Fowler, B.J., Cho, W.G., Kleinman, M.E., Ponicsan, S.L., Hauswirth, W.W., Chiodo, V.A., et al. (2011). DICER1 deficit induces Alu RNA toxicity in age-related macular degeneration. *Nature* Vol.471, No.7338, (March 2011), pp. 325-330, ISSN 0028-0836

Kang, K. W., Lee, S. J., Park, J. W., & Kim, S. G. (2002). Phosphatidylinositol 3-kinase regulates nuclear translocation of NF-E2-related factor 2 through actin rearrangement in response to oxidative stress. *Molecular pharmacology* Vol.62, No.5, (November 2002), pp. 1001-1010, ISSN 0026-895X

Kang, K. W., Ryu, J. H., & Kim, S. G. (2000). The essential role of phosphatidylinositol 3-kinase and of p38 mitogen-activated protein kinase activation in the antioxidant response element-mediated rGSTA2 induction by decreased glutathione in H4IIE hepatoma cells. *Molecular pharmacology* Vol.58, No.5, (November 2000), pp. 1017-1025, ISSN 0026-895X

Kaspar, J.W. & Jaiswal, A.K. (2011) Tyrosine phosphorylation control nuclear export of Fyn, allowing Nrf2 activation of cytoprotective gene expression. *FASEB Journal* (March 2011), pp 1076-1087, ISSN 0892-6638.

Katsuoka, F., Motohashi, H., Ishii, T., Aburatani, H., Engel, J.D., & Yamamoto, M. (2005). Genetic evidence that small maf proteins are essential for the activation of antioxidant response element-dependent genes. *Molecular and Cell Biololgy* Vol.25, No.18, (September 2005), pp. 8044-8051, ISSN 0270-7306

Kensler, T.W., Wakabayashi, N., & Biswal, S. (2007). Cell survival responses to environmental stresses via the Keap1-Nrf2-ARE pathway. *Annual Review of Pharmacology and Toxicology* Vol.47, (2007), pp. 89-116, ISSN 0362-1642

Klionsky, D.J. (2007) Autophagy: from phenomenology to molecular understanding in less than a decade. *Nature Review Molecular &Cell Biology* Vol.8, (November 2007), pp. 931-937, ISSN 1471-0072

Kobayashi, A., Kang, M.I., Okawa, H., Ohtsuji, M., Zenke, Y., Chiba, T., Igarashi, K., and Yamamoto, M. (2004). Oxidative stress sensor Keap1 functions as an adaptor for Cul3-based E3 ligase to regulate proteasomal degradation of Nrf2. *Molecular and Cell Biology* Vol.24, No.16, (August 2004), pp. 7130-7139, ISSN 0270-7306

Komatsu, M., Kurokawa, H., Waguri, S., Taguchi, K., Kobayashi, A., et al. (2010) The selective autophagy substrate p62 activates the stress responsive transcription factor Nrf2 through inactivation of Keap1. *Nature Cell Biology* Vol.12, No.3, (March 2010), pp. 213-224, ISSN 1465-7392

Kong, L., Tanito, M., Huang, Z., Li, F., Zhou, X., Zaharia, A., Yodoi, J., McGinnis, J.F., & Cao, W. (2007). Delay of photoreceptor degeneration in tubby mouse by sulforaphane. *Journal of Neurochemistry* Vol.101, No.4, (May 2007), pp. 1041-1052, ISSN 0022-3042

Lee, J. M., Hanson, J. M., Chu, W. A., & Johnson, J. A. (2001). Phosphatidylinositol 3-kinase, not extracellular signal-regulated kinase, regulates activation of the antioxidant-responsive element in IMR-32 human neuroblastoma cells. *Journal of biological chemistry* Vol.276, No.23, (June 2001), pp. 20011-20016, ISSN 0021-9258

Lee, J.-H., Yu, W.H, Kuma A., Lee, S., Mohan, P.S., Peterhoff, C.M., Wolfe, D.M., Martinez-Vicente, M., Massey, A.C., Sovak, G., Uchiyama, Y., Westaway, D., Cuervo, A.M. & Nixon, R.A. (2010) Lysosomal proteolysis and autophagy require presenilin 1 and are disrupted by Alzheimer-related PS1 mutations. *Cell* Vol.141, No.7, (June 2010), pp 1146-1158, ISSN 0092-8674

Lee, P. P., Feldman, Z. W., Ostermann, J., Brown, D. S., & Sloan, F. A. (2003). Longitudinal prevalence of major eye diseases. *Archives of Ophthalmology* Vol.121, No.9, (September 2003), pp. 1303-1310, ISSN 0003-9950

Levine, B., Mizushima, N. & Virgin, H.W. (2011) Autophagy in immunity and inflammation. *Nature* Vol.469, (January 2011), pp. 323-335, ISSN 0028-0836

Mandal, M. N. A., Patlolla, J. M. R., Zheng, L., Agbaga, M. P., Tran, J. T. A., Wicker, L., Asus-Jacobi, A., Elliott, M. H., Rao, C. V., & Anderson, R. E. (2009). Curcumin protects retinal cells from light-and oxidant stress-induced cell death. *Free Radical Biology and Medicine* Vol.46, No.5, (March 2009), pp. 672-679, ISSN 0891-5849

Marzec, J. M., Christie, J. D., Reddy, S. P., Jedlicka, A. E., Vuong, H., Lanken, P. N., Aplenc, R., Yamamoto, T., Yamamoto, M., Cho, H. Y., & Kleeberger, S. R. (2007). Functional polymorphisms in the transcription factor NRF2 in humans increase the risk of acute lung injury. *Faseb Journal* Vol.21, No.9, (July 2007), pp. 2237-2246, ISSN 0892-6638 1546-1726

Martinez-Vicente, M., Talloczy, Z., Wong, E., Tang, G., Koga, H., et al. (2010) Cargo recognition failure is responsible for inefficient autophagy in Huntington's disease. *Nature Neuroscience* Vol.13, (April 2010), pp. 567-576, ISSN

McLeod, D. S., Grebe, R., Bhutto, J., Merges, C., Baba, T., & Lutty, G. A. (2009) Relationship between RPE and choriocapillaris in age-related macular degeneration. *Investigative Ophthalmology & Visual Science* Vol.50, No. 10, (October 2009), pp 4982-4991, ISSN 0146-0404

McMahon, M., Thomas, N., Itoh, K., Yamamoto, M., & Hayes, J. D. (2004). Redox-regulated turnover of Nrf2 is determined by at least two separate protein domains, the redox-sensitive Neh2 degron and the redox-insensitive Neh6 degron. *Journal of Biological Chemistry* Vol.279, No.30, (July 2004), pp. 31556-31567, ISSN 0021-9258

Mitchell, P., Wang, J. J., Smith, W., & Leeder, S. R. (2002). Smoking and the 5-year incidence of age-related maculopathy - The Blue Mountains Eye Study. *Archives of Ophthalmology* Vol.120, No.10, (October 2002), pp. 1357-1363, ISSN 0003-9950

Moiseyev, G., Takahashi, Y., Chen, Y., Gentleman, S., Redmond, T. M., Crouch, R. K., & Ma, J. X. (2006). RPE65 is an iron(II)-dependent isomerohydrolase in the retinoid visual cycle. *Journal of Biological Chemistry* Vol.281, No.5, (February 2006), pp. 2835-2840, ISSN 0021-9258

Moriarty-Craige, S.E., Ha, K.N., Sternberg, P. Jr., Lynn, M., Bressler, S., Gensler, G. & Jones, D.P. (2007) Effects off long-term zinc supplementation on plasma thiol metabolites and redox status in patients with age-related macular degeneration. *American Journal of Ophthalmology* Vo.143, No.2, (February 2007), pp. 206-211, ISSN 0002-9394

Motohashi, H., Katsuoka, F., Engel, J. D., & Yamamoto, M. (2004). Small Maf proteins serve as transcriptional cofactors for keratinocyte differentiation in the Keap1-Nrf2 regulatory pathway. *Proceedings of the National Academy of Sciences of the United States of America* Vol.101, No.17, (April 2004), pp. 6379-6384, ISSN 0027-8424

Mullins, R. F., Johnson, M. N., Faidley, E. A., Skeie, J. M., & Huang, J. (2011) Choriocapillaris vascular dropout related to density of drusen in human eyes with early age-related macular degeneration. *Investigative Ophthalmology & Visual Science* Vol.52, No. 3, (March 2011), pp 1606-1612, ISSN 0146-0404

Mullins, R. F., Russell, S. R., Anderson, D. H., & Hageman, G. S. (2000). Drusen associated with aging and age-related macular degeneration contain proteins common to extracellular deposits associated with atherosclerosis, elastosis, amyloidosis, and dense deposit disease. *Faseb Journal* Vol.14, No.7, (May 2000), pp. 835-846, ISSN 0892-6638

Nagai, N., Thimmulappa, R. K., Cano, M., Fujihara, M., Izumi-Nagai, K., Kong, X. O., Sporn, M. B., Kensler, T. W., Biswal, S., & Handa, J. I. (2009). Nrf2 is a critical modulator of the innate immune response in a model of uveitis. *Free Radical Biology and Medicine* Vol.47, No.3, (August 2009), pp. 300-306, ISSN 0891-5849

Nelson, K. C., Armstrong, J. S., Moriarty, S., Cai, J. Y., Wu, M. W. H., Sternberg, P., & Jones, D. P. (2002). Protection of retinal pigment epithelial cells from oxidative damage by oltipraz, a cancer chemopreventive agent. *Investigative Ophthalmology & Visual Science* Vol.43, No.11, (November 2002), pp. 3550-3554, ISSN 0146-0404

Nelson, K.C., Carlson, J, Newman, M.L., Sternberg, P. Jr., Jones, D.P., Kavanagh, T.J., Diaz, D., Cai, J. & Wu M. (1999) Effect of dietary inducer dimethylfumarate on glutathione in cultured human retinal pigment epithelial cells. *Investigative Ophthalmology & Visual Science* Vol.40, No. 9, (August 1999), pp 1927-1935, ISSN 0146-0404

Niture, S.K., Jain, A.K., Shelton, P.M. & Jaiswal, A.K. (2011) Src subfamily kinases regulate nuclear export and degradation of the transcription factor Nrf2 to switch off Nrf2-mediated antioxidant activation of cytoprotective gene expression. *Journal of Biological Chemistry.* in press, (June 2011), ISSN 0021-9258

Okawa, H., Motohashi, H., Kobayashi, A., Aburatani, H., Kensler, T. W., & Yamamoto, M. (2006). Hepatocyte-specific deletion of the keap1 gene activates Nrf2 and confers potent resistance against acute drug toxicity. *Biochemical and Biophysical Research Communications* Vol.339, No.1, (January 2006), pp. 79-88, ISSN 0006-291X

Organisciak, D. T., Wang, H. M., Li, Z. Y., & Tso, M. O. M. (1985). The Protective Effect of Ascorbate in Retinal Light Damage of Rats. *Investigative Ophthalmology & Visual Science* Vol.26, No.11, (November 1985), pp. 1580-1588, ISSN 0146-0404

Osburn, W. O., & Kensler, T. W. (2008). Nrf2 signaling: An adaptive response pathway for protection against environmental toxic insults. *Mutation Research-Reviews in Mutation Research* Vol.659, No.1-2, (July-August 2008), pp. 31-39, ISSN 1383-5742

Pearson, K.J., Lewis, K.N., Price, N.L., et al. (2008) Nrf2 mediates cancer protection but not prolongevity induced by caloric restriction. *Proceedings of the National Academy of Sciences of the United States of America* Vol.105, No.7, (February 2008), pp. 2325-2330, ISSN 0027-8424

Pi, J., Bai, Y., Reece, J. M., Williams, J., Liu, D., Freeman, M. L., Fahl, W. E., Shugar, D., Liu, J., Qu, W., Collins, S., & Waalkes, M. P. (2007). Molecular mechanism of human Nrf2 activation and degradation: role of sequential phosphorylation by protein kinase CK2. *Free Radical Biology & Medicine* Vol.42, No.12, (June 15 2007), pp. 1797-1806, ISSN 0891-5849

Pitha-Rowe, I., Liby, K., Royce, D., & Sporn, M. (2009). Synthetic Triterpenoids Attenuate Cytotoxic Retinal Injury: Cross-talk between Nrf2 and PI3K/AKT Signaling through Inhibition of the Lipid Phosphatase PTEN. *Investigative Ophthalmology & Visual Science* Vol.50, No.11, (November 2009), pp. 5339-5347, ISSN 0146-0404

Pool-Zobel, B., Veeriah, S., & Bohmer, F. D. (2005). Modulation of xenobiotic metabolising enzymes by anticarcinogens - focus on glutathione S-transferases and their role as targets of dietary chemoprevention in colorectal carcinogenesis. *Mutation Research-Fundamental and Molecular Mechanisms of Mutagenesis* Vol.591, No.1-2, (December 2005), pp. 74-92, ISSN 0027-5107

Pryor, W. A., Prier, D. G., & Church, D. F. (1983). Electron-Spin Resonance Study of Mainstream and Sidestream Cigarette-Smoke - Nature of the Free-Radicals in Gas-Phase Smoke and in Cigarette Tar. *Environmental Health Perspectives* Vol.47, (January 1983), pp. 345-355, ISSN 0091-6765

Rada, P., Rojo, A. I., Chowdhry, S., McMahon, M., Hayes, J. D., & Cuadrado, A. (2011). SCF/{beta}-TrCP promotes glycogen synthase kinase 3-dependent degradation of the Nrf2 transcription factor in a Keap1-independent manner. *Molecular and Cellular Biology* Vol.31, No.6, (March 2011), pp. 1121-1133, ISSN 1098-5549

Ramkumar, H. L., Chan, C. C., & Zhang, J. (2010). Retinal ultrastructure of murine models of dry age-related macular degeneration (AMD). *Progress in Retinal and Eye Research* Vol.29, No.3, (May 2010), pp. 169-190, ISSN 1350-9462

Rangasamy, T., Cho, C. Y., Thimmulappa, R. K., Zhen, L. J., Srisuma, S. S., Kensler, T. W., Yamamoto, M., Petrache, I., Tuder, R. M., & Biswal, S. (2004). Genetic ablation of Nrf2 enhances susceptibility to cigarette smoke-induced emphysema in mice. *Journal of Clinical Investigation* Vol.114, No.9, (November 2004), pp. 1248-1259, ISSN 0021-9738

Rosenfeld, P. J., Brown, D. M., Heier, J. S., Boyer, D. S., Kaiser, P. K., Chung, C. Y., & Kim, R. Y. (2006). Ranibizumab for neovascular age-related macular degeneration. *New England Journal of Medicine* Vol.355, No.14, (October 2006), pp. 1419-1431, ISSN 0028-4793

Saint-Geniez, M., Kurihara, T., Sekiyama, E., Maldonado, A. E., & D'Amore, P. A. (2009). An essential role for RPE-derived soluble VEGF in the maintenance of the choriocapillaris. *Proceedings of the National Academy of Sciences of the United States of America* Vol.106, No.44, (November 2009), pp. 18751-18756, ISSN 0027-8424

Salazar, M., Rojo, A. I., Velasco, D., de Sagarra, R. M., & Cuadrado, A. (2006). Glycogen synthase kinase-3beta inhibits the xenobiotic and antioxidant cell response by direct phosphorylation and nuclear exclusion of the transcription factor Nrf2. *Journal of Biological Chemistry* Vol.281, No.21, (May 2006), pp. 14841-14851, ISSN 0021-9258

Sasaki, H., Sato, H., Kuriyama-Matsumura, K., Sato, K., Maebara, K., Wang, H. Y., Tamba, M., Itoh, K., Yamamoto, M., & Bannai, S. (2002). Electrophile response element-mediated induction of the cystine/glutamate exchange transporter gene expression. *Journal of Biological Chemistry* Vol.277, No.47, (November 2002), pp. 44765-44771, ISSN 0021-9258

Sato, H., Tamba, M., Ishii, T., & Bannai, S. (1999). Cloning and expression of a plasma membrane cystine/glutamate exchange transporter composed of two distinct proteins. *Journal of Biological Chemistry* Vol.274, No.17, (April 1999), pp. 11455-11458, ISSN 0021-9258

Shen, G., Hebbar, V., Nair, S., Xu, C., Li, W., Lin, W., Keum, Y. S., Han, J., Gallo, M. A., & Kong, A. N. (2004). Regulation of Nrf2 transactivation domain activity. The differential effects of mitogen-activated protein kinase cascades and synergistic stimulatory effect of Raf and CREB-binding protein. *Journal of Biological Chemistry* Vol.279, No.22, (May 2004), pp. 23052-23060, ISSN 0021-9258

Sherratt, P. J., Huang, H. C., Nguyen, T., & Pickett, C. B. (2004). Role of protein phosphorylation in the regulation of NF-E2-related factor 2 activity. *Methods in Enzymology* Vol.378, (2004), pp. 286-301, ISSN 0076-6879

Shibata, T., Iuchi, Y., Okada, F., Kuwata, K., Yamanobe, T., Bannai, S., Tomita, Y., Tomita, Y. & Fujii J. (2009) Aggravation of ischemia-reperfusion-triggered acute renal failure in xCT-deficient mice. *Archives of Biochemistry and Biophysic* Vol.490, No.1, (October 2009),pp. 63-69, ISSN 0003-9861

Shibata, T., Ohta, T., Tong, K.I., Kokubu, A., Odogawa, R., Tsuta, K., Asamura, H., Yamamoto, M. & Hirohashi S. (2008). Cancer related mutations in NRF2 impair its recognition by Keap1-Cul3 E3 ligase and promote malignancy. *Proceedings of the*

National Academy of Sciences of the United States of America   Vol.105,   No.36, (September 2008), pp. 13568-13573, ISSN 0027-8424

Smith, W., Assink, J., Klein, R., Mitchell, P., Klaver, C. C. W., Klein, B. E. K., Hofman, A., Jensen, S., Wang, J. J., & de Jong, P. T. V. M. (2001). Risk factors for age related macular degeneration - Pooled findings from three continents. *Ophthalmology* Vol.108, No.4, (April 2001), pp. 697-704, ISSN 0161-6420

Sparrow, J. R., Fishkin, N., Zhou, J. L., Cai, B. L., Jang, Y. P., Krane, S., Itagaki, Y., & Nakanishi, K. (2003). A2E, a byproduct of the visual cycle. *Vision Research* Vol.43, No.28, (December 2003), pp. 2983-2990, ISSN 0042-6989

Sun, Z., Huang, Z., & Zhang, D. D. (2009). Phosphorylation of Nrf2 at multiple sites by MAP kinases has a limited contribution in modulating the Nrf2-dependent antioxidant response. *PLoS One* Vol.4, No.8, (August 2009), pp. e6588, ISSN 1932-6203

Tanito, M., Masutani, H., Kim, Y. C., Nishikawa, M., Ohira, A., & Yodoi, J. (2005). Sulforaphane induces thioredoxin through the antioxidant-responsive element and attenuates retinal light damage in mice. *Investigative Ophthalmology & Visual Science* Vol.46, No.3, (March 2005), pp. 979-987, ISSN 0146-0404

Tomobe, K., Shinozuka, T., Kuroiwa, M. & Nomura Y. (2011) Age-related changes of Nrf2 and phosphorylated GSH-3β in a mouse model of accelerated aging (SAMP8). *Archives of Gerontology and Geriatrics* Article in Press, ISSN 0167-4943

Tso, M. O. M., Woodford, B. J., & Lam, K. W. (1984). Distribution of Ascorbate in Normal Primate Retina and after Photic Injury - a Biochemical, Morphological Correlated Study. *Current Eye Research* Vol.3, No.1, (January 1984), pp. 181-191, ISSN 0271-3683

Tso, M. O. M., Zhang, C., Abler, A. S., Chang, C. J., Wong, F., Chang, G. Q., & Lam, T. T. (1994). Apoptosis Leads to Photoreceptor Degeneration in Inherited Retinal Dystrophy of Rcs Rats. *Investigative Ophthalmology & Visual Science* Vol.35, No.6, (May 1994), pp. 2693-2699, ISSN 0146-0404

Uno, K., Prow, T. W., Bhutto, I. A., Yerrapureddy, A., McLeod, D. S., Yamamoto, M., Reddy, S. P., & Lutty, G. A. (2010). Role of Nrf2 in retinal vascular development and the vaso-obliterative phase of oxygen-induced retinopathy. *Experimental Eye Research* Vol.90, No.4, (April 2010), pp. 493-500, ISSN 0014-4835

Wagner, C. A., Lang, F., & Broer, S. (2001). Function and structure of heterodimeric amino acid transporters. *American Journal of Physiology-Cell Physiology* Vol.281, No.4, (October 2001), pp. C1077-C1093, ISSN 0363-6143

Wakabayashi, N., Slocum, S. L., Skoko, J. J., Shin, S., & Kensler, T. W. (2010). When NRF2 Talks, Who's Listening? *Antioxidants & Redox Signaling* Vol.13, No.11, (December 2010), pp. 1649-1663, ISSN 1523-0864

Wang, A. L., Lukas, T. J., Yuan, M., Du, N., Tso, M. O., & Neufeld, A. H. (2009). Autophagy and Exosomes in the Aged Retinal Pigment Epithelium: Possible Relevance to Drusen Formation and Age-Related Macular Degeneration. *PLoS One* Vol.4, No.1, (January 8 2009), pp. e4160, ISSN 1932-6203

Wang, L., Chen, Y., Sternberg, P., & Cai, J. (2008). Essential roles of the PI3 kinase/Akt pathway in regulating Nrf2-dependent antioxidant functions in the RPE. *Investigative Ophthalmology & Visual Science* Vol.49, No.4, (April 2008), pp. 1671-1678, ISSN 0146-0404

Wei, Y., Gong, J., Yoshida, T., Eberhart, C.G., Xu, Z., Kombairaju P., Spron, M.B., Handa, J.T. & Duh, E.J. (2011) Nrf2 has a protective role against neuronal and capillary degeneration in retinal ischemia-reperfusion injury. *Free Radical Biology & Medicine* Vol.51, No.1 (July 2011), pp 216-224, ISSN 0891-5849

Winkler, B.S. (2008) An hypothesis to account for the renewal of outer segments in rod and cone photoreceptor cells: renewal as a surrogate antioxidant. *Investigative Ophthalmology & Visual Science* Vol.49, No.8, (August 2008), pp. 3259-3261, ISSN 0146-0404

Wu, Y. L., Yanase, E., Feng, X. D., Siegel, M. M., & Sparrow, J. R. (2010). Structural characterization of bisretinoid A2E photocleavage products and implications for age-related macular degeneration. *Proceedings of the National Academy of Sciences of the United States of America* Vol.107, No.16, (April 20 2010), pp. 7275-7280, ISSN 0027-8424

Xue, L. L., Gollapalli, D. R., Maiti, P., Jahng, W. J., & Rando, R. R. (2004). A palmitoylation switch mechanism in the regulation of the visual cycle. *Cell* Vol.117, No.6, (June 11 2004), pp. 761-771, ISSN 0092-8674

Yoh, K., Itoh, K., Enomoto, A., Hirayama, A., Yamaguchi, N., Kobayashi, M., Morito, N., Koyama, A., Yamamoto, M., & Takahashi, S. (2001). Nrf2-deficient female mice develop lupus-like autoimmune nephritis. *Kidney International* Vol.60, No.4, (October 2001), pp. 1343-1353, ISSN 0085-2538

Young, R. W. (1967). The renewal of photoreceptor cell outer segments. *The Journal of Cell Biology* Vol.33, No.1, (April 1967), pp. 61-72, ISSN 0021-9525

Young, R. W., & Bok, D. (1969). Participation of the retinal pigment epithelium in the rod outer segment renewal process. *The Journal of Cell Biology* V ol.42, No.2, (August 1969), pp. 392-403, ISSN 0021-9525

Yu, R., Chen, C., Mo, Y. Y., Hebbar, V., Owuor, E. D., Tann, T. H., & Kong, A. N. T. (2000). Activation of mitogen-activated protein kinase pathways induces antioxidant response element-mediated gene expression via a Nrf2-dependent mechanism. *Journal of Biological Chemistry* Vol.275, No.51, (December 2000), pp. 39907-39913, ISSN 0021-9258

Yu, R., Mandlekar, S., Lei, W., Fahl, W. E., Tan, T. H., & Kong, A. N. (2000). p38 mitogen-activated protein kinase negatively regulates the induction of phase II drug-metabolizing enzymes that detoxify carcinogens. *Journal of Biological Chemistry* Vol.275, No.4, (January 2000c), pp. 2322-2327, ISSN 0021-9258

Zhang, J., Hosoya, T., Maruyama, A., Nishikawa, K., Maher, J. M., Ohta, T., Motohashi, H., Fukamizu, A., Shibahara, S., Yamamoto, M., & Itoh, K. (2007). Nrf2 Neh5 domain is differentially utilized in the transactivation of cytoprotective genes. *Biochemical Journal* Vol.404, (June 2007), pp. 459-466, ISSN 0264-6021

Zhao, Z. Y., Chen, Y., Wang, J., Sternberg, P., Freeman, M. L., Grossniklaus, H. E., & Cai, J. Y. (2011). Age-Related Retinopathy in NRF2-Deficient Mice. *PLoS One* Vol.6, No.4, (April 2011), pp. e19456 ISSN 1932-6203

Zhou, J. L., Jang, Y. P., Kim, S. R., & Sparrow, J. R. (2006). Complement activation by photooxidation products of A2E, a lipofuscin constituent of the retinal pigment epithelium. *Proceedings of the National Academy of Sciences of the United States of America* Vol.103, No.44, (October 2006), pp. 16182-16187, ISSN 0027-8424

Zipper, L. M., & Mulcahy, R. T. (2000). Inhibition of ERK and p38 MAP kinases inhibits binding of Nrf2 and induction of GCS genes. *Biochemical and Biophysical Research Communications* Vol.278, No.2, (November 2000), pp. 484-492, ISSN 0006-291X

9

Mechanisms of RDH12-Induced Leber Congenital Amaurosis and Therapeutic Approaches

Anne Kasus-Jacobi[1], Lea D. Marchette[1], Catherine Xu[1],
Feng Li[1], Huaiwen Wang[1] and Mark Babizhayev[2]
[1]Oklahoma University Health Sciences Center
[2]Innovative Vision Products, Inc.
USA

To Finley: You made this work very special to us.

1. Introduction

Retinal dystrophies are characterized by the degeneration of vision-supporting photoreceptor cells of the retina, leading to irreversible blindness. It is a heterogeneous group of diseases that can be caused by mutations on more than 150 identified genes with diverse functions (http://www.sph.uth.tmc.edu/Retnet/home.htm). Retinal dystrophies can be classified based on whether the rod or the cone photoreceptor cells are affected first, and based on the onset and progression of vision loss [1]. Leber congenital amaurosis (LCA) is in clear contrast with other inherited retinal dystrophies in that both rod and cone photoreceptor cells are affected from the onset of the disease [1]. The second major characteristic of LCA is that the progression to complete blindness is fast, making it the most devastating form of inherited retinal dystrophies [1]. In most cases, visual handicap is diagnosed before one year of age and progresses to legal blindness in early adulthood [2]. Other signs of the disease are an extinguished or severely reduced scotopic and photopic electroretinogram, absent or diminished pupillary response to light, and nystagmus (roaming eye movements) [3]. It is a rare disease, affecting approximately 1:30,000 people worldwide but it is the first cause of inherited blindness in children [2].

During the past 15 years, our understanding of the genetic basis of LCA has greatly progressed [1]. Today, 14 different genes causing LCA have been identified [1]. Together they are responsible for approximately 75% of LCA cases, the remaining 25% of LCA cases being caused by mutations in unidentified genes. The identified LCA-causing genes are expressed in various cell types of the retina and are involved in a wide variety of developmental and physiological pathways [1]. Because the disease is induced by mutation on a single gene, LCA patients are potentially good candidates for gene replacement therapy. In recent years, exciting results have been obtained in clinical trials for LCA caused by mutations on the *RPE65* gene (LCA2), representing 3 to 16% of LCA cases [4]. Several other LCA-causing genes have received proof-of-concept validation for gene therapy in animal models [1]. We can anticipate that in the following years, patients with LCA induced by mutations on these genes will undergo clinical trials for gene replacement therapy.

In this chapter, we will concentrate on LCA13 caused by mutations in the *RDH12* gene. This gene encodes for an enzyme of the short-chain dehydrogenase/reductase superfamily. It was named retinol dehydrogenase 12 (RDH12) based on its similarity with the RDH11 enzyme (Figure 1) [5]. Gene replacement therapy is not currently available for LCA13 patients and may not be for several years. Thus, any alternative therapeutic approach would be beneficial. We will review our and other's findings regarding the function of RDH12, providing new insight into the mechanism of RDH12-induced LCA. We will discuss how understanding the role of RDH12 is allowing the development of alternative therapeutic strategies to gene replacement therapy for patients with LCA13. Finally, we will describe our encouraging preliminary results obtained in a mouse line with disrupted *Rdh12* gene, using an imidazole-containing peptide derivative, which could be rapidly developed into an effective therapeutic strategy to preserve retinal structure and function in LCA13 patients.

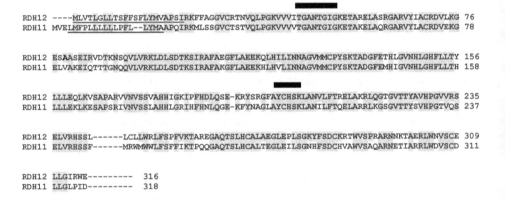

Fig. 1. **Alignment of human RDH12 and RDH11 sequences.** Residue numbers are shown on the *right*. Identical residues are *boxed*. *Overbars* denote the two signature sequences for the superfamily of short-chain dehydrogenases/reductases [6]. GenBank™ accession numbers for human RDH12 and RDH11 are NP_689656 and CAG33461, respectively. Stretches of NH2-terminal hydrophobic residues predicted to be inserted in the membrane are underlined.

2. RDH12 and Leber Congenital Amaurosis

In 2004, mutations in the *RDH12* gene were found in a subset of LCA patients [7, 8]. Since then, more than 30 *RDH12* mutations have been found in the homozygous or compound heterozygous state in LCA13 patients [7-11]. LCA13 is inherited in an autosomal recessive manner and represents about 4% of all LCA cases [2]. LCA13 appears to share a common clinical picture with other types of LCA characterized by a poor visual function in early life, followed by a progressive decline due to both rods and cones degeneration [9].

Interestingly, when compared with the RPE65-mutant retina that has a relatively well preserved structure with a disproportionate loss of photoreceptor function (as measured in 4 LCA2 patients; ages 17, 19, 19 and 23), the structure of RDH12-mutant retina appears disrupted at much younger ages (measured in 4 LCA13 patients; ages 8, 11, 13 and 21) [12].

A number of RDH12 mutations leading to LCA have been biochemically evaluated by expressing the mutants in cultured cells and by measuring the enzymatic activities of the recombinant enzymes [7-11]. These studies have shown that mutations in RDH12 result in decreased or abolished enzymatic activity due to a lower affinity for the substrate or a lower affinity for the coenzyme and/or to a decreased specific activity. In addition, most of RDH12 mutations resulted in low steady-state levels of the mutant proteins in cells [11, 13]. It was hypothesized that these mutants could be recognized as misfolded and targeted for accelerated degradation by the ubiquitin-proteasome system [13]. These studies strongly suggest that the loss of RDH12 function is the primary event causing the development of LCA13 phenotype (i.e. rapid loss of photoreceptor function and disruption of retinal structure). Thus, to determine the triggering event in LCA13 pathogenesis, and because RDH12 is an enzyme, the fundamental question is: what is the nature of the RDH12 substrate?

3. Enzymatic activity of RDH12

RDH12 is an oxidoreductase enzyme of the short-chain dehydrogenase/reductase superfamily [5]. Its substrate and coenzyme specificities have been elucidated *in vitro* [5, 14]. RDH12 was found to reduce all-*trans* retinal and other retinaldehydes (in *cis* configurations) to corresponding retinols, using the reduced form of nicotinamide adenine dinucleotide phosphate as cofactor [5, 14]. In addition, various aldehyde-containing molecules, including 4-hydroxynonenal (4-HNE), were found to be reduced by RDH12 to corresponding alcohols [14]. Thus, RDH12 has a double substrate specificity for all-*trans* retinal (and other retinaldehydes) and for 4-HNE (and other toxic aldehydes). In addition, the possibility that RDH12 could have other -yet unknown- substrates cannot be ruled out.

The existence of two groups of substrates for RDH12 suggests that this enzyme could have two distinct physiological functions *in vivo*. As mentioned, mutations of RDH12 associated with LCA resulted in a decreased enzymatic activity of RDH12, inhibiting the reduction of all-*trans* retinal and 4-HNE to the corresponding alcohols *in vitro* [7, 10, 11, 15].

4. Possible RDH12 function(s) in the retina

RDH12 is abundantly expressed in rod and possibly cone photoreceptor cells in the retina [16-19]. These cells are photosensitive; they detect the presence of photons through the 11-*cis* retinal chromophore bound to opsin protein (forming the photosensitive rhodopsin). When photobleaching of rhodopsin occurs, light isomerizes 11-*cis* retinal to all-*trans* retinal, which then dissociates from opsin. This photoisomerization is the initial event that triggers the visual transduction pathway, activation of second order neurons, and eventually transmission of the signal to the brain. Under constant illumination, 11-*cis* retinal has to be replaced (recycled) and all-*trans* retinal has to be removed from the surrounding of opsin so that photoreceptor cells continue to have an optimum sensitivity to light. The retinoid or visual cycle is the multi-step biochemical pathway that allows the recycling of 11-*cis*-retinal. The retinol dehydrogenases RDH8 (expressed in photoreceptor cells) and RDH5 (located in retinal pigment epithelium cells) were shown to directly participate in this essential pathway for maintenance of normal vision [20]. A possible function for RDH12 could thus be to reduce all-*trans* retinal, duplicating the RDH8 function, to keep photoreceptor cells in a state of high sensitivity to light.

We proposed another possible function for RDH12 in photoreceptor cells, in relation with its ability to reduce 4-HNE [15]. Reactive oxygen species formed within the mitochondria as byproducts of the electron transport chain can directly attack polyunsaturated fatty acids and initiate an auto-amplified chain reaction of lipid oxidation in cellular membranes. This causes the degradation of polyunsaturated fatty acids into a variety of oxidized products, including short- and medium-chain reactive aldehydes such as malondialdehyde, 4-hydroxyhexenal, and 4-HNE [21]. 4-HNE is the oxidation product of ω-6 arachidonic and linoleic fatty acids and is the most abundant and toxic end-product of lipid oxidation found in tissues [21-23]. It reacts readily with histidine, cysteine, and lysine to form Michael's adduct with these residues [24]. Oxidative modification of protein by 4-HNE leads to a variety of effects including inhibition of enzymatic activities; inhibition of protein functions; targeting of modified proteins for degradation; inhibition of protein, RNA, and DNA synthesis; cell cycle arrest; and apoptosis [21, 22, 25, 26]. When 4-HNE is reduced to the corresponding alcohol dihydroxynonene, its ability to form toxic adduct with proteins is abolished. Thus, we proposed that a possible function for RDH12 in the retina could be to detoxify 4-HNE by reducing it to dihydroxynonene [15].

When there is a loss of enzymatic function in cells, the substrate of the inactivated enzyme accumulates while the product of the reaction decreases. The next question is then whether it is the accumulation of substrate(s) or the disappearance of product(s), or both, that triggers the LCA13 phenotype. All-*trans* retinol, the product of all-*trans* retinal reduction, is not absolutely required for visual function because it is constantly supplied to the retinal pigment epithelium cells from the circulating blood. Therefore the most probable hypothesis is that accumulation of the substrate (all-*trans* retinal) rather than lack of product (all-*trans* retinol) might cause the retinal phenotype in LCA13 patients. Dihydroxynonene, the product of 4-HNE reduction, is not known to mediate any crucial biological function therefore in this scenario also, it seems that accumulation of the toxic substrate (4-HNE) rather than lack of product (dihydroxynonene) would cause the LCA13 phenotype.

5. Utilization of the *Rdh12* knockout mouse to determine the physiological substrate of RDH12

Identifying possible substrates for an enzyme *in vitro* is not enough to demonstrate that they are physiological substrates. *In vivo*, other considerations such as the localization and concentration of substrate relative to that of the enzyme are very important. Locations of the enzyme and substrate have to overlap and the substrate concentration has to be within a specific range for the enzymatic reaction to take place *in vivo*. The next step is thus to determine if there is accumulation of all-*trans* retinal and/or 4-HNE in the retina, in absence of RDH12. Mice with disrupted *Rdh12* gene have been generated [16, 19] and they have been useful to determine what substrate of RDH12 accumulates in the retina.

After bleaching of rhodopsin, a moderate delay in all-*trans* retinal clearance was found in the *Rdh12* knockout retina [19, 27, 28]. To explain the existing but surprisingly small delay in all-*trans* retinal clearance, it has been argued that RDH12 is located only in the inner segment of photoreceptor cells, while rhodopsin is located only in the outer segment. Thus, it was proposed that instead of participating directly (with RDH8) to the reduction of all-*trans* retinal released in the outer segment, RDH12 could reduce only a small portion of all-*trans* retinal overflowing to the inner segment after bleaching of rhodopsin [27, 28].

In our study, we found that retinas of both albino [15] and pigmented *Rdh12* knockout mice (Figure 2) accumulated more 4-HNE-modified proteins than the corresponding wild-type animals on the same genetic background. As shown in Figure 2, pigmented knockout mice have significantly more retinal 4-HNE-protein adduct than the wild-type when exposed to bright light, a condition that induces oxidative damage. Similarly, in the BALB/c albino mice, 4-HNE-protein adduct was 60% higher in *Rdh12* knockout than in wild-type retinas in 2-month old animals raised under dim cyclic light [15]. These results support the hypothesis that 4-HNE is a physiological substrate of RDH12 in rod inner segments.

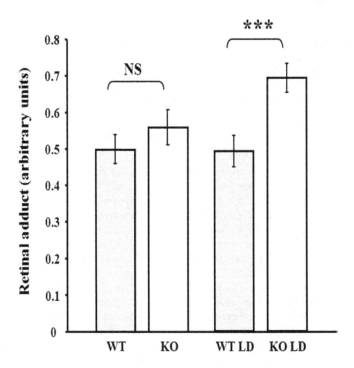

Fig. 2. **RDH12 protects against light-induced adduct formation in pigmented mouse retina.** Graph shows results for 6 mice per group. Littermates of wild-type and *Rdh12*

knockout mice were raised under dim (5-10 lux) cyclic light for 8 weeks. Control wild-type (WT) and knockout (KO) mice were killed 5 h after the (dim) light started. Light damaged (WT LD and KO LD) mice were killed after 48 h exposure to bright light (3,000 lux), without prior dilation of the pupils. Dissected retinas were homogenized in T-PER buffer (Pierce), according to the manufacturer's instructions. Protein concentrations were measured and dot blot analyses were carried out as described to quantify retinal adduct [15]. Equal aliquots (5 μg) of retinal protein were applied to a 96-well dot blot apparatus (Bio-Rad) and then transferred to a nitrocellulose membrane by vacuum filtration. Sample loading was monitored by staining the membrane with Ponceau red (Sigma). Membranes were blotted over night with a 1:1000 dilution of anti-HNE antibody coupled with horseradish peroxidase (abcam). Signals were quantified using SuperSignal West Femto Chemiluminescent Substrate (Pierce) and the digital Kodak Image Station 4000R. Error bars denote SEM and Student's t test was used for significance. NS, not significant ($p>0.05$); ***, $p<0.0001$.

The conclusion of these studies is that at least two physiological substrates of RDH12 coexist in photoreceptor cells; namely all-*trans* retinal and 4-HNE. The clearance of both of these substrates is delayed in the *Rdh12* knockout retina and it is now of crucial importance to determine which one, or if they can both, trigger the LCA13 phenotype.

6. Limitations of the *Rdh12* knockout mouse model to determine what substrate mediates photoreceptor damage

The main limitation to further determine whether accumulation of all-*trans* retinal or accumulation of 4-HNE is the triggering event in LCA13 is that, unlike LCA13 patients, the *Rdh12* knockout mouse does not develop a retinal phenotype [16, 19]. Thus the *Rdh12* knockout mouse is not an appropriate model for LCA13. We propose two possible explanations for the differences between mouse and human phenotypes.

6.1 Perhaps in mouse -but not in human- another enzyme is compensating for the loss of RDH12

In addition to RDH12, RDH11 and RDH13 are located in the inner segment of mouse photoreceptors. RDH11 and 12 are integral membrane proteins. Both enzymes are inserted in the membrane through a stretch of ~20 NH2-terminal hydrophobic residues (Figure 1) [5, 29]. RDH13 does not contain this stretch of hydrophobic residues and is a peripheral membrane protein. In previous studies, we showed that RDH11 is localized in the Golgi apparatus in spermatocytes [29] and in various cultured cells (unpublished observation). We performed a subcellular fractionation of mouse retinal tissues through ultracentrifugation on sucrose gradient [30]. RDH12 was found in Golgi- and endoplasmic reticulum-enriched fractions and RDH11 was detected only in the Golgi-enriched fractions [31]. Another study showed that RDH13 is a mitochondrial enzyme, localized within the intermembrane space, and associated with the inner mitochondrial membrane [32]. These different subcellular localizations suggest a specific role for RDH13 in the mitochondria, another specific role for RDH12 in the endoplasmic reticulum, but a possible redundant function for RDH11 and RDH12 in the Golgi. In the *Rdh12* knockout mouse photoreceptors, RDH11 may functionally compensate for RDH12 because these enzymes have overlapping localization and they have similar enzymatic activities and substrate specificities [17]. In humans on the other hand, RDH11 may not be expressed in photoreceptor cells [5] and thus may not compensate for the loss of RDH12 activity, possibly explaining the more dramatic phenotype in LCA13 patients.

6.2 Perhaps bright light is triggering the phenotype resulting from disruption of RDH12 enzymatic activity

Patients with LCA13 show an early disruption of their retinal structure [12]. The distorted laminar architecture of RDH12-mutant retinas seems to be a specific feature of some subtypes of LCA [12]. It has been suggested that such dysplastic retinal response could be triggered by some forms of photoreceptor damage induced by environmental conditions [12]. For example, light exacerbates the retinal dysplasia in a mouse model of LCA caused by *CRB1* mutations (LCA8) [33, 34]. Interestingly, the *Rdh12* knockout mice do not have a retinal phenotype when they are raised under a controlled dim (5-10 lux) cyclic light environment [15, 16, 19]. However, when they are challenged by exposure to bright light (3,000 lux for the *Rdh12* knockout mice under the BALB/c background), the *Rdh12*-null photoreceptors appear significantly more sensitive than the wild-type cells to light-induced apoptosis [15, 19]. Since *Rdh12* knockout photoreceptors degenerate only after exposure to bright light but do not have a spontaneous degeneration when raised under controlled dim cyclic light, it is possible that similarly, the LCA13 patients have retinal degeneration because they are regularly exposed to very bright light intensities (i.e. outdoor light during a sunny day). Anticipation of dysplastic retinal response and greater understanding of the pathway that triggers it could lead to specific therapy to prevent this process in LCA13 patients. Without such prevention, the amount of salvageable retina might quickly become so low that any gene replacement therapy would not be worth attempting.

It is likely that the compensation by other RDHs combined with the controlled lighting environment, and anatomical differences between mouse and human retinas explain the absence of retinal phenotype in the *Rdh12* knockout mouse, as opposed to the dramatic phenotype in LCA13 patients. In any case, it is difficult to use the *Rdh12* knockout mice to determine what substrate of RDH12 accumulating in absence of enzyme induces a retinal phenotype, because there is no phenotype. Retinal damage can be induced by exposure to bright light but this treatment exacerbates the production of both substrates of RDH12 simultaneously so it is impossible to distinguish which one triggers the hypersensitivity of *Rdh12*-null photoreceptor cells to light-induced damage. In addition, we cannot exclude the alternative possibility that the hypersensitivity to light of the *Rdh12*-null photoreceptors is not the specific result of accumulation of RDH12 substrate(s) but rather due to a non-specific effect of the gene inactivation.

7. Alternative strategy to determine what substrate mediates photoreceptor damage

An alternative strategy is to experimentally induce the production of all-*trans* retinal and 4-HNE simultaneously by exposure of the *Rdh12* knockout mice to bright light, while at the same time decreasing the level of 4-HNE using a molecule that can specifically scavenge 4-HNE and lower its concentration in the retina (Figure 3). This strategy allowed us to distinguish the relative participation of each substrate to the photoreceptor hypersensitivity to light.

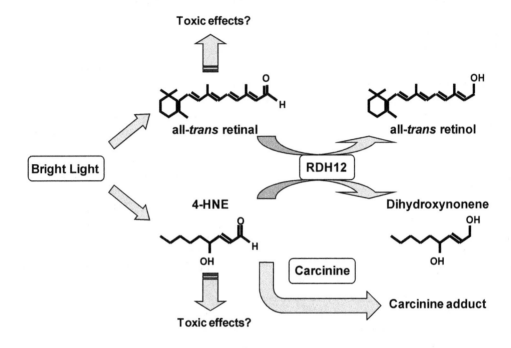

Fig. 3. **Experimental strategy to determine what substrate of RDH12 mediates photoreceptor hypersensitivity to light-induced damage.** Exposure to bright light exacerbates the production of both substrates (all-*trans* retinal and 4-HNE) simultaneously. In absence of RDH12, both substrates accumulate so it is impossible to distinguish which one triggers the hypersensitivity of photoreceptor cells to light-induced damage. Carcinine scavenges 4-HNE, forming 4-HNE-carcinine adduct, and thus can be used to lower 4-HNE independently of all-*trans* retinal. This allowed us to dissociate the effects of 4-HNE and all-*trans* retinal in the *Rdh12* knockout mouse retina.

Carcinine (β-alanyl-L-histamine) is a natural imidazole-containing peptide derivative that has antioxidant properties and can scavenge reactive aldehydes produced by lipid peroxidation [35, 36], thus preventing them from reacting with cellular proteins (manuscript submitted for publication). We have shown that intravitreal injection and systemic administration of carcinine protect wild-type photoreceptors from light-induced damage (manuscript submitted for publication). Photoreceptors are the first retinal cell type to show signs of damage after exposure to bright light. Light-induced apoptosis of photoreceptor cells is preceded by an increase of oxidative modification of retinal proteins [17, 37] and can be blocked by various types of antioxidants [38-40] including carcinine (manuscript submitted for publication).

We used carcinine to lower 4-HNE independently of all-*trans* retinal and dissociate the effects of these two molecules in mouse retina. Incubation of carcinine with all-*trans* retinal *in vitro* does not lead to any modification of the all-*trans* retinal molecule as determined by high-performance liquid chromatography analysis (unpublished observation) but incubation with 4-HNE leads to the formation of an adduct between carcinine and 4-HNE as determined by high-performance liquid chromatography and mass spectrometry (manuscript submitted for publication). Thus, carcinine is not expected to lower the retinal level of all-*trans* retinal or other retinoids under normal conditions or during exposure to bright light.

As shown in Figure 4A, without carcinine treatment (phospate buffered saline-injected eye), exposure of wild-type mice to bright light induces a decrease of rod-mediated visual function by approximately 50% for both a- and b-waves (black bars). As expected, the *Rdh12* knockout mice are more sensitive than the wild-type to light-induced damage, as shown by the 80 to 90% decrease of rod-mediated visual function for both a- and b-waves under the same conditions of light exposure (white bars). This result is consistent with previously published studies showing hypersensitivity of these knockout mice to light-induced damage [15].

Carcinine is expected to prevent light-induced damage mediated by oxidative stress and lipid peroxidation in photoreceptors. As shown in Figure 4A, with carcinine treatment (carcinine-injected eye), exposure of wild-type mice to bright light induce the decrease of rod-mediated visual function to about 25% loss instead of 50% loss without carcinine. In the *Rdh12* knockout mice, carcinine completely prevents the decrease of rod-mediated visual function. The remaining rod-mediated visual function after light damage goes from 10% without carcinine to 100% with carcinine, demonstrating a considerably beneficial effect of carcinine in these mice. The reason(s) why carcinine seems to protect more efficiently *Rdh12* knockout than wild-type photoreceptors is unknown. However, we can speculate that the disruption of *Rdh12* creates a "mild stress" in photoreceptors, inducing maybe some alternative protective mechanisms. The combination of enhanced compensatory protection and carcinine protection could be a possible explanation for this apparent higher efficiency of carcinine in the knockout than in the wild-type photoreceptors.

As shown in Figure 4B, cone-mediated visual function is more affected in the knockout than in the wild-type mouse by exposure to bright light (in phospate buffered saline -injected eye), and complete protection was provided by carcinine in both wild-type and knockout mice (carcinine-injected eye).

The fact that carcinine completely prevents light-induced damage in the *Rdh12* knockout mouse photoreceptors strongly suggests that the damage induced by light is mostly -if not only- mediated by oxidative stress and lipid peroxidation products accumulating in the *Rdh12* knockout photoreceptor cells. However, a mirror experiment in which all-*trans* retinal is specifically lowered independently of 4-HNE would further confirm our conclusion, if there was no protection. To specifically lower all-*trans* retinal independently of 4-HNE, a possible approach could be to overexpress the RDH8 enzyme in the *Rdh12* knockout photoreceptors because, as we have shown before, 4-HNE is not a substrate of RDH8 [29].

A- Rod response after light-induced damage

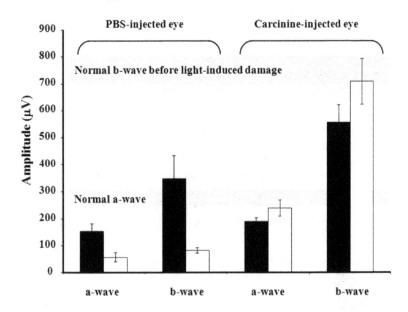

B- Cone response after light-induced damage

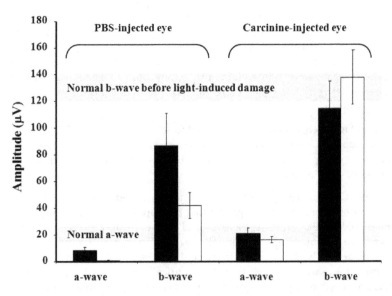

Fig. 4. **Carcinine protects visual function against light-induced damage in wild-type and** *Rdh12* **knockout mice.** BALB/c mice were raised in dim cyclic light for 8 weeks. Each

mouse was injected intravitreally in one eye with 1 μl phospate buffered saline (PBS) and in the other eye with 1 μl of 2 M carcinine diluted in PBS. Mice were returned in dim cyclic light for 48 h before light damage was initiated. Light damage was then induced in mice by 5 h exposure to 4,000 lux of white fluorescent light. After light exposure, mice are returned in dim cyclic light for 7 days to allow the retina to clear all dead cells. A. Scotopic electroretinographies were performed using saturating flash intensity. The a- and b-wave amplitudes of wild-type (black bars) and *Rdh12* knockout (white bars) are plotted to quantify rod-mediated visual function. B. Photopic ERGs were then performed to measure cone-mediated visual function. The a- and b-wave amplitudes are plotted to quantify cone-mediated visual function. Graphs show averaged results from 7 mice and error bars indicate SEM. Grey boxes show normal a- and b-waves recorded from PBS-injected eyes in mice that were not exposed to bright light.

8. Could decrease clearance of 4-HNE have toxic effects in photoreceptors?

Effects of 4-HNE in cells and its association with disease states have been increasingly well documented [23, 41]. Studies have shown that low, basal levels of the lipid aldehyde are present in cells (<5 μM), and at these concentrations, 4-HNE acts as a signaling molecule [42, 43]. It can activate cell growth and survival as well as stress response mechanisms, such as mitogen activated protein kinases, detoxification mechanisms, and inflammatory response, and by this way prepare the cells to overcome acute stress (protective effects) [41]. Under conditions of oxidative stress, 4-HNE concentrations increase above physiological levels; in membranes it accumulates at concentrations of 10 μM to 5 mM in response to oxidative insult [22, 23]. At such concentrations, the protective effect is lost; 4-HNE forms adduct with proteins inactivating their physiological functions, and activates intra cellular pathways promoting cell death [22, 23, 41].

The presence of 4-HNE-derived epitopes, including 4-HNE-protein adduct, has been reported in a growing number of diseases, including diabetes, cardiovascular, autoimmune, and neurodegenerative diseases, such as Alzheimer's disease, Parkinson's disease and amyotrophic lateral sclerosis [23]. The consistently growing evidence of increased 4-HNE tissue/blood levels in a great variety of human diseases certainly suggests a pathogenetic involvement of the aldehyde in their clinical expression and possible progression [41]. Recent studies have implicated 4-HNE in the pathogenesis of atherosclerosis and Alzheimer's disease [22, 41].

Oxidative stress, which induces lipid peroxidation and 4-HNE production, has been abundantly described to induce photoreceptor cell death [44-47]. Whether toxicity is mediated by 4-HNE and other lipid peroxidation products is unknown. We hypothesize that 4-HNE-mediated toxicity is inducing the rapid loss of vision in LCA13 patients. This hypothesis is based on the following evidences: (1) in cell culture, enzymatically active RDH12 protects against 4-HNE-induced cell death, while enzymatically inactive RDH12 does not [15, 37]. (2) Photoreceptor cells are particularly predisposed to oxidative stress because the retina has a high oxygen consumption, is chronically exposed to light, and contains several photosensitizers. This leads to an active production of reactive oxygen species. Furthermore, photoreceptors have a high content in polyunsaturated fatty acids, making their membranes particularly susceptible to lipid oxidation induced by reactive oxygen species. (3) In photoreceptor cells, 4-HNE production is induced by exposure to bright light, specifically in the inner segment, the compartment where RDH12 is located [15, 37]. (4) Disruption of RDH12 induces accumulation of 4-HNE-modified proteins in mouse retina, correlated with a hypersensitivity to acute light damage [15].

Taken together these results show a correlation between accumulation of 4-HNE in photoreceptor inner segments and loss of visual function, suggesting a possible cause-effect relationship. The cause-effect relationship has not been demonstrated but the mechanisms of 4-HNE toxicity have been abundantly documented in other cells types and disease states.

In LCA13 patients, it is likely that the loss of retinal structure and function is triggered by accumulation of RDH12 substrate(s). Two physiological substrates of RDH12 have been identified *in vitro* and *in vivo*. In absence of RDH12, accumulation of each of these substrates could theoretically mediate unwanted effects in photoreceptor cells.

9. Carcinine – A possible therapeutic agent for LCA13?

If 4-HNE is indeed involved in the LCA13 disease mechanism, then carcinine would clearly be beneficial based on its antioxidant and 4-HNE scavenging activities. Additionally, we recently found that carcinine has another effect that might be of significant interest for LCA13.

9.1 Carcinine protects RDH12 from degradation

In a previous study, we have shown that exposure to bright light induces a specific decrease of RDH12 protein level in the mouse retina while the closely related RDH11 protein remains stable [17]. This effect is not accompanied by a decrease of the *Rdh12* mRNA level so we hypothesized that the protein reduction was due to increased degradation rather than decreased production of RDH12 [17]. We further hypothesized that RDH12, like any other protein could be modified by 4-HNE (or maybe even more so because it has specific affinity for this molecule) and targeted for degradation [17]. Bright light would increase the endogenous production of 4-HNE and modification of RDH12, and the adduct would be quickly degraded. If not compensated by an increase in RDH12 synthesis, this would result in a net decrease of RDH12.

We used mouse retinal explants to test this hypothesis (Figure 5). Incubation of mouse retinas in a media containing 4-HNE leads to a 40% decrease of RDH12 in 4 h, while RDH12 level remains stable in retinas incubated in the same media without 4-HNE (Figure 5A). Total 4-HNE-modified proteins were then immunoprecipitated with anti-HNE antibody and immunoblotted using an RDH12 antibody. RDH12 was immunoprecipitated by the anti-HNE antibody (Figure 5B), demonstrating the modification of RDH12 by 4-HNE. The 4-HNE-RDH12 adduct accumulates first (at 1 and 2 h incubation with 4-HNE) and then decreases (at 4 and 6 h incubation with 4-HNE), supporting the hypothesis that the adduct is targeted for degradation. When compared with the total amount of 4-HNE-modified protein, the modification of RDH12 does not seem to happen significantly faster than the modification of the other proteins (Figure 5C). This result invalidates the idea that the specific affinity of RDH12 for 4-HNE would increase the rate of adduct formation. By contrast, the decrease of 4-HNE-RDH12 adduct is significantly faster than the decrease of the total amount of 4-HNE-modified protein (Figure 5C). This result suggests that RDH12 is particularly unstable (compared with other proteins) when subjected to oxidative modification.

A.

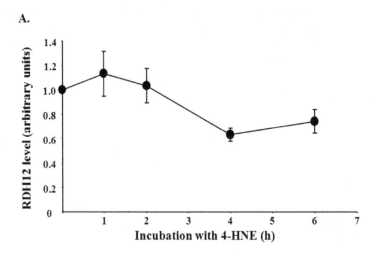

B.

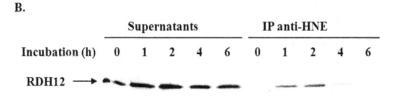

C.

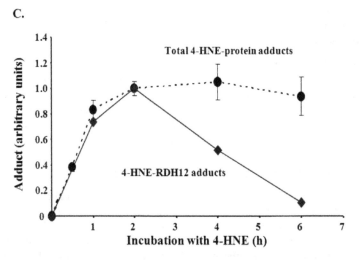

Fig. 5. **4-HNE modifies RDH12 and induces its degradation in retinal explants.** Retinas were dissected from 4- to 6-weeks-old pigmented wild-type mice. Retinas were incubated in Dulbecco's modified Eagle's medium, with or without 200 μM 4-HNE, at 37°C under 5% CO_2.

At indicated times, 6 retinas were removed from incubation, immediately washed in phosphate buffered saline, and frozen in liquid nitrogen for subsequent protein preparation. Frozen retinas were homogenized in T-PER buffer (Pierce), according to the manufacturer's instructions. A. Protein concentrations were measured and immunoblot analysis using anti-RDH12 antibody was performed using 30 µg of protein. The levels of RDH12 in retinal explants incubated with 4-HNE were expressed relative to those of RDH12 in retinal explants incubated without 4-HNE, arbitrarily defined as 1.0. B. Immunoprecipitation of 4-HNE-modified proteins was carried out as follow: equal amounts of protein were pooled from 6 retinas. 100 µg of pooled protein were incubated with 5 µl of anti-HNE antibody coupled with biotin (abcam) over night at 4oC, in a volume of 100 µl T-PER. 50 µl of streptavidin agarose resin (Pierce) was then added to each sample and incubated for 1 h at 4oC. After 3 washes with 1 ml T-PER, proteins were eluted in 50 µl Laemmli buffer and immunoblot analysis of supernatant and immunoprecipitated proteins were carried out with the anti-RDH12 antibody. C. Dot blot quantification of total 4-HNE-protein adduct was carried out as described in Fig. 2. with 2.5 µg of protein. The results from B were quantified and plotted on the same graph. At each time point the amounts of adducts are expressed relative to the highest level of adduct, arbitrarily defined as 1.0. Signals were detected using SuperSignal West Pico chemiluminescent or West Femto Maximum Signal Substrate (Pierce) and quantified using Kodak Molecular Imaging Software.

Interestingly, following intravitreal injection (Figure 6A) or systemic administration of carcinine (Figure 6B), the RDH12 protein level in mouse retina is stabilized and completely resistant to light-induced degradation. *In vivo*, the amount of 4-HNE-RDH12 adduct was undetectable (unpublished observation) so we could not determine whether carcinine was protecting RDH12 because it was opposing the 4-HNE-modification of RDH12 or through another mechanism. Absence of detectable 4-HNE-RDH12 adduct *in vivo* might be explained by the fact that endogenous production of 4-HNE as well as formation and degradation of adduct is an ongoing process, by contrast with the single dose of 4-HNE applied to the retinal explants creating a detectable "pulse" of 4-HNE-RDH12 adduct.

The stabilization of RDH12 protein by carcinine could enhance its therapeutic benefits for LCA13 patients. As discussed before, the RDH12 mutants associated with LCA are not only poorly active, but are also particularly unstable. The stabilizing effect of carcinine could keep the level of mutant RDH12 high enough to allow residual RDH12 enzymatic activity in photoreceptor cells. This, in addition with 4-HNE scavenging and antioxidant properties, could preserve the retinal structure and function in LCA13 patients.

9.2 Carcinine can be administered topically for chronic treatment

Treatment with carcinine would have to be started at the time of diagnosis and applied chronically to protect against 4-HNE and oxidative damage, which are ongoing processes in cells. We have investigated various modes of administration that could be compatible with a chronic treatment and measured the resulting level of carcinine in the retina (manuscript submitted for publication and unpublished results). Interestingly, topical administration through eye drop leads to detectable levels of carcinine in the retina (Figure 7). This result suggests that carcinine migrates from the cornea to the retina, following topical administration. The mechanisms of migration (simple diffusion versus transport) as well as the routes of migration (trans-corneal versus trans-conjonctival penetration, migration through the vitreous humor or by lateral diffusion through the sclera, etc) are currently under investigation. The possibility to administer carcinine through eye drops is promising because it is a non-invasive and particularly easy route of administration, compatible with chronic treatment.

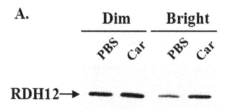

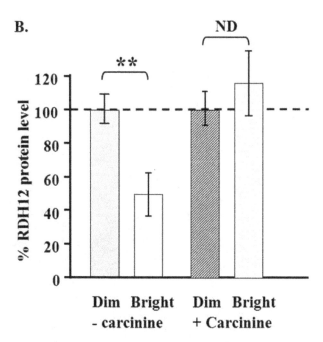

Fig. 6. **Carcinine protects RDH12 from light-induced degradation in mouse retina.** BALB/c mice were raised in dim cyclic light for 8 weeks before carcinine treatment. A. Mice were injected with carcinine or PBS and exposed to bright light as described in Fig. 4. For each group, 10 µg protein extract from 6 mice were pooled (60 µg final) and immunoblotted with anti-RDH12 antibody. B. Carcinine was administered through gavage (0 or 20 mg / mouse/ day) once a day for 5 days before light exposure. Mice were then exposed to bright white fluorescent light (3,000 lux) for 4h. Retinas were immediately frozen and proteins were extracted from one retina from each mouse (4 mice per group) using T-PER reagent. Protein

extracts from each mouse were individually quantified by immunoblot. RDH12 levels were
normalized to β-actin first and expressed relative to the level of RDH12 in retinas of dim
untreated mice, defined as 100%. Graph shows average and SEM values for 4 mice per group.
Student's *t* test was used for significance; NS, not significant (>0.05); **=p<0.001.

A.

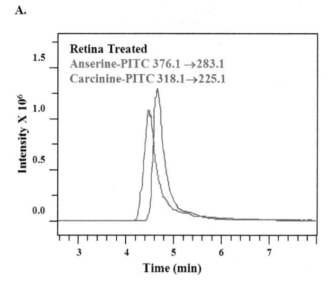

B.

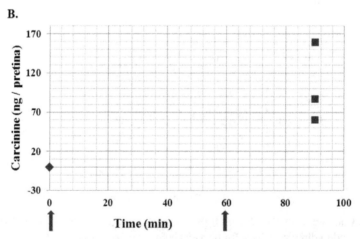

Fig. 7. **Topical administration of carcinine leads to detectable levels in the retina.**
Mice received carcinine (0.2 M) dissolved in Can-C eye drop solution (Innovative Vision
Products, Inc). To analyze and quantify retinal carcinine, 2 retinas were homogenized in 1ml of
cold 0.01M HCl with polytron. One μg of internal standard anserine was added to the samples.
Samples were extracted with acetonitrile and derivatized with phenylisothiocyanate (PITC).
Samples were analyzed by high-performance liquid chromatography / mass spectrometry

(Michrom Bioresources Paradigm MSRB capillary HPLC, Bruker Daltonics HCT Ultra Ion trap MS). High-performance liquid chromatography was run on column Magic MS C18, 5m, 200 A, 0.5 x 150 mm with Solvent A (0.09% formic acid, 0.01% TFA, 2% acetonitrile, 97.9% water) and Solvent B (0.09% formic acid, 0.0085% TFA, 95% acetonitrile, 4.9% water). An isocratic program (15% B for 10 min) was used. The flow rate was 20 ml/min and detection wavelength was 215 nm. An ion trap mass spectrometer (HCT Ultra PTM discovery system, Bruker Daltonics) equipped with an electrospray ion source and operating under an Esquire data analysis system was used. The spray voltage was set at 4 kV in the positive mode. The heater temperature was maintained at 300 °C. A, 0.2 M carcinine was administered in Can-C eye drop solution at 0 min and mice were killed 30 min later to collect retinas. B, Another set of mice received 0.2 M carcinine at 0 and 60 min (indicated by arrows) and were killed 30 min following the second administration (at 90 min) to collect retinas.

A. Dim cyclic light

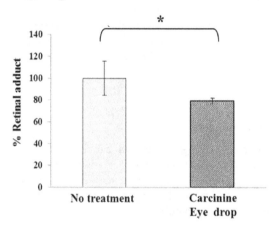

B. Bright light

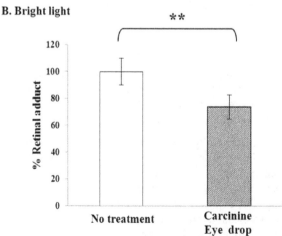

Fig. 8. **Carcinine decreases total 4-HNE-modified protein in mouse retina.** BALB/c mice were raised in dim cyclic light for 8 weeks before carcinine treatment. 0.2 M carcinine was

administered in Can-C eye drop solution (1 drop each 60 min, for 6 h) and mice were kept in dim light (A) or exposed to bright light (3,000 lux) for 4 h, starting right after administration of the second drop (B). Immediately after exposure to bright light, retinas were collected. Whole retinal homogenates were prepared and equal aliquots (10 μg) of retinal homogenates were analyzed by dot blot using anti-HNE coupled with HRP to quantify total 4-HNE-protein adduct. Five mice were used in each group, and the mean and SEM are plotted. Values were compared using Student's t test for significance; *=$p<0.05$; **=$p<0.001$.

9.3 Carcinine decreases the amount of 4-HNE-protein adduct in the retina

After administration of carcinine through eye drop, we found that the total amount of protein modified by 4-HNE in mouse retina is significantly decreased, both under dim and bright light (Figure 8). This result suggests that carcinine can scavenge 4-HNE *in vivo* after topical administration through eye drop. This implies that carcinine levels within the retina are adequate and that carcinine can enter the retinal cells to scavenge 4-HNE produced endogenously. Thus, carcinine could prevent the accumulation of toxic 4-HNE in RDH12-mutant retinas. We predict that carcinine, administered through eye drops, will prevent light-induced retinal damage in the wild-type and *Rdh12* knockout but these experiments have not been completed at this time.

10. Future directions

10.1 Developing therapeutic strategies

As shown by our preliminary experiments with carcinine, it is possible to start developing appropriate therapeutic strategies from the information already available on the function of RDH12. As discussed, exposure to bright light, as well as increased all-*trans* retinal levels, and increased oxidative damage particularly through 4-HNE modification are suspected to play a role in the disease mechanism. Accordingly, protection against these triggers can be developed with the goal to protect the retinal structure at least long enough to allow LCA13 patients to be eligible for gene replacement therapy.

10.1.1 Protection from light-induced damage

As discussed, the *Rdh12* knockout photoreceptors are more sensitive than the wild-type photoreceptors to light damage in mouse and exposure to bright light might be a trigger for the early dysplastic retinal response in LCA13 patients. Therefore, protection against light-induced retinal damage is an appropriate strategy.

Physical protection from bright light by wearing sun glasses should be encouraged for patients with LCA13. Compounds such as retinoid-like small molecules that provide chemical protection against light-induced retinal damage could also be beneficial [48, 49]. A number of studies have identified that photobleaching of rhodopsin is the essential trigger for retinal light damage [50, 51]. Genetically-modified mice that lack the opsin apoprotein or that have the opsin apoprotein but lack the ability to generate 11-*cis*-retinal are both protected against light damage [50-52]. A steady state rhodopsin level is achieved by the balance between its bleaching and regeneration. Therefore, the rate of rhodopsin regeneration is an important factor in light damage susceptibility. Fast regeneration of functional rhodopsin after bleaching increases retinal sensitivity to light damage, whereas slowing the flux of retinoids through the visual cycle increases the resistance of photoreceptors to light-induced insult. For example, slowing rhodopsin regeneration and inhibiting the visual cycle with 13-*cis*-retinoic acid prevents light damage in albino rats [53]. More recently, it has been shown that retinylamine provides efficient protection from light damage through a similar mechanism [48].

Most of the small molecules inhibiting the visual cycle are structurally similar to retinoids [49]. However, we recently identified α-phenyl-N-*tert*-butyl nitrone, a commonly used free radical spin trap, as another type of compound with no structural similarity with retinoids that interferes with rhodopsin regeneration during continuous illumination and protects against light-induced retinal degeneration [54]. The advantage that α-phenyl-N-*tert*-butyl nitrone may have over these retinol-related compounds is that it is not structurally similar nor a derivative of any of the visual cycle components and therefore may not have adverse effect by interacting with retinoid receptors and other components of the visual cycle.

10.1.2 Protection from oxidative damage

Because oxidative damage is likely to contribute to the LCA13 disease mechanism, compounds that inhibit oxidative damage or enhance endogenous protection against oxidative damage would be appropriate candidates for LCA13 treatment.

A wide variety of antioxidants are available as oral supplementations. Specific advantages of carcinine would be to combine antioxidant and 4-HNE scavenging activities. Thus, carcinine can offer an additional line of defense against oxidative damage by decreasing 4-HNE, a secondary product of oxidative stress that mediates and amplify the oxidative damage triggered by reactive oxygen species and that was shown to accumulate in mouse retina in absence of RDH12.

In addition, the main limitation for therapeutic utilization of antioxidants in retinal diseases is usually the poor targeting of the posterior segment of the eye (choroid, retinal pigmented epithelium, and retina) due to anatomical and physiological barriers that normally protect the eye. Most molecules cannot reach the posterior segment tissues upon topical administration in the form of eye drops. Periocular or intravitreal injections are more efficient routes of administration but they are invasive procedures, which are not compatible with a chronic preventive treatment. Oral supplementation of antioxidants is usually preferred but oral bioavailability and the necessity to cross the blood-retinal barrier limits the amount of compound reaching the target tissues, and therefore limits the prevention of oxidative damage in these tissues.

Carcinine is one of the very few compounds that can reach posterior segment tissues upon topical administration (less than 10 of such compounds have been reported to date) [55]. This method of administration represents the great advantages of being non-invasive, safer because it is used locally no systemic side effects are expected, and cheaper because it is used locally the amount needed is smaller than with systemic administration than any other methods. It is also compatible with a chronic treatment that could be administered by the patients themselves, or by their parents.

Drugs that upregulate the body's natural defense against oxidative stress would also be appropriate. Reactive oxygen species are constantly generated in cells as unwanted byproducts of aerobic metabolism. A wide variety of enzymatic as well as non-enzymatic cellular defense systems prevents and repair reactive oxygen species-induced damage to tolerable levels. Under ideal circumstances, the rate of production of oxidative damage should be comparable to that of its removal or repair. In LCA13, absence of the cellular defense mediated by RDH12 could perhaps be compensated by the enhancement of other cellular cytoprotective mechanisms through dietary or pharmaceutical manipulations. A wide variety of dietary polyphenols and other classes of phytochemicals have been reported to induce the expression of enzymes involved in cellular antioxidant defenses and detoxification mechanisms [56]. Such compounds would be appropriate candidates for LCA13 treatment as well.

11. Conclusion

Although generally described in the literature as an enzyme involved in all-*trans* retinal reduction, in this chapter we presented evidences for an additional detoxification role of RDH12 in photoreceptor inner segments, reducing the 4-HNE produced by lipid oxidation that takes place constantly in mouse retina. Loss of this function in patients with inherited retinal dystrophy due to mutations in *RDH12* might contribute to the dramatic and early onset loss of retinal structure and function in these individuals. Our preliminary experiments with carcinine show that this compound might be beneficial in LCA13 because it has antioxidant, 4-HNE scavenging, and RDH12 stabilizing effects in the retina. In addition, we showed that carcinine can be conveniently administered through eye drops to target the retina. Additional therapeutic strategies are developed for protection against bright light and all-*trans* retinal toxicity. Finally, the recent impressive clinical accomplishment of gene therapy for LCA2 patients laid the ground for using similar approaches to treat various types of LCA, including LCA13.

12. Acknowledgment

The authors thank Dr. Debra A. Thompson for her critical review of this manuscript. This work was supported by grants from the National Center for Research Resources (P20RR017703), the National Eye Institute (R21EY018907 and P30EY012190), the Oklahoma Center for the Advancement of Science and Technology, the University of Oklahoma College of Medicine Alumni Association, and by an unrestricted Grant from Research to Prevent Blindness, Inc. to the Ophthalmology Department of the University of Oklahoma Health Sciences Center.

13. References

[1] den Hollander, A.I., et al., *Lighting a candle in the dark: advances in genetics and gene therapy of recessive retinal dystrophies.* J Clin Invest, 2010. 120(9): p. 3042-53.

[2] Weleber, R.G., P.J. Francis, and K.M. Trzupek, *Leber Congenital Amaurosis.* GeneReviews, 2010.

[3] den Hollander, A.I., et al., *Leber congenital amaurosis: genes, proteins and disease mechanisms.* Prog Retin Eye Res, 2008. 27(4): p. 391-419.

[4] Stein, L., et al., *Clinical gene therapy for the treatment of RPE65-associated Leber congenital amaurosis.* Expert Opin Biol Ther, 2011. 11(3): p. 429-39.

[5] Haeseleer, F., et al., *Dual-substrate specificity short chain retinol dehydrogenases from the vertebrate retina.* J Biol Chem, 2002. 277(47): p. 45537-46.

[6] Kavanagh, K.L., et al., *Medium- and short-chain dehydrogenase/reductase gene and protein families : the SDR superfamily: functional and structural diversity within a family of metabolic and regulatory enzymes.* Cell Mol Life Sci, 2008. 65(24): p. 3895-906.

[7] Janecke, A.R., et al., *Mutations in RDH12 encoding a photoreceptor cell retinol dehydrogenase cause childhood-onset severe retinal dystrophy.* Nat Genet, 2004. 36(8): p. 850-4.

[8] Perrault, I., et al., *Retinal dehydrogenase 12 (RDH12) mutations in leber congenital amaurosis.* Am J Hum Genet, 2004. 75(4): p. 639-46.

[9] Schuster, A., et al., *The phenotype of early-onset retinal degeneration in persons with RDH12 mutations.* Investigative ophthalmology & visual science, 2007. 48(4): p. 1824-31.

[10] Sun, W., et al., *Novel RDH12 mutations associated with Leber congenital amaurosis and cone-rod dystrophy: biochemical and clinical evaluations.* Vision research, 2007. 47(15): p. 2055-66.

[11] Thompson, D.A., et al., *Retinal degeneration associated with RDH12 mutations results from decreased 11-cis retinal synthesis due to disruption of the visual cycle.* Hum Mol Genet., 2005. 14(24): p. 3865-75.

[12] Jacobson, S.G., et al., *RDH12 and RPE65, visual cycle genes causing leber congenital amaurosis, differ in disease expression.* Invest Ophthalmol Vis Sci, 2007. 48(1): p. 332-8.

[13] Lee, S.A., O.V. Belyaeva, and N.Y. Kedishvili, *Disease-associated variants of microsomal retinol dehydrogenase 12 (RDH12) are degraded at mutant-specific rates.* FEBS Lett. 584(3): p. 507-10.

[14] Belyaeva, O.V., et al., *Biochemical properties of purified human retinol dehydrogenase 12 (RDH12): catalytic efficiency toward retinoids and C9 aldehydes and effects of cellular retinol-binding protein type I (CRBPI) and cellular retinaldehyde-binding protein (CRALBP) on the oxidation and reduction of retinoids.* Biochemistry, 2005. 44(18): p. 7035-7047.

[15] Marchette, L.D., et al., *Retinol dehydrogenase 12 detoxifies 4-hydroxynonenal in photoreceptor cells.* Free Radic Biol Med, 2009.

[16] Kurth, I., et al., *Targeted disruption of the murine retinal dehydrogenase gene Rdh12 does not limit visual cycle function.* Molecular and cellular biology, 2007. 27(4): p. 1370-9.

[17] Kanan, Y., et al., *Retinol dehydrogenases RDH11 and RDH12 in the mouse retina: expression levels during development and regulation by oxidative stress.* Investigative ophthalmology & visual science, 2008. 49(3): p. 1071-8.

[18] Kanan, Y., et al., *Retinoid processing in cone and Muller cell lines.* Exp Eye Res, 2008. 86(2): p. 344-54.

[19] Maeda, A., et al., *Retinol dehydrogenase (RDH12) protects photoreceptors from light-induced degeneration in mice.* The Journal of biological chemistry, 2006. 281(49): p. 37697-704.

[20] Parker, R.O. and R.K. Crouch, *Retinol dehydrogenases (RDHs) in the visual cycle.* Exp Eye Res, 2010. 91(6): p. 788-92.

[21] Esterbauer, H., *Cytotoxicity and genotoxicity of lipid-oxidation products.* Am J Clin Nutr, 1993. 57(5): p. 779S-785S; discussion 785S-786S.

[22] Petersen, D.R. and J.A. Doorn, *Reactions of 4-hydroxynonenal with proteins and cellular targets.* Free Radic Biol Med, 2004. 37(7): p. 937-45.

[23] Uchida, K., *4-Hydroxy-2-nonenal: a product and mediator of oxidative stress.* Prog Lipid Res, 2003. 42(4): p. 318-43.

[24] Uchida, K. and E.R. Stadtman, *Modification of histidine residues in proteins by reaction with 4-hydroxynonenal.* Proceedings of the National Academy of Sciences of the United States of America, 1992. 89(10): p. 4544-8.

[25] Esterbauer, H., R.J. Schaur, and H. Zollner, *Chemistry and biochemistry of 4-hydroxynonenal, malonaldehyde and related aldehydes.* Free Radic Biol Med, 1991. 11(1): p. 81-128.

[26] Awasthi, Y.C., et al., *Role of 4-hydroxynonenal in stress-mediated apoptosis signaling.* Molecular aspects of medicine, 2003. 24(4-5): p. 219-30.

[27] Maeda, A., et al., *Limited Roles of Rdh8, Rdh12 and Abca4 on All-Trans-Retinal Clearance in Mouse Retina.* Invest Ophthalmol Vis Sci, 2009.

[28] Chrispell, J.D., et al., *Rdh12 activity and effects on retinoid processing in the murine retina.* J Biol Chem, 2009. 284(32): p. 21468-77.

[29] Kasus-Jacobi, A., et al., *Characterization of mouse short-chain aldehyde reductase (SCALD), an enzyme regulated by sterol regulatory element-binding proteins.* J Biol Chem, 2003. 278(34): p. 32380-9.

[30] Subramaniam, V.N., et al., *Biochemical fractionation and characterization of proteins from Golgi-enriched membranes.* The Journal of biological chemistry, 1992. 267(17): p. 12016-21.

[31] Saadi, A., et al., *Role of photoreceptor retinol dehydrogenases in detoxification of lipid oxidation products.* Studies on Retinal and Choroidal Disorders, To be published in 2012.

[32] Belyaeva, O.V., et al., *Human retinol dehydrogenase 13 (RDH13) is a mitochondrial short-chain dehydrogenase/reductase with a retinaldehyde reductase activity.* Febs J, 2007. 275(1): p. 138-47.

[33] Mehalow, A.K., et al., *CRB1 is essential for external limiting membrane integrity and photoreceptor morphogenesis in the mammalian retina.* Hum Mol Genet, 2003. 12(17): p. 2179-89.

[34] van de Pavert, S.A., et al., *Crumbs homologue 1 is required for maintenance of photoreceptor cell polarization and adhesion during light exposure.* J Cell Sci, 2004. 117(Pt 18): p. 4169-77.

[35] Babizhayev, M.A., *Biological activities of the natural imidazole-containing peptidomimetics n-acetylcarnosine, carcinine and L-carnosine in ophthalmic and skin care products.* Life Sci, 2006. 78(20): p. 2343-57.

[36] Babizhayev, M.A., et al., *L-carnosine (beta-alanyl-L-histidine) and carcinine (beta-alanylhistamine) act as natural antioxidants with hydroxyl-radical-scavenging and lipid-peroxidase activities.* Biochem J, 1994. 304 (Pt 2): p. 509-16.

[37] Tanito, M., et al., *Protein modifications by 4-hydroxynonenal and 4-hydroxyhexenal in light-exposed rat retina.* Investigative ophthalmology & visual science., 2005. 46(10): p. 3859-68.

[38] Organisciak, D.T., et al., *Protection by dimethylthiourea against retinal light damage in rats.* Investigative ophthalmology & visual science, 1992. 33(5): p. 1599-609.

[39] Tanito, M., et al., *Cytoprotective effect of thioredoxin against retinal photic injury in mice.* Investigative ophthalmology & visual science, 2002. 43(4): p. 1162-7.

[40] Tanito, M., et al., *Attenuation of retinal photooxidative damage in thioredoxin transgenic mice.* Neuroscience letters, 2002. 326(2): p. 142-6.

[41] Poli, G., et al., *4-hydroxynonenal: a membrane lipid oxidation product of medicinal interest.* Med Res Rev, 2008. 28(4): p. 569-631.

[42] Tanito, M., M.P. Agbaga, and R.E. Anderson, *Upregulation of thioredoxin system via Nrf2-antioxidant responsive element pathway in adaptive-retinal neuroprotection in vivo and in vitro.* Free Radic Biol Med, 2007. 42(12): p. 1838-50.

[43] Forman, H.J., *Reactive oxygen species and alpha,beta-unsaturated aldehydes as second messengers in signal transduction.* Ann N Y Acad Sci, 2010. 1203: p. 35-44.

[44] Cingolani, C., et al., *Retinal degeneration from oxidative damage.* Free Radic Biol Med, 2006. 40(4): p. 660-9.

[45] He, X., et al., *Iron homeostasis and toxicity in retinal degeneration.* Prog Retin Eye Res, 2007. 26(6): p. 649-73.

[46] Hollyfield, J.G., *Age-related macular degeneration: the molecular link between oxidative damage, tissue-specific inflammation and outer retinal disease: the Proctor lecture.* Invest Ophthalmol Vis Sci, 2010. 51(3): p. 1275-81.

[47] Kutty, R.K., et al., *Induction of heme oxygenase 1 in the retina by intense visible light: suppression by the antioxidant dimethylthiourea.* Proceedings of the National Academy of Sciences of the United States of America, 1995. 92(4): p. 1177-81.

[48] Maeda, A., et al., *Effects of potent inhibitors of the retinoid cycle on visual function and photoreceptor protection from light damage in mice.* Mol Pharmacol, 2006. 70(4): p. 1220-9.

[49] Travis, G.H., et al., *Diseases caused by defects in the visual cycle: retinoids as potential therapeutic agents.* Annual review of pharmacology and toxicology, 2007. 47: p. 469-512.

[50] Humphries, M.M., et al., *Retinopathy induced in mice by targeted disruption of the rhodopsin gene.* Nat Genet, 1997. 15(2): p. 216-9.

[51] Grimm, C., et al., *Protection of Rpe65-deficient mice identifies rhodopsin as a mediator of light-induced retinal degeneration.* Nat Genet, 2000. 25(1): p. 63-6.

[52] Redmond, T.M., et al., *Rpe65 is necessary for production of 11-cis-vitamin A in the retinal visual cycle.* Nat Genet, 1998. 20(4): p. 344-51.

[53] Sieving, P.A., et al., *Inhibition of the visual cycle in vivo by 13-cis retinoic acid protects from light damage and provides a mechanism for night blindness in isotretinoin therapy.* Proc Natl Acad Sci U S A, 2001. 98(4): p. 1835-40.

[54] Mandal, M.N., et al., *PBN ({alpha}-phenyl-N-tert-butyl nitrone) Prevents Light-induced Degeneration of the Retina by Inhibiting RPE65 Isomerohydrolase Activity.* J Biol Chem.

[55] Gaudana, R., et al., *Ocular drug delivery.* AAPS J, 2010. 12(3): p. 348-60.

[56] Surh, Y.J., J.K. Kundu, and H.K. Na, *Nrf2 as a master redox switch in turning on the cellular signaling involved in the induction of cytoprotective genes by some chemopreventive phytochemicals.* Planta Med, 2008. 74(13): p. 1526-39.

Part 2

Eye Plastics and Orbital Disorders

10

Eyelid and Orbital Infections

Ayub Hakim

Department of Ophthalmology, Western Galilee - Nahariya Medical Center, Nahariya, Israel

1. Introduction

The major infections of the ocular adnexal and orbital tissues are preseptal cellulitis and orbital cellulitis. They occur more frequently in children than in adults. In Schramm's series of 303 cases of orbital cellulitis, 68% of the patients were younger than 9 years old and only 17% were older than 15 years old.

Orbital cellulitis is less common, but more serious than preseptal. Both conditions happen more commonly in the winter months when the incidence of paranasal sinus infections is increased. There are specific causes for each of these types of cellulitis, and each may be associated with serious complications, including vision loss, intracranial infection and death. Studies of orbital cellulitis and its complication report mortality in 1- 2% and vision loss in 3-11%. In contrast, mortality and vision loss are extremely rare in preseptal cellulitis.

1.1 Definitions

Preseptal and orbital cellulites are the most common causes of acute orbital inflammation. Preseptal cellulitis is an infection of the soft tissue of the eyelids and periocular region that is localized anterior to the orbital septum outside the bony orbit. Orbital cellulitis (3.5 per 100,00) is an infection of the soft tissues of the orbit that is localized posterior to the orbital septum and involves the fat and muscles contained within the bony orbit. Both types are normally distinguished clinically by anatomic location.

1.2 Pathophysiology

The soft tissues of the eyelids, adnexa and orbit are sterile. Infection usually originates from adjacent non-sterile sites but may also expand hematogenously from distant infected sites when septicemia occurs. Preseptal cellulitis usually originates from skin infection with or without local trauma. It may also originate from structures inside the eyelid that are connected to the surface and become infected such as external and internal hordeolom. Chalazion is an example of internal hordeolom and these are all infected glands with surface connections. Glands with even partial preseptal location such as the lacrimal gland, in which the palpebral lobe is located preseptally, may also cause preseptal cellulitis.

Orbital cellulitis occurs in the following three situations:

- Spreading of an infection from the periorbital structures, usually from the paranasal sinuses, but also from the face, the globe and the lacrimal sac.

- Direct inoculation of the orbit from surgical trauma.
- Hematogenous spread from distant sites (bacteremia).

In case of local cutaneous infection, preseptal cellulitis can arise from the spread of a contiguous anterior eyelid infection such as a chalazion, local trauma resulting in infection such as insect bite, or a foreign body. The skin and, in some instances, the sinuses and lacremal mucosa, are colonized by various microorganisms. Orbital cellulitis following trauma is the consequence of a direct exposure of the orbital contents to these microorganisms. Open periorbital fractures, as well as closed fractures involving the sinuses or the nasal bone, may be a risk factor for orbital infections.

Orbital cellulitis, in contrast, usually arises from spread of infection from the paranasal sinuses. The ethmoid sinus is the most common source that extends to the orbit in children. In adults, pansinusitis is often accompanied by orbital cellulitis and its spread is believed to be caused through the ethmoid or frontal sinuses. The ethmoid sinus separeated from the orbit medially by the thinnest orbital bone – lamina papyracea. Often, the lamina contains congenital dehiscences through which sinus infections can easily spread into the orbit. This may support the frequency of orbital cellulitis secondary to ethmoiditis. The anterior and posterior ethmoidal foramina may also serve as potential passages for infection.

The orbital roof borders the frontal sinus. It is a diploeic bone and is thicker than the lamina papiracea. Infection may spread more easily through the valveless facial veins. Since the frontal sinus is adjacent to the anterior cranial fossa, it may serve as an intermediary for the spread of infection.

The orbital floor that borders the maxillary antrum also contain congenital dehiscences through which infection from the maxillary sinus can enter and facilitate infection spreading.

The posterior medial wall of the orbit borders the sphenoid sinus. Isolated sphenoiditis is rare. The sphenoid may be involved secondary to ethmoiditis. Sphenoethmoidal sinusitis has distinct clinical characteristics. Marked visual loss with or without ophthalmoplegia usually precedes the findings of proptosis and inflammatory orbital signs. This condition is rare due to the thick bony barrier and firm attachment of periorbita to the posterior orbital wall.

One dehiscence or more is often present in orbital walls, particularly in the thin-walled lamina papyracea and this facilitates the spread of infection to the orbit. Posteriorly, the optic nerve within the optic canal is adjacent to the lateral wall of the sphenoidal sinus. Dehiscence can also be found in the lateral wall of the sphenoidal sinus adjacent to the optic canal. The free valveless venous communication between the orbit and the sinus is another reason predisposing the orbit to the spread of adjacent sinus infection.

However, not all orbital cellulitis infections caused by sinus disease are secondary to acute sinusitis. Orbital fracture involving sinuses may allow spreading of an existing chronic sinus infection. Open fractures may also result in orbital cellulitis due to direct contact with the environment. Foreign bodies, such as a glass, wood or orbital floor implants, can cause orbital cellulitis. Infection can extend to the orbit from the eye, teeth, middle ear, or in neglected cases of preseptal cellulitis, from the eyelids and face.

Uncomplicated eyelid, strabismus, cataract surgery, glaucoma valve and retinal surgery may all expose the orbit to infection. Orbital implants that are imbedded and other foreign bodies, such as Molteno valve implant, may carry a risk for infection, especially if they are colonized or exposed. Orbital cellulitis secondary to keratitis may develop after radial keratotomy.

Advanced carries with secondary infection, poor dental work or an infected root or dental cyst can cause orbital cellulitis. Extraction of maxillary premolars, molars or canines exposes the patient to orbital infection. The most common pathway for odontico-orbital infections is through the paranasal sinuses. The apices of maxillary molars and premolars are in close proximity to the floor of the maxillary sinus and are, in fact, in direct contact with the maxillary mucosa. Direct fistula to the antrum may be caused by a floor fracture during dental extraction or maxillary mucosa disruption. Infection spreading from the sinus to the orbit can occur through congenital dehiscences in the medial orbital wall or through communication between the venous plexus of the maxillary mucosa and the ophthalmic veins, thereby causing thrombophlebitis.

Another pathway for the spread of infection is the thin buccal cortical plate of the alveolar processes.

Finally orbital cellulitis can occur secondarily from embolic spread in subacute bacterial endocarditis and from other distant organs.

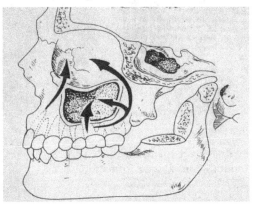

Pathway for odontico-orbital infections

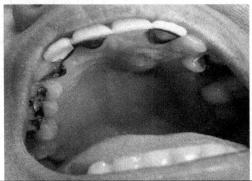

Dental abscess.Predisposing factors:poor dental care, advanced caries, root treatment, following dental extraction.

1.3 Classification

In 1970, chandler described a spectrum of progressive infectious changes in orbital cellulitis.

Chandler's Classification:

Stage I – Preseptal cellulitis

Ocasionally, edema may spread secondarily to preseptal cellulitis posterior to the septum without infection. In these cases chemosis may be present, but the extraocular movements and visual acuity remain intact.

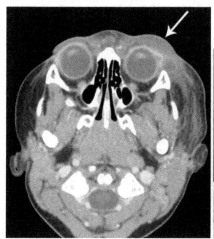 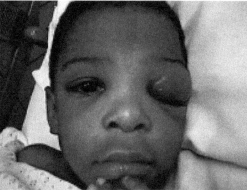

Stage II – Orbital cellulitis

Diffuse edema of orbital contents, with leukocytosis, fever, proptosis and impaired extraocular motility without discrete abscess formation.

Examples are shown in the images below:

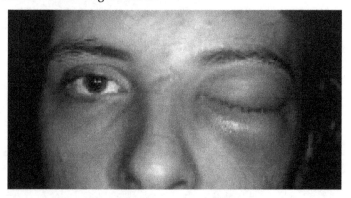

A male with left orbital cellulitis presented with proptosis, ophthalmoplegia, and edema and erythema of the eyelids. The patient also exhibited pain on eye movement, fever, headache, and malaise.

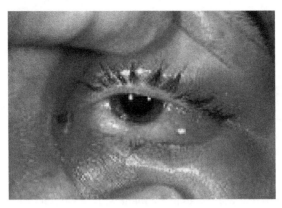

A male with left orbital cellulitis with proptosis, ophthalmoplegia, and edema and erythema of the eyelids. The patient also exhibited chemosis and resistance to retropulsion of the globe.

Stage III - Subperiosteal abscess

The globe is often displaced and limited in the field of gaze of the abscess.

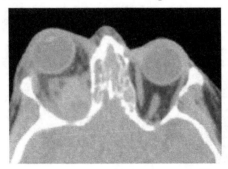

An axial computed tomography scan in a patient with a right orbital infection caused by streptococcus pneumoniae and a right superior orbital subperiosteal abscess that resulted in blindness.

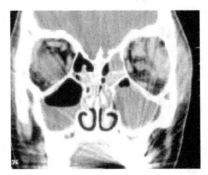

A coronal computed tomography scan of a child with pansinusitis as well as a left orbital and subperiosteal abscess.

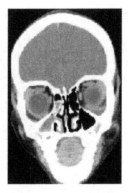

A coronal computed tomography scan in a patient with sickle cell disease. In this image, the patient has a left subperiosteal bleeding that mimiced the appearance of an infectious subperiosteal abscess.

Stage IV – Intraorbital abscess, purulent collection:

These patients have severe proptosis, chemosis, ophthalmoplegia and often visual loss.

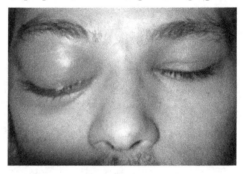

Frontal view of the patient with a right orbital abscess showing periorbital redness, swelling and proptosis.

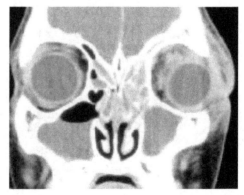

Coronal computed tomography scan in a pediatric patient with pansinusitis sinusitis and left orbital abscess.

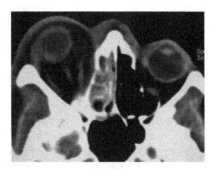

Axial computerized tomography scan shows a right classic proptosis associated with an abscess of the orbit, as well as displacement of the medial orbital tissues and tenting of the posterior.

Stage V – Cavernous sinus thrombosis (septic abscess)

In these instances, the orbital signs evolve in the fellow eye (bilateral) and other central nervous system signs supervene.

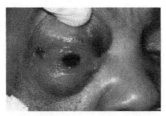

Carotid caverous fitula

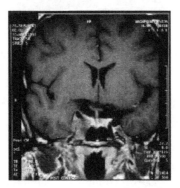

A T1 weighted coronal MRI demonstrating asymmetry between the caverenous sinuses with obliteration of the right cavernous sinus.

2. Preseptal cellulitis

Preseptal cellulitis is more common than orbital cellulitis. It can present with swelling and erythema of tissues surrounding the orbit, with or without fever. Preseptal cellulitis most commonly occurs from a contiguous infection of the soft tissues of the face and eyelids secondary to local trauma, foreign bodies or insect or animal bites. It is rare for untreated preseptal cellulitis to progress to orbital cellulitis by local extension. Defining the exact location of inflammation is essential for proper diagnosis and treatment.

2.1 Symptoms and signs

Patients with preseptal cellulitis often have a short history (days) of painless swelling of the eyelids. A history of early upper respiratory tract infection, trauma, insect or animal bite, conjunctivitis, or chalazion may be disclosed. Fever is an inconstant feature. The eyelid characteristically is erythematous, edematous, tender and warm. Vision and pupillary response are always unaffected and proptosis, globe displacement and limitation in ocular motility are never present. Concurrent preseptal cellulitis was discovered in the presence of many systemic diseases including, varicella, asthma, nasal polyposis and neutropenia. Preseptal cellulitis is more common among children than in adults.

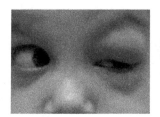 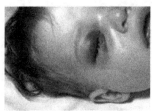 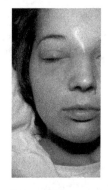

Preseptal cellulitis is more common in children than in adults.

swelling and erythema of soft tissues surrounding the orbit.

Eyelid swelling, erythema, local warmth, tenderness.no proptosis, limited ocular motility or optic nerve involvement.

2.2 Microbiology

The most common inciting microorganisms include *Streptococcus pneumoniae*, *Staphylococcus aureus*, other Streptococcus species and anaerobes. *Haemophilus infuenzae* type B was the most common cause in children under four years old. However, routine vaccination with conjugate *Haemophilus influenzae* vaccines since 1985 has dramatically decreased this infection in young children. Less commonly implicated microorganisms include Acinetobacter spp., *Nocardia brasiliensis*, *Bacillus anthracis*, *Pseudomonas aeruginosa*, *Neisseria gonorrhoea*, Proteus spp., *Pasteurella multocida*, *Mycobacterium tuberculosis* and Trichophyton spp.

2.3 Differential diagnosis

Conditions that might masquerade as preseptal cellulitis include allergic edema (anaphylactoid reaction) of the eyelids, severe blepharitis with scruffs (seborrheic), collarets(staphylococcal), sleeves(demodex) with or without erythema but no local warmth. The meibomianitis is characterised with eyelid swelling, pouting of meibomian gland orisices and discharge from orifices but no local warmth.

In addition dacryoadenitis, blunt trauma, thyroid eye disease, leukemic infiltrates, blepharochalasis syndrome and autoimmune inflammatory disorder such as lupus. Other disorders of less resemblance include orbital tumors/pseudotumours (, orbital vasculitis, necrotising fascitis and others.

2.4 Management

Treatment regimens cover the most likely organisms to cause infection in this setting and according to case series. Outpatient treatment should include broad-spectrum oral antibiotics and close observation. The author came to a conclusion that most cases of preseptal cellulitis can be safely managed as outpatients with oral antibiotics and follow-up until improvement is documented. If the condition does not improve or deteriorates 48 hours or more after oral antibiotic treatment, the patients should be admitted for intravenous antibiotic treatment and close observation. The average time of hospitalization is four days.

The appropriate antibiotics in adults include Amoxicillin–clavulinate (Augmentin) 875 mg every 12 h, and in children 90 mg/kg/day amoxicillin and 6.4 mg/Kg/day of clavulanate divided to two doses. Another option includes Cefpodoxime (Vantin) 200 mg every 12 h in adults, and 10 mg/kg/d divided every 12 h in children with maximum daily dose of 400 mg. Cefdinir (Omnicef) 600 mg daily in adults, and 14 mg/kg/d divided every 12 h in children with maximum daily dose 600 mg is another option.

Pediatric patients under 1 year of age and all more severe cases require the same approach as patients with orbital cellulitis, namely, intravenous broad-spectrum antibiotics and hospital observation .Blood cultures should be obtained if the systemic fever increases. The recommended duration of antimicrobial therapy is for 7-10 days. Occasionally, patients will continue to have local signs of cellulitis at end of treatment. Oral antibiotic therapy is recommended to be continued in these patients until resolution of the erythema. Children with preseptal cellulitis, no orbital involvement, and who do not appear toxic can be treated with intramuscular or oral antibiotics on a daily basis as outpatients. Preseptal cellulitis in adults can be managed on outpatient basis with oral antibiotics with frequent monitoring for progression.

3. Orbital cellulitis

Orbital cellulitis occurs in three settings:

i.   Extension of infection from periorbital structures, such as the face, lacrimal sac and globe, but particularly from the paranasal sinuses. Acute sinusitis is complicated by orbital cellulitis in 1-3% of cases and the coexisting sinusitis is present in 73-94% of patients with orbital cellulitis. Ethmoid sinusitis and pansinusitis are most likely to progress to orbital cellulitis. The first ocular sign of sinusitis may be preseptal inflammation only. This can then quickly progress to the classic clinical picture of orbital cellulitis. Other causes include – orbital trauma, with fracture or a foreign body, dacryocystitis, and infection of teeth, middle ear or face.

ii.   Direct inoculation from accidental trauma or from surgery. Orbital cellulitis is uncommon complication of ophthalmic surgery, being reported after strabismus surgery, blepharoplasty, radial keratotomy, retinal surgery and following peribulbar anesthesia. A special case is fungal orbital cellulitis, a relatively rare condition occurring in two principal forms – 1. Subacute infection due to genera of Zygomacetes (mucormycosis). 2. A more chronic orbital infection caused by species of Aspergillus. The distinction between these two may be difficult on clinical observation alone.
iii. Hematogenous spread (endogenous from bacteremia). The microorganisms responsible for most cases are aerobic non-spore forming bacteria.

3.1 Symptoms and signs

Orbital cellulitis as preseptal cellulitis can present with swelling and erythema. The cardinal signs and symptoms are proptosis, ophthalmoplegia and globe displacement. Pain on eye movement, vision loss (indicates orbital apex involvement), diplopia, conjunctival chemosis and elevated intraocular pressure are common but variable accompanying signs.

3.2 Microbiology

S. aureus and Streptococci are the most commonly identified organisms in culture-positive orbital cellulitis. Less common causes are H. influenza and non-spore forming anaerobes. However, many other common and rare bacterial pathogens include Eikenella corrodens, Aeromonas hydrophilia, P. aeroginosa, fungal and mycobacterial pathogens, including Scedosporium apospermum, M. tuberculosis and Mycobacterium avium complex. The prognosis of aspergillosis is poor. More than 80% of reported patients have died from this causative.

3.3 Differential diagnosis

Conditions that may mimic orbital cellulitis include:

*   Anaphylactoid reaction can be characterised with eyelid swelling and erythema but no local warmthand no proptosis, limited ocular motility or optic nerve involvement.
*   Cavernous sinus syndrome that is characterised by proptosis, complete ophthalmoplegia, optic nerve involvement, V2 involvement, evolve to bilateral condition and usually in debilitated patients (diabetics, drug abusers, HIV).
*   The orbital apex syndrome is characterised with complete external ophthalmoplegia, optic nerve and V1 involvement with/without proptosis.
*   Superior orbital fissure syndrome is a condition that is characterised with complete external ophlmoplegia, V1 involvement with or without proptosis.
*   The orbital compartment syndrome and the orbital tumors can present with proptosis, limited ocular motility, optic nerve involvement and increased intraocular pressure but no local warmth.

3.4 Diagnosis

There have been no controlled trials examining the utility of radiologic studies (e.g. computed tomography scanning, orbital ultrasound, or magnetic resonance imaging) in the diagnosis of orbital cellulitis or in distinguishing preseptal from orbital cellulitis.

Computed Tomography scanning (CT)

CT can confirm extension of inflammation into the orbit, detect coexisting sinus disease, and identify an orbital or subperiosteal abscess. Whether every patient with suspected orbital cellulitis needs a CT scan is controversial. Some experts suggest that a CT scan be performed only in those patients who deteriorate or fail to respond to 48 hours of IV antibiotics, as the majority of patients with orbital cellulitis do well with conservative medical management. It is suggested that patients with suspected orbital cellulitis – those with proptosis, globe displacement, limitation of eye movements, double vision, vision loss, and those patients in whom the physician cannot accurately assess vision – usually patients less than one year of age, at presentation have a baseline CT scan.

Orbital Ultrasunography(US)

US provides higher-resolution details of orbital contents and is useful when sequential follow-up of an abscess or drained abscess is required. However, orbital sonography is not widely available and is dependent on the expertise of the sonographer.

Magnetic Resonance Imaging (MRI)

MRI is superior to CT in the resolution of soft tissue disease. However, it is not usually performed because of the need for sedation in pediatric patients and because MRI is rarely immediately available.

Microbiologic studies

The causative microorganism in orbital cellulitis may be difficult to identify due to normal flora contaminants, mixed infection, and prior antibiotic therapy. Cultures for aerobic and anaerobic organisms may be obtained from blood, sinus aspirates, and abscess. Because blood cultures are usually negative, some clinicians obtain cultures of eye secretions or pharyngeal culture. However, these cultures are likely to be contaminated with normal oropharyngeal flora and should not guide the choice of antibiotic therapy. Microbiologic data limited to microorganisms recovered by surgical drainage from orbital abscesses or involved sinuses and/or positive blood culture are the most reliable information. It is recommended that in patients with suspected orbital cellulitis, blood cultures should be obtained before the initiation of antibiotic treatment. If surgery is performed, culture of abscess material or sinus contents should be sent for aerobic, anaerobic and fungal cultures.

3.5 Complications

The complications of bacterial orbital cellulitis may be orbital or intracranial. Orbital complications of orbital cellulitis include subperiosteal or orbital abscess formation in 7-9%, permanent globe displacement, limited ocular motility that may cause diplopia, and vision loss in 1%. Orbital abscess may be clinically indistinguishable from orbital cellulitis. Proptosis and globe displacement tends to be more severe with orbital abscess than in orbital cellulitis, and patients are more likely to be systemically ill. The diagnosis of orbital abscess is confirmed by imaging or at surgery. The identification of an orbital abscess on the baseline CT scan is important since these patients almost always require surgery. Intracranial complications, which are encountered in 4% of orbital cellulitis secondary to sinusitis include meningitis in 2%, cavernous sinus thrombosis in 1%, intracranial abscess formation, epidural or subdural abscess or parenchymal brain abscess in 1%, and carotid artery occlusion. Intracranial involvement may be heralded by ophthalmoplegia, changes in mental status, contralateral cranial nerve palsy, or bilateral orbital cellulitis. Cavernous sinus thrombosis has become relatively rare in developed countries because of prompt and adequate treatment of most cases of acute sinusitis, but it still poses a major threat. The mortality rate of cavernous sinus thrombosis may exceed 50%.

Permanent vision loss may occur because of:

1. Corneal ulcer and perforation secondary to exposure or neurotrophic keratitis.
2. Destruction of intraocular tissues following neovascular or inflammatory glaucoma, endophthalmitis, septic uveitis or retinitis and exudative retinal detachment.
3. Various other mechanisms affecting the globe or posterior orbit, such as secondary glaucoma due to elevated orbital pressure, infectious optic neuritis or inflammatory optic neuritis , pressure effects the optic nerve, thrombophlebitis of ocular veins and central retinal artery occlusion.

Blindness can result from elevated intraorbital pressure causing optic neuropathy or extension of the infection to the optic nerve from the sphenoid sinus.

3.6 Management

Prompt administration of appropriate antibiotics is the key for successful treatment of orbital cellulitis. After appropriate workup, all periorbital and orbital infections should be treated with broad-spectrum antimicrobial agents. There have been no controlled trials examining the required duration of antimicrobial therapy in orbital cellulitis. Treatment regimens are based upon coverage of the most likely organisms to cause infection in this setting and treatment of case series. The initial empiric antibiotic treatment should consist of parenteral broad-spectrum therapy. Infection due to methicillin-resistant *S. aureus* is best treated with vancomycin, clindamycin and cefotaxime.

Fungal orbital cellulitis occurs and is primarily due to mucor and aspergillums species. It requires antifungals, such as amphotericin. Corticosteroids may be helpful in bacterial infections, but they should not be started before surgery and until the patient has been on appropriate antibiotics for 2-3 days to ascertain eradication of the microbial agents.

If secondary glaucoma develops, ocular anti-hypertensive agents should be initiated promptly. Prompt diagnosis and therapy are important since delayed intervention can result in sustained vision loss.

3.6.1 Antibiotic treatment

Due to increasing incidence of Methicillin-resistant *S. Aureus,* empiric therapy with Vancomycin (Vancocin) (15 mg/kg IV every 12 hours in adults, 10 to 15 mg/kg IV every 6 hours in children, maximum daily dose of 4gr) is recommended. If susceptibility testing reveals Methicillin-sensitive *S. aureus,* Vancomycin should be replaced with Nafcilin (Unipen), or Oxacillin (Bactocill) - (both agents are dosed at 2gr IV every 4 hours in adults, and 200 mg/kg per day IV in 4-6 divided doses in children, maximum daily dose of 12gr) since these agents have better CNS penetration than vancomycin.

One of the following should be added:

1. Ampicillin-sulbactam (Unasyn) 3gr IV every 6 hours in adults, 300 mg/kg per day in 4 divided doses in children, maximum daily dose of 12 gr.
2. Ticarcillin-clavulanate (Ticar), which covers most of the Gram-negative bacteria as well as Gram-positive organisms, including atypical *H. influenza*, and has also excellent anaerobic coverage. The dosage is 3.1gr IV every 4 hours in adults, 200-300 mg of ticarcillin component per kg per day in 4-6 divided doses in children of less than 60 kg. The maximum daily dose of ticarcillin component is 18 gr.
3. Piperacillin-Tazobactam 4.5gr IV every 6 hours in adults, 240 mg/kg per day in 3 divided doses in children, with a maximum daily dose of 16gr of piperacillin component.
4. Ceftriaxone (Rocephin) is effective agpenicillinase-producing *S. aureus*, most Gram–positive organisms, and most Gram-negative organisms except for Pseudomonas. Ceftriaxone also crosses the blood-brain barrier; therefore, it is an excellent choice if there is a suspicion of concurrent intracranial infection. 2gr IV every 12 hours in adults, 80-100 mg/kg per day in 2 divided doses in children, maximum dose of 4gr daily may be given.
5. Cefotaxime (Claforan), a third-generation cephalosporin that covers most of the common sinus pathogens with the exception of *Clostridium difficile*, may be given 2gr IV every 4 hours in adults, 150-200 mg/kg per day in 3-4 equally divided doses in children, with a maximum daily dose of 12gr.

Patients allergic to penicillin and/or cephalosporins may be treated with a combination of vancomycin and a flouroquinolon. For patients over 17 years of age, ciprofloxacin 500 mg twice a day or levofloxacin 500 mg daily may be prescribed. Flouroquinilones are not recommended for use in pediatric patients as first-line therapy for any infection because of the musculoskeletal side effects - The mildest side effects include muscle pain, called fibromyalgia. A more serious side effect, though also less common, is tendon damage. Fluoroquinolones can, in high doses, cause tendon damage, which can ultimately lead to rupture of the Achilles tendon (in addition gastrointestinal effects predominating (nausea, vomiting, diarrhea, or abdominal pain in 1.0%–5.0% of thepatients), followed byeffects onthecentral nervous system (dizziness, headache, and/or insomnia in 0.1%–0.3% of the patients) and skin (0.5%–2.2% of the patients). Elevation in levels of hepatic enzymes occurred in 1.8%–2.5% of thepatients, azotemia in 0.2%–1.3%, and eosinophilia in 0.2%–2.0%. Initial antibiotic therapy should be administered IV under hospitalization. Generally switching to oral therapy is done after the patient is afebrile and skin findings have begun to resolve, which usually take 3-5 days.

The duration of treatment depends on the response. Patients should be treated with parenteral antibiotics until they show clear evidence of clinical improvement as manifested by decrease in orbital congestive signs such as proptosis, gaze limitation, cellulitis and edema. Intravenous therapy should continue for a minimum of 3 days. Then oral antibiotic therapy may be instituted for a total course of 10 days to 3 weeks, depending on the severity of infection. Associated bacteremia, however, should be treated with 7-10 days of IV therapy.

As aforesaid, the oral regimen should be tailored based upon the results of the cultures. If the results are not available, reasonable empiric oral antibiotic choices include 1. amoxicillin

– clavulinate – 875 mg twice daily for adults or children over 40 kg, and 45 mg/kg/day divided every 12 hours for children over 3 moths and under 40 kg or 2. fluoroquinolone – (levofloxacin 750 mg once daily in adults). Linezolid (ZYVOX) - (600 mg twice daily in adults and children over 12 years of age, 10 mg/kg three times daily for children under 11 years) should be added if MRSA is suspected.

Careful follow-up is indicated in all patients who present with orbital cellulitis. This should include twice-daily examinations with attention to visual acuity, confrontation visual fields, exophthalmometry, motility and pupillary examination.

3.6.2 Antifungals

(Amphotericin B- Ambisome) 1 mg/kg IV q24h or Voriconazole (VFEND, Pfizer) 6 mg/kg IV q12h for 2 doses, then 4 mg/kg IV q12h or Voriconazole 200-300 mg PO q12h

Antifungal is the treatment of choice for fungal orbital cellulitis. It is administered IV and may be appropriately administered before laboratory confirmation of fungal infection in cases of severe infection and debilitated patients (diabetes mellitus, drug abusers, human immunodeficiency disease, metastatic cancer, prolonged administration of antibiotics and/ or corticosteroids).

3.6.3 Surgery

The timing for surgical intervention is critical. In cases of orbital cellulitis without abscess formation, in which visual acuity is 20/60 (Snellen notation), 6/15 (metric equivalent) or less, or declines with appropriate medical management, orbital exploration should be emergent. In cases in which the acuity is better than 20/60, the patient should be followed, expectantly, and frequently while more conservative management is initiated.

Orbital surgery is indicated if the patient:

1. Fails to respond
2. Deteriorates clinically despite treatment
3. Has worsening visual acuity or develops afferent pupillary defect
4. Develops an abscess, except selected pediatric cases with medial subperiosteal abscess, which may be successfully treated medically.

In patients older than 14 years of age, the author favours the latter approach because the risks of surgery are negligible compared with the visual and life-threatening risks of no intervention. In patients 9 years of age or younger, 25% of the subperiosteal abscesses are likely to resolve with antibiotic therapy alone. Several indications have been suggested for drainage of subperiosteal abscesses. These include age of 9 years or older, large abscess, frontal sinusitis, non-medial abscesschronic sinusitis, dental infection, optic nerve involvement, suspicion of anaerobic infection and recurrence after drainage. All other cases may be managed conservatively by intravenous antibiotics.

4. References

Abbott RL, Shekter WB: Necrotizing erysipelas of the eyelids. Ann Ophthalmol 11:381, 1979

Abou-Rayyah Y, Rose GE, Konrad H, et al. Clinical, radiological and pathological examination of periocular dermoid cyst:evidence of inflammation from an early age. Eye (Lond) 2002;16:507.

Adams WG, Deaver KA, Cochi SL, et al: Decline of childhood *Haemophilus influenzae* type b (Hib) disease in the Hib vaccine era. JAMA 269:221, 1993

Agarwal M, Biswas J, S K, Shanmugam MP. Retinoblastoma presenting as orbital cellulitis: report of four cases with a review of the literature. Orbit 2004;23:93.

Ailal F,Bousfiha A, Jouhad Z, et al. (Orbital cellulitis in children: a retrospective study of 33). Med trop (Mars) 2004; 64:359.

Allan BP,Egbert MA, Myall RW. Orbital abscess of odontologic origin. Case report and review of the literature. Int J Oral Maxillofac surg 1991;20:268.

Allen MV, Cohen KL, Grimson BS. Orbital cellulitis secondary to dacryocystitis following blepharoplasty. Ann Ophthalmol 1985; 17:498.

Ambati BK, Ambati J, Azar N, Stratton L, Schmidt EV: Periorbital and orbital cellulitis before and after the advent of haemophilus influenzae type B vaccination. Ophthalmology 107:1450, 2000

Antoine GA, Grundfast KM: Periorbital cellulitis. Int J Pediatr Otorhinolaryngol 13:273, 1987

Arjmand EM, Lusk RP, Muntz HR. Pediatric sinusitis and subperiosteal orbital abscess formation:diagnosis and treatment. Otolaryngol Head Neck Surg 1993;109:886.

Ataullah S, Sloan B. Acute dacryocystitis presenting as an orbital absvess. Clin Experiment ophthalmol 2002;30:44.

Bach MC, Knowland M, Schuyler WBJ: Acute orbital myositis mimicking orbital cellulitis. Ann Intern Med 109:243, 1988

Barkin RM, Todd JK: Periorbital cellulitis in children. Pediatrics 62:390, 1978

Barman Balfour JA, Lamb HM: Moxifloxacin, a review of its potential in the management of community-acquired respiratory tract infections. Drugs 59:115, 2000

Barone SR, Aiuto LT. Periorbital and orbital cellulitis in the Haemophilus influenzae vaccine era. J Pediatr Ophthalmol Strabismus 1997; 34:293.

Batson OV: Relationship of the eye to the paranasal sinuses. Arch Ophthalmol 16:322, 1936

Bergin DJ, Wright JE: Orbital cellulitis. Br J Ophthalmol 70:174, 1986

Botting AM, McIntosh D, Mahadevan M. Paediatric pre- and post-septal peri-orbital infections are different diseases. A retrospective review of 262 cases. Int J Pediatr Otorhinolaryngol 2008; 72:377.

Brannan PA, Kersten RC, Hudak DT, et al. Primary Nocardia brasiliensis of the eyelid. Am J Ophthalmol 2004; 138:498.

Brenner DJ, Elliston CD, Hall EJ, Berdon WE: Estimated risks of radiation-induced fatal cancer from pediatric CT. AJR 176:289, 2001

Brook I, Frazier EH. Microbiology of subperiosteal orbital abscess and associated maxillary sinusitis. Laryngoscope 1996; 106:1010.

Bullock JD, Fleishman JA: The spread of odontogenic infections to the orbit: diagnosis and management. J Oral Maxillofac Surg 43:749, 1985

Caça I, Cakmak SS, Unlü K, et al. Cutaneous anthrax on eyelids. Jpn J Ophthalmol 2004; 48:268.

Carter BL, Bankoff MS, Fisk JD: Computed tomographic detection of sinusitis responsible for intracranial and extracranial infections. Radiology 147:739, 1983

Casteel I, DeBleecker C, Demaerel P, et al: Orbital myositis following an upper respiratory tract infection: contribution of high resolution CT and MRI. J Belg Radiol 74:45, 991

Catalano RA, Smoot CN: Subperiosteal orbital masses in children with orbital cellulitis: time for a reevaluation? J Pediatr Ophthalmol Strabismus Surg 27:141, 1990

Chalumeau M, Tonnelier S, d'Athis P, et al: Fluoroquinolone safety in pediatric patients: a prospective, multicenter, comparative cohort study in France. Pediatrics 111:714, 2003

Chandler JR, Langenbrunner DJ, Stevens ER: The pathogenesis of orbital complications in acute sinusitis. Laryngoscope 80:1414, 1970

Chaudhry IA, Shamsi FA, Elzaridi E, et al. Inpatient preseptal cellulitis: experience from a tertiary eye care centre. Br J Ophthalmol 2008; 92:1337.

Chaudhry IA, Shamsi FA, Elzaridi E, et al. Outcome of treated orbital cellulitis in a tertiary eye care center in the middle East. Ophthalmology 2007; 114:345.

Chou SY, Tsai CC, Kau SC, et al. Aeromonas hydrophila orbital cellulitis in a patient with myelodysplastic syndrome. J Chin Med Assoc 2004; 67:51.

Claudia F E Kirsch, MD, Roger Turbin, MD, Devang Gor, MD, Barton F Branstetter IV, MD, Bernard D Coombs, MB, ChB, PhD, C Douglas Phillips, MD, Robert M Krasny, MD, James G Smirniotopoulos, MD (Orbital Infection Imaging) - Updated: May 27, 2011.

David G Hunter , MD, PhD, Michele Trucksis, Phd, MD, Stephen B Calderwood, MD, Morven S Edwards, MD, Jonathan Trobe, MD, Anna R Thorner, MD, Uptodate review version 19.2:2011 May.

Donahue Sp, Khoury JM, Kowalski RP: Common ocular infections. Drugs 52:526, 1996

Duane's Ophthalmology, William, M.D. Tasman, Edward A., M. Jaeger, Publisher: Lippincott Williams & Wilkins, ISBN: 0781725879 DDC: 617 Edition: Hardcover; 2000-09

Dudin A, Othman A. Acute periorbital swelling: evaluation of management protocol. Pediatr Emerg Care 1996; 12:16.

Eustis HS, Mafee MF, Walton C, Mondonca J: MR imaging and Ct of orbital infections and complications in acute rhinosinusitis. Radiol Clin North Am 36:1165, 1998

Filips RF, Liudahl JJ. Asymptomatic posterior orbital cellulitis resulting from ethmoid/maxillary sinusitis. J Am Optom Assoc 1997; 68:55.

Forstot SL, Ellis PP: Nontraumatic rupture of the globe secondary to orbital cellulitis. Am J Ophthalmol 88:262

Frederick J, Braude AI: Anaerobic infection of the paranasal sinuses. N Engl J Med 290:135, 1974

Galetta SL, Wulc AE, Goldberg HI, et al: Rhinocerebral mucormycosis: management and survival after carotid occlusion. Ann Neurol 28:103, 1990.

Gamble RE: Acute inflammations of the orbit in children. Arch Ophthalmol 10:483, 1933

Ganesh A, Venugopalan P. Preseptal orbital cellulitis following oral trauma. J Pediatr Ophthalmol Strabismus 2000; 37:315.

Gans H, Sekula J, Wlodyka J: Treatment of acute orbital complications. Arch Ophthalmol 100:329, 1974

Garcia GH, Harris GJ, Criteria for nonsurgical management of subperiosteal abscess of the orbit: analysis of outcomes 1988-1998. Ophthalmology 2000;107:1454-6.

Gellady AM, Shulman ST, Ayoub EM: Periorbital and orbital cellulitis in children. Pediatrics 61:272, 1978

Givner LB. Periorbital versus orbital cellulitis. Pediatr Infect Dis J 2002; 21:1157.

Gold SC, Arrigg PG, Hedges TR: Computerized tomography in the management of acute orbital cellulitis. Ophthalmic Surg 18:753, 1987

Goldberg F, Berne AS, Oski FA: Differentiation of orbital cellulitis from preseptal cellulitis by computed tomography. Pediatrics 62:1000, 1978

Goldfarb MS, Hoffman DS, Rosenberg S: Orbital cellulitis and orbital fractures. Ann Ophthalmol 19:97, 1987

Goodwin WJ, Weinshall M, Chandler JR: The role of high resolution computerized tomography and standardized ultrasound in the evaluation of orbital cellulitis. Laryngoscope 92:728, 1982

Greenberg MF, Pollard ZF. Medical treatment of pediatric subperiosteal orbital abscess secondary to sinusitis. J AAPOS 1998; 2:351.

Grossniklaus HE, Wojno TH: Leukemic infiltrate appearing as periorbital cellulitis. Arch Ophthalmol 108:484, 1990

Hajek M:Complications involving the orbit and visual organ. In Pathology and Treatment of Inflammatory Disease of the Nasal Accessory Sinuses. vol 2, 1926578–606

Handler LC, Davey IC, Hill JC, Lauryssen C: The acute orbit: differentiation of orbital cellulitis from periosteal abscess by computerized tomography. Neuroradiology 33:15, 1991

Harr DL, Quencer RM, Abrams GW: Computed tomography and ultrasound in the evaluation of orbital infection and pseudotumor. Radiology 142:395, 1982

Harris GJ. Age as a factor in the bacteriology and response to treatment of subperiosteal abscess of the orbit. Trans Am Ophthalmol Soc 1993; 91:441.

Harris GJ. Subperiosteal abscess of the orbit. Age as a factor in the bacteriology and response to treatment. Ophthalmology 1994; 101:585.

Harris GJ: Subperiosteal abscess of the orbit. Arch Ophthalmol 101:751, 1983

Hawkins DB, Clark RW: Orbital involvement in acute sinusitis. Clin Pediatr 16:464, 1977

Haynes R, Cramblett H: Acute ethmoiditis. Am J Dis Child 114:261, 1967

Hegde V, Smith G, Choi J, Pagliarini S. A case of gonococcal kerato-conjunctivitis mimicking orbital cellulitis. Acta Ophthalmol Scand 2005; 83:511.

Hemady R, Zimmerman A, Katzen BW, Karesh JW. Orbital cellulitis caused by Eikenella corrodens. Am J Ophthalmol 1992; 114:584.

Hirsch M, Lifschitz T: Computerized tomography in the diagnosis and treatment of orbital cellulitis. Pediatr Radiol 18:302, 1988

Hofbauer JD, Gordon LK, Palmer J. Acute orbital cellulitis after peribulbar injection. Am J Ophthalmol 1994; 118:391.

Hornblass A, Herschorn BJ, Stern K, Grimes C: Orbital abscess. Surv Ophthalmol 29:169, 1984

Howe L, Jones NS. Guidelines for the management of periorbital cellulitis/abscess. Clin Otolaryngol Allied Sci 2004; 29:725.

Hubert L: Orbital infection due to nasal sinusitis. NY State J Med 37:1559, 1937

Hutcheson KA, Magbalon M. Periocular abscess and cellulitis from Pasteurella multocida in a healthy child. Am J Ophthalmol 1999; 128:514.

Israele V, Nelson JD: Periorbital and orbital cellulitis. Pediatr Infect Dis J 6:404, 1987

Jacobs D, Galetta S. Diagnosis and management

Jain A, Rubin PAD: Orbital cellulitis in children. Int Ophthalmol Clin 41:71, 2001

Janakarajah N, Sukumaran K: Orbital cellulitis of dental origin: case report and review of the literature. Br J Oral Maxillofac Surg 23:140, 1985

Jarrett WH, Gutman FA: Ocular complications of infection in the paranasal sinuses. Arch Ophthalmol 81:683, 1969

Jarrett WH, Gutman FA: Ocular complications of infection in the paranasal sinuses. Arch Ophthalmol 81:683, 1969

John N Harrington, MD, FACS, Brian A Phillptts, MD, Franisco Talavera, PharmD, PhD, Mark T Duffy, MD, PhD, Lance L Brown, OD, MD. Chief Editor:Hampton Roy Sr, MD, Medscape review version (Preseptal and Orbital cellulitis), Oct 10 2011.

Jones J, Katz SE, Lubow M. Scedosporium apiospermum of the orbit. Arch Ophthalmol 1999; 117:272.

Karesh J, Lakhanpal V, Haney P, et al: Metastatic anaerobic orbital subperiosteal abscess: value of CT scanning. J Pediatr Ophthalmol Strabismus 19:52, 1982

Karkos PD, Karagama Y, Karkanevatos A, Srinivasan V. Recurrent periorbital cellulitis in a child. A random event or an underlying anatomical abnormality? Int J Pediatr Otorhinolaryngol 2004; 68:1529.

Kaufman SJ: Orbital mucopyoceles: two cases and a review. Surv Ophthalmol 25:253, 1981

Komolafe OO, Ashaye AO. Combined central retinal artery and vein occlusion complicating orbital cellulitis. Niger J Clin Pract 2008; 11:74.

Krohel GB, Kraus HR, Winnick J: Orbital abscesses: presentation, diagnosis, therapy, and sequelae. Ophthalmology 89:492, 1982

Krohel GB, Krauss HR, Christensen RE, Minckler D: Orbital abscess. Arch Ophthalmol 98:274, 1980

Kyprianou I, D'Souza A, Saravanappa N, et al. Referral patterns in paediatric orbital cellulitis. Eur J Emerg Med 2005; 12:6.

Langham-Brown JJ, Rhys-Williams S: Computed tomography of acute orbital infection: the importance of coronal sections. Clin Radiol 40:471, 1989

Lasko B, Lau CY, Saint-Pierre C, et al: Efficacy and safety of oral levofloxacin compared with clarithromycin in the treatment of acute sinusitis in adults: a multicentre, double blind, randomized study. J Int Med Res 26:281, 1998

Lemke BN, Gonnering RS, Harris J, Weinstein JM: Orbital cellulitis with periorbital elevation. Ophthalmic Plast Reconstruct Surg 3:1, 1987

Mair MH, Geley T, Judmaier W, Gassner I. Using orbital sonography to diagnose and monitor treatment of acute swelling of the eyelids in pediatric patients. AJR Am J Roentgenol 2002; 179:1529.

Malik NN, Goh D, McLean C, Huchzermeyer P. Orbital cellulitis caused by Peptostreptococcus. Eye (Lond) 2004; 18:643.

Maniglia AJ, Kronberg FG, Culbertson W: Visual loss associated with orbital and sinus disease. Laryngoscope 94:1050, 1984

Manning SC: Endoscopic management of medial subperiosteal orbital abscess. Arch Otolaryngol Head Neck Surg 119:789, 1993

Mathews D, Mathews JP, Kwartz J, Inkster C. Preseptal cellulitis caused by Acinetobacter lwoffi. Indian J Ophthalmol 2005; 53:213.

McKinley SH, Yen MT, Miller AM, Yen KG. Microbiology of pediatric orbital cellulitis. Am J Ophthalmol 2007; 144:497.

McLeod SD, Flowers CW, Lopez PF, et al. Endophthalmitis and orbital cellulitis after radial keratotomy. Ophthalmology 1995; 102:1902.

Miller J. Acinetobacter as a causative agent in preseptal cellulitis. Optometry 2005; 76:176.

Mills R. Orbital and periorbital sepsis. J Laryngol Otol 1987; 101:1242.

Mills RP, Kartush JM. Orbital wall thickness and the spread of infection from the paranasal sinuses. Clin Otolaryngol Allied Sci 1985; 10:209.

Milstone AM, Ruff AJ, Yeamans C, Higman MA. Pseudomonas aeruginosa pre-septal cellulitis and bacteremia in a pediatric oncology patient. Pediatr Blood Cancer 2005; 45:353; discussion 354.

Molarte AB, Isenberg SJ: Periorbital cellulits in infancy. J Pediatr Ophthalmol Strabismus 26:232, 1989

Morell A, Skvaril F, Hitzig WH, Barandum S: IgG subclasses: development of the serum concentrations in "normal" infants and children. J Pediatr 80:960, 1972

Morgan PR, Morrison WV: Complications of frontal and ethmoidal sinusitis. Laryngoscope 90:661, 1980

Nageswaran S, Woods CR, Benjamin DK Jr, et al. Orbital cellulitis in children. Pediatr Infect Dis J 2006; 25:695.

Newell FW, Leveille AS: Management and complications of bacterial periorbital and orbital cellulitis. Metab Pediatr Syst Ophthalmol 6:209, 1982

Noel LP, Clarke WN, Peacocke TA: Periorbital and orbital cellulitis in childhood. Can J Ophthalmol 16:178, 1981Jackson K, Baker SR: Clinical implications of orbital cellulitis. Laryngoscope 96:568, 1986

Okamoto Y, Hiraoka T, Okamoto F, Oshika T. A case of subperiosteal abscess of the orbit with central retinal artery occlusion. Eur J Ophthalmol 2009; 19:288.

Osguthorpe JD, Hochman M. Inflammatory sinus diseases affecting the orbit. Otolaryngol Clin North Am 1993; 26:657.

Partamian LG, Jay WM, Fritz KJ: Anaerobic orbital cellulitis. Ann Ophthalmol 15:123, 1983

Patil B, Agius-Fernandez A, Worstmann T. Hyaluronidase allergy after peribulbar anesthesia with orbital inflammation. J Cataract Refract Surg 2005; 31:1480.

Patt BS, Manning SC. Blindness resulting from orbital complications of sinusitis. Otolaryngol Head Neck Surg 1991; 104:789.

Patt BS, Manning SC: Blindness resulting from orbital complications of sinusitis. Otolaryngol Head Neck Surg 104:789, 1991

Pelton RW, Smith ME, Patel BC, Kelly SM. Cosmetic considerations in surgery for orbital subperiosteal abscess in children: experience with a combined transcaruncular and transnasal endoscopic approach. Arch Otolaryngol Head Neck Surg 2003; 129:652.

Powell KR: Orbital and periorbital cellulitis. Pediatr Rev 16:163, 1995

Quick CA, Payne E: Complicated acute sinusitis. Laryngoscope 82:1248, 1972

R Gentry Wilkerson, MD, Richard H Sinert, DO, Zach Kassutto, MD, FAAP, Elizabeth Fiedler, MD, Edmond A Hooker II, MD, DrPH, FAAEM, Francisco Talavera, PharmD, PhD, Douglas Lavenburg, MD, John D Halamka, MD, MS, Robert E O'Connor, MD, MPH (Chief Editor), eMedicine review (Periorbital infections),jul 10 2011.

Ragab A, Samaka RM. Department of ORL Head and Neck Surgery, Menoufyia University Hospital, (Is pyogenic ethmoidal osteitis the cause of complicated rhinosinusitis with subperiosteal orbital abscess?).PubMed, Eur Arch Otorhinolaryngol. 2010 Aug;267(8):1231-7. Epub 2010 Jan 13.

Rahbar R, Robson CD, Petersen RA, et al. Management of orbital subperiosteal abscess in children. Arch Otolaryngol Head Neck Surg 2001; 127:281.

Raina UK, Jain S, Monga S, et al. Tubercular preseptal cellulitis in children: a presenting feature of underlying systemic tuberculosis. Ophthalmology 2004; 111:291.

Raja NS, Singh NN. Bilateral orbital cellulitis due to Neisseria gonorrhoeae and Staphylococcus aureus: a previously unreported case. J Med Microbiol 2005; 54:609.

Rees TD, Craig SM, Fisher Y: Orbital abscess following blepharoplasty. Plast Reconstr Surg 73:126, 1983

Reynolds DJ, Kodsi SR, Rubin SE, Rodgers IR. Intracranial infection associated with preseptal and orbital cellulitis in the pediatric patient. J AAPOS 2003; 7:413.

Robbins JB, Schneerson R, Argaman M, Handzel ZT: Haemophilus influenzae type b: disease and immunity in humans. Ann Intern Med 78:259, 1973

Robie F, O'Neal R, Kelsey DS: Periobital cellulitis. J Pediatr Ophthalmol 14:354, 1977

Rubin SE, Rubin LG, Zito J, et al: Medical management of orbital subperiosteal abscess in children. J Pediatr Ophthalmol Strabismus Surg 26:21, 1989

Rubinstein A, Riddell CE. Posterior scleritis mimicking orbital cellulitis. Eye (Lond) 2005; 19:1232.

Rubinstein JB, Handler SD. Orbital and periorbital cellulitis in children. Head Neck Surg 1982; 5:15.

Rubinstein JB, Handler SD: Orbital and periorbital cellulitis in children. Head Neck Surg 5:15, 1982

Rudloe TF, Harper MB, Prabhu SP, et al. Acute periorbital infections: who needs emergent imaging? Pediatrics 2010; 125:e719.

Rumelt S, Rubin PAD. Potential sources of orbital cellulitis. Int Ophthalmol Clin 36:207, 1996

Russo G, Di Pietro M, La Spina M. Ocular involvement in neuroblastoma: not always metastasis. Lancet Oncol 2004; 5:324.

Ruttum MS, Ogawa G. Adenovirus conjunctivitis mimics preseptal and orbital cellulitis in young children. Pediatr Infect Dis J 1996; 15:266.

Ryan JT, Preciado DA, Bauman N, et al. Management of pediatric orbital cellulitis in patients with radiographic findings of subperiosteal abscess. Otolaryngol Head Neck Surg 2009; 140:907.

Saini JS, Mohan K, Khandalavala B: Wooden foreign bodies of the orbit. Orbit 8:139, 1989

Schmitt NJ, Beatty RL, Kennerdell JS. Superior ophthalmic vein thrombosis in a patient with dacryocystitis-induced orbital cellulitis. Ophthal Plast Reconstr Surg 2005; 21:387.

Schramm VL Jr, Curtin HD, Kennerdell JS. Evaluation of orbital cellulitis and results of treatment. Laryngoscope 1982; 92:732.

Schramm VL, Curtin HD, Kennerdell JS: Evaluation of orbital cellulitis and results of treatment. Laryngoscope 92:732, 1982

Schramm VL, Myers EN, Kennerdell JS: Orbital complications of acute sinusitis: Evaluation, management, and outcome. Trans Am Acad Otolaryngol 86:221, 1978

Schur PH, Rosen F, Norman ME: Immunoglobulin subclasses in normal children. Pediatr Res 13:181, 1979

Schwartz G. Department of Emergency Medicine, Vanderbilt University Medical Center, (Etiology, Diagnosis, and Treatment of Orbital Infections) – PubMed, Curr Infect Dis Rep. 2002 Jun;4(3):201-205

Scott PM, Bloome MA: Lid necrosis secondary to streptococcal periorbital cellulitis. Ann Ophthalmol 4:461, 1981

Sears JM, Gabriel HM, Veith J. Preseptal cellulitis secondary to Proteus species: a case report and review. J Am Optom Assoc 1999; 70:661.

Shapiro ED, Wald ER, Broznski BA: Periorbital cellulitis and paranasal sinusitis: A reappraisal. Pediatr Infect Dis J 1:91, 1982

Shields CL, Shields JA, Honavar SG, Demirci H. Primary ophthalmic rhabdomyosarcoma in 33 patients. Trans Am Ophthalmol Soc 2001; 99:133.

Shields JA, Shields CL, Suvarnamani C, et al: Retinoblastoma manifesting as orbital cellulitis. Am J Ophthalmol 112:442, 1991

Siber GR, Schur PH, Aisenberg AC, et al: Correlation between serum IgG-2 concentrations and the antibody response to bacterial polysaccharide antigens. N Engl J Med 303:178, 1980

Silver HS, Fucci MJ, Flanagan JC, Lowry LD: Severe orbital infection as a complication of orbital fracture. Arch Otolaryngol Head Neck Surg 118:845, 1992

Sirbaugh PE. A case of orbital pseudotumor masquerading as orbital cellulitis in a patient with proptosis and fever. Pediatr Emerg Care 1997; 13:337.

Slavin ML, Glaser JS: Acute severe irreversible visual loss with sphenoethmoiditis: 'posterior' orbital cellulitis. Arch Ophthalmol 105:345, 1987

Smith AT, Spencer JT: Orbital complications resulting from lesions of the sinuses. Ann Otol Rhinol Laryngol 57:5, 1948

Smith TF, O'Day D, Wright PF: Clinical implications of preseptal (periorbital) cellulitis in childhood. Pediatrics 62:1006, 1978

Sobol SE, Marchand J, Tewfik TL, et al. Orbital complications of sinusitis in children. J Otolaryngol 2002; 31:131.

Sorin A, April MM, Ward RF. Recurrent periorbital cellulitis: an unusual clinical entity. Otolaryngol Head Neck Surg 2006; 134:153.

Spires JR, Smith RJH: Bacterial infections of the orbital and perirobital soft tissues in children. Laryngoscope 96:763, 1986

Stammberger H: Endoscopic endonasal surgery: concepts in treatment of recurring rhinosinusitis. Otolaryngol Head Neck Surg 94:143, 1986

Stammberger H: Functional Endoscopic Sinus Surgery. p 68. Philadelphia: BC Decker, 1991

Starkey CR, Steele RW. Medical management of orbital cellulitis. Pediatr Infect Dis J 2001; 20:1002.

Swift AC, Charlton G. Sinusitis and the acute orbit in children. J Laryngol Otol 1990; 104:213.

Tannenbaum M, Tenzel J, Byrne SF, et al: Medical management of orbital abscess. Surv Ophthalmol 30:211, 1986

Thatcher DB: Necrotic choroidal melanoma presenting with severe inflammation. Surv Ophthalmol 12:247, 1967

Towbin R, Han BK, Kaufman RA, Burke M: Postseptal cellulitis: CT in diagnosis and management. Radiology 158:735, 1986

Uehara F, Ohba N: Diagnostic imaging in patients with orbital cellulitis and inflammatory pseudotumor. Int Ophthalmol Clin 42:133, 2002

Uzcátegui N, Warman R, Smith A, Howard CW. Clinical practice guidelines for the management of orbital cellulitis. J Pediatr Ophthalmol Strabismus 1998; 35:73.

Uzcategui N, Warman R, Smith A, Howard CW: Clinical practice guidelines for the management of orbital cellulitis. J Pediatr Ophthalmol Strabismus 35:73, 1998

Vail DT: Orbital complications in sinus disease: a review. Am J Ophthalmol 14:202, 1931

Varma D, Metcalfe TW. Orbital cellulitis after peribulbar anaesthesia for cataract surgery. Eye (Lond) 2003; 17:105.

Velazquez AJ, Goldstein MH, Driebe WT. Preseptal cellulitis caused by trichophyton (ringworm). Cornea 2002; 21:312.

von Noorden GK: Orbital cellulitis following extraocular muscle surgery. Am J Ophthalmol 74:627, 1972

Watters EC, Wallar H, Hiles DA, Michaels RH: Acute orbital cellulitis. Arch Ophthalmol 94:785, 1976

Weakley DR. Orbital cellulitis complicating strabismus surgery: a case report and review of the literature. Ann Ophthalmol 1991; 23:454.

Weber AL, Mikulis DK. Inflammatory disorders of the paraorbital sinuses and their complications. Radiol Clin North Am 1987; 25:615.

Weiss A, Friendly D, Eglin K, et al: Bacterial periorbital and orbital cellulitis in childhood. Ophthalmology 90:195, 1983

Welsh LW, Welsh JJ: Orbital complications of sinus disease. Laryngoscope 84:848, 1974

Westfall CT, Shore JW: Isolated fractures of the orbital floor: risk of infection and the role of the antibiotic prophylaxis. Ophthalmic Surg 22:409, 1991

Whitnall SE: The Anatomy of the Human Orbit and Accessory Organ of Vision. 2nd ed, pp 29–35.New York: Oxford University Press, 1932

Williamson-Nobel FA: Diseases of the orbit and its contents secondary to pathological conditions of the nose and paranasal sinuses. Ann R Coll Surg 15:46, 1954

Wilson ME, Paul TO: Orbital cellulitis following strabismus surgery. Ophthalmic Surg 18:92, 1987

Wulc AE, Adams JL, Dryden RM: Cerebrospinal fluid leakage complicating orbital exenteration. Arch Ophthalmol 107:827, 1989

Wulc, AC. Orbital infections. In: Duane's Ophthalmology 1999 CD ROM edition, Volume 2, Chapter 34.Williams BJ, Harrison HC: Subperiosteal abscesses of the orbit due to sinusitis in childhood. Aust NZ J Ophthalmol 19:29, 1991

Younis RT, Lazar RH, Bustillo A, Anand VK. Department of Otolaryngology, University of Miami School of Medicine, (Orbital infection as a complication of sinusitis: are diagnostic and treatment trends changing?) PubMed, Ear Nose Throat J. 2002 Nov;81(11):771-5.

Younis RT, Lazar RH, Bustillo A, Anand VK: Orbital infection as a complication of sinusitis: are diagnostic and treatment trends changing. Ear, Nose, Throat J 81:771, 2002

Youssef Z, Pennefather PM, Watts MT. Orbital cellulitis vs allergic reaction to hyaluronidase as the cause of periorbital oedema. Eye (Lond) 2005; 19:691.

Zhanel GG, Ennis K, Vercaine L, et al: A critical review of the fluoroquinolones. Drugs 62:13, 2002

Ziakas NG, Boboridis K, Gratsonidis A, et al. Wegener's granulomatosis of the orbit in a 5-year-old child. Eye (Lond) 2004; 18:658.

Zimmerman RA, Bilaniuk LT: CT of orbital infection and its cerebral complications. AJR 134:45, 198

11

Extended Applications of Endoscopic Sinus Surgery to the Orbit and Pituitary Fossa

Balwant Singh Gendeh
Department of Otorhinolaryngology – Head and Neck Surgery
UKM Medical Center, Jalan Yaacob Latif, Bandar Tun Razak, Kuala Lumpur
Malaysia

1. Introduction

There has been significant evolution over time from external headlight sinus surgery to endoscopic sinus surgery(ESS). ESS was pioneered by Messenklinger, who discovered that the sinuses had a predetermined mucociliary clearance pattern towards the natural ostium irrespective of additional openings into the sinuses. This philosophy of opening the natural ostium of the diseased sinus was then popularized by Stammberger and Kennedy. ESS is now accepted as the surgical management of choice for chronic sinusitis. Furthermore, as our knowledge of the anatomy of the sinuses has improved, other anciliary surgeries such as endoscopic lacrimal surgery, orbital decompression, applications to the pterygopalatine and infratemporal fossa, approaches from the sphenoid/sella extending the cribriform, parasellar and clival region have evolved. Moreover, innovation in instrumentation has led to the acceptance of endoscopic management of benign endonasal tumors and more recently, on endoscopic management of malignant tumors of the nose and sinuses.

The current interest in ESS stems from several developments. The first is the advent of compact, multi-angled telescopes that allow excellent visualization of the nasal cavity for examination and of the sinuses during procedures, including such areas as the maxillary ostia and the frontal recess. Secondly, is the acceptance and appreciation of the great work of Messerklinger(1967) demonstrating that the anterior ethmoids are usually the key to persistent sinusitis. Thirdly, is the advent in radiological imaging. Endoscopic diagnostic examinations in conjunction with modern imaging methods, particularly CT scan, have proven to be an ideal combination and have been accepted as the "Standard of Care' for sinus disease. The CT scan can clearly identify anterior ethmoids disease which can easily be missed on a plain paranasal sinus X-ray. These developments make it possible to diagnose more accurately and treat sinusitis refractory to non-invasive therapy.

The technique of ESS was developed in Europe by Messerklinger and Wigand, who had two different goals designed for extremes of disease. The Messerklinger technique advocated in 1985 is an anterior to posterior approach which involves only the anterior ethmoids and the maxillary sinus ostium and can be extended into the posterior ethmoids, sphenoid and the frontal sinus anteriorly if necessary. Thus, the Messerklinger technique is ideal for patient with anterior ethmoid disease with or without maxillary or frontal sinus disease. On the contrary, the Wigand approach advocated in 1978 is posterior-to-anterior and routinely involves all the sinuses on the ipsilateral side and is ideal for patient with pan-sinusitis who has or is apt to fail the more limited Messerklinger approach. Both techniques are based on the assumption that the sinus mucosa is most likely reversibly diseased and will return to normal once ventilation has been established. No attempt is made to eradicate the sinus mucous membrane, as in the Caldwell-Luc procedure, but rather to reestablish drainage so the mucosa can return to normal and restore its proper function.

Although telescopes give the surgeon a clearer and magnified view of the nose and sinuses, the picture on the video monitor is not three-dimentional and depth perception and orientation can be difficult. Consequently there is a risk of getting lost and this may result in an injury to the orbit, its contents, the optic nerve and the intracranial cavity. To reduce this risk, surgeons should ensure that they are thoroughly familiar with the anatomy and the anatomical variations that can occur in the nose and sinuses. Therefore, radiological imaging is essential prior to surgical intervention.

A significant development for soft-tissue removal was the development of "through-cutting" instrumentation. Powered instrumentation using soft tissue shavers (Metronic, Xomed, USA) offer another significant advancement to the endoscopic sinus surgeon but with some risk to the orbit and cranium in inexperienced hands (Fig 1). Setliff and Parsons were the first to report the use of soft-tissue shavers in endoscopic sinus surgery (Setliff , 1994). ESS with its minimally invasive technique often reduces pain, bleeding and length of hospital stay and avoids external incision and thus reduces surgical cost compared to conventional techniques. Endoscopic surgery cannot replace every conventional external approach and we should never be embarrassed to employ or convert to these conventional approaches when necessary (Gendeh et al, 2007). However, not all cases are suitable for an endoscopic approach and the surgeon must be experienced in the full range of surgical options, the patho-physiology and natural history of disease processes, if optimum results are to be achieved. This is particularly true in the controversial area of sinonasal neoplasia.

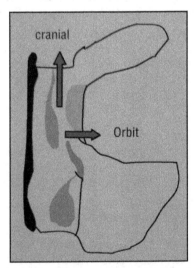

Fig. 1. Diagrammatic coronal section of paranasal sinuses showing the anatomical proximity of orbit and cranium to the nasal cavity in utilization of powered instrumentation and the risk involved.

This chapter will briefly outline the future trends in endoscopic skull base surgery. The Expanded Endonasal Approach(EEA) is a an extended endoscopic transnasal approach, providing access to the entire skull base from the epicenter, the sphenoid sinus.

It is important to define the word "endoneurosurgery" (Kassam et al, 2007). This is a new and emerging field and represents the use of the endoscope as the sole and only tool used to visualize the entire neural axis. In the case of EEA, only the endoscope is used to access the ventral skull via a completely transnasal route. As a joint team effort, this extended applications beyond the sphenoid sinus/sella needs a lot of surgical skills, planning and coordination for proper patient selection and optimal care. The EEA provides surgical access to the ventral skull base to resect a wide variety of intra-dural and extra-dural pathologies and allows the reconstruction of the resulting defect using a naso-septal flap. The evolution of these techniques has been enabled by technological advances including the design of specific endonasal instrumentation, surgical navigation technology and the development of new biomaterials for reconstruction. The incidence of tumor recurrence will be very much reduced with this minimally invasive ventral skull base technique. The use of powered instruments with navigational fusion imaging is most beneficial especially in revision cases.

2. Endoscopic dacryocystorhinostomy

Dacryocystorhinostomy(DCR) involves the formation of a bypass from the lacrimal sac into the nose. It is essential that with proper history and examination including syringing and probing, a correct diagnosis is made. Syringing and probing is performed only in congenital and acquired nasolacrimal duct obstruction (NLDO) and are indications for the procedure. They are not performed in acute and chronic dacryocystitis.

2.1 Indications (Table 1)

The main indication is when there is distal outflow obstruction to the nasolacrimal system which can clearly be demonstrated on a dacrocystogram. Endoscopic surgery is not indicated for obstruction of a punctum or a canaliculus for which there are other procedures. Often distal obstruction is mixed with varying degree of proximal obstruction and this need to be explained when counseling the patient. Syringing and probing is helpful in defining the site of obstruction. It is expected that in congenital and acquired NLDO, the epiphora would resolve and in acute and chronic dacryocysitis, the infection would be resolved without recurrences.

1.	Primary acquired NLDO
2.	Secondary acquired NLDO
	a. Infectious causes of secondary acquired lacrimal duct obstruction
	b. Inflammatory causes of secondary lacrimal obstruction
	c. Neoplastic causes of lacrimal obstruction
	d. Traumatic causes of lacrimal obstruction
	e. Mechanical causes of lacrimal obstruction

Table 1. Indications for Endonasal DCR(EDCR)

A dacrocystogram (Fig 2) is indicated if there is any mass within the sac and scintigraphy helps to define a functional problem. A functional problem is one issue for which a dacryocystogram is helpful. Lacrimal sac mass is another indication for dacryocystogram. A bloody discharge from the punctum is a symptom that needs investigating to exclude malignancy in the sac. The common symptoms are epiphora, recurrent dacryocystitis or swelling from a mucocele. It is unusual for intranasal pathology like Wegener granulomatosis and sarcoidosis to be the causative factor. Nasolacrimal duct obstruction can occur following a middle-third facial fracture. Distal nasolacrimal obstruction can be secondary to endoscopic sinus surgery if the Stammberger Rhinoforce Antrum Punch (Stortz, Germany) used to remove the uncinate process is placed too far forward.

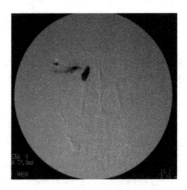

Fig. 2. A dacrocystogram showing distal obstruction of right nasolacrimal system on failure of penetration of dye into the inferior meatus in a patient with unilateral unresolving tearing.

2.2 Contraindications (Table 2)

A contraindication to DCR is the presence of a benign or malignant lesion in the lacrimal system or the surrounding tissues and active Wegener granulomatosis. Other causes are lacrimal sac diverticulum,, canalicular stenosis, lacrimal calculi and extensive midfacial trauma.

1.	Known or suspected lacrimal system neoplasm
2.	Large lateral lacrimal sac diverticulum
3.	Common canalicular stenosis
4.	Lacrimal system stones
5.	Extensive midfacial trauma

Table 2. Contraindications for Endonasal DCR(EDCR)

2.3 Anatomy and pre-operative assessment

The lacrimal system comprises the lacrimal gland and its drainage system which commences with a punctum in each eyelid for 1mm at right angles to the lid margin. It continues as the upper and lower canaliculus which run parallel to the lid margin and then join to form a common canaliculus that drains into the lacrimal sac (Fig 3). Inferiorly the sac forms the nasolacrimal duct, which drains into the inferior meatus about 1cm posterior to the anterior end of the inferior turbinate (Fig 4). The lacrimal sac sits in the lacrimal fossa which is a very thin bone. Unlike its anterior margin, the anterior lacrimal crest, is made of very dense bone. In about 8% of patients, an anterior ethmoidal air cell lies medial to the lacrimal fossa which needs to be transverse before a rhinostomy can be created.

Topical anesthetic drops such as amethocaine are placed in the eye followed by dilatation of the upper and lower puncta performed with punctual dilator. The puncta are initially dilated with the instrument perpendicular to the lid margin, rotating it for the first 1 mm with the lid margin taut, before turning it medially parallel to the lid. Upon dilatation of the punctum, a "0" Bowman probe is passed through the dilated punctum and angled medially. As the probe enters the common canaliculus, a slight resistance may be felt as a "soft stop" and as it touches the medial wall of the sac, there is a "hard stop". The probe is then angled vertically down to feel whether there is any sac pathology or distal obstruction. This is a description for probing in children, which is preferably performed under general anaesthesia. It is avoided in adults because of the intolerable pain. Rigid 0.7 mm dacryocystoscopes can be used to inspect the fine obstructing membranes that can be found at the medial aspect of the upper and lower canaliculi (Wormald, 2002). These proximal membranes are the main cause of proximal obstruction, and a DCR is not indicated if this is the site of the obstruction. For surgeons becoming familiar with intranasal anatomy or a history of previous sinonasal surgery, it may be helpful to introduce a 20-gauge fiberoptic endoilluminator(Stortz, Germany) through the superior or inferior canaliculus after punctual dilator. The endoilluminator is then advanced gently until a hard stop signifying the lacrimal bone is identified (Woog, 2004). The location of the lacrimal sac may then be visualized endoscopically by transillumination (Fig 5 a, b).

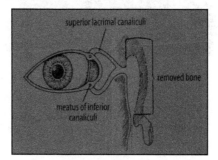

Fig. 3. Diagrammatic anatomical picture of nasolacrimal drainage system

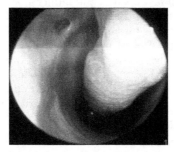

Fig. 4. Endoscopic view of a right nasolacrimal duct opening into an inferior meatus

Distal obstruction is diagnosed by probing and then syringing to see whether the fluid can initially pass through the canaliculi into the nose. If it refluxes through the other punctum, it indicates that there is distal obstruction. On the contrary, if there is reflux through the same punctum, then there is canalicular or common canalicular stenosis and this can be confirmed by gentle probing. There are many causes of dysfunction that requires a different treatment than DCR. The most common site of distal obstruction is where the sac becomes the duct. Some surgeons will offer a DCR to patients with a functional blockage where there is free flow on syringing but on scintigraphy the pump system does not work. Only 70-75% of the tears are drained through the inferior canaliculus. Lester-Jones Pyrex tube is required only in bi-canalicular extensive obstruction that cannot be managed by other procedures such as forced probing and silicone intubation.

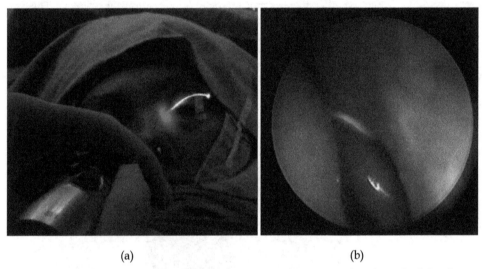

(a)   (b)

Fig. 5. A picture showing a fiber-optic endoilluminator being introduced via the left inferior cannaliculus to illuminate the nasolacrimal sac(a) and a zero degree endoscopic view identifying the location of the illuminated lacrimal sac(b) in the same patient.

2.4 Surgical technique

Upon nasal decongestion with neuropatties and infilteration with lidocaine and adrenaline, a 15 scalpel blade is used for initial mucosal incisions. The first incision is made horizontally 1 cm above the axilla of the middle turbinate, commencing 3 mm posterior to the axilla and coming forward 1 cm onto the frontal process of the maxilla. The blade is then turned vertically and incision made about two thirds of the vertical height of middle turbinate, stopping just above the insertion of the inferior turbinate into the lateral nasal wall. The blade is then turned horizontally and the inferior insertion commenced at the insertion of the uncinate process and brought forward to meet the vertical incision.

A suction Freer's dissector (Stortz, Germany) is used to elevate the mucosal flap, ensuring that the tip of the sucker always maintains contact with the bone. Meanwhile the bone should be palpable so that the junction of the soft lacrimal bone and hard bone of the frontal process can be identified. The thin lacrimal bone is 2 to 5 mm wide before the insertion of the uncinate process is reached. The dissection stops at the uncinate. A round knife (Stortz, Germany) is used to flake the soft lacrimal bone away from the postero-inferior region of the sac.

A forward-bitting Hajek Koeffler punch (Stortz, Germany) is used to remove the lower portion of the frontal process of the maxilla (Fig 6). The tip of the punch is used to push the lacrimal sac away where the lacrimal bone has to be removed. The punch is engaged in the hard bone of the frontal process and this bone is removed. Care should be taken not to grasp the sac as the punch is closed during bone removal. Removal of the frontal process of the maxilla uncovers the antero-inferior portion of the lacrimal sac. Bony removal with punch is continued as far superiorly as possible until the bone becomes too thick for the punch to engage. At this juncture the 15 degree curved 2.9 mm rough diamond burr(Medtronic Xomed, Jacksonville, Florida, USA) is attached to the micro-debrider and used to remove the rest of the bone up to the superior mucosal incision (Jones,1998). Often, an agger nasi cell is present and the mucosa of this cell will be exposed as the sac is followed superiorly above the axilla of the middle turbinate thus exposing the frontal recess (Fig 7). The diamond burr can be brought into light contact with the lacrimal sac lining without damaging the sac. A cutting burr will remove the bone faster but may cause significant damage to the sac wall with development of hole in the sac wall.

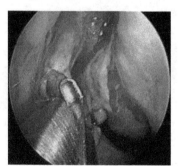

Fig. 6. Intraoperative endoscope view showing right dacrocystorhinostomy with initial removal of the thin lacrimal bone with Hajek Koffler sphenoid punch and subsequently the hard frontal process of maxilla with a microdrill

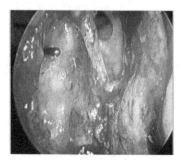

Fig. 7. Intraoperative endoscopic view showing a right dacrocystorhinostomy with wide exposure of the nasolacrimal sac with visible end of eye probe and removal of agger nasi cell exposing the frontal recess

Next, the inferior punctum is dilated with a punctum dilator and a Bowman's canalicular probe is passed into the sac. If the tip of the probe is not seen to move behind the thin sac wall, the probe is not in the lumen. The exposed sac is incised vertically with a DCR minisickle knife (Metronic Xomed, USA). Belucci scissors (Stortz, Germany) are used to make upper and lower releasing incisions in the posterior flap which is rolled out on the lateral nasal wall. The sac should now be completely marsupialized and lie flat on the lateral nasal wall. Approximating the lacrimal and nasal mucosa should result in a first intention healing rather than a secondary intention healing and should reduce the formation of granulation tissue and scarring. The puncta are dilated and Silastic lacrimal intubation tubes(O'Donoghue tubes) are placed through the upper and lower puncta and retrieved endonasally. Ligar clips are placed to secure the tubes in place (Fig 8). Before placing the clips ensure a loop of tubing is pulled in the medial canthus of the eye so that the tubes are not tight. If the loop is tight the tubes can cheese-wire through the punctum (Khairullah and Gendeh, 2011). A square of Gelfoam(Pharmacia NSW, Sydney, Australia) or Merogel (Metronic Xomed) is slid up the tubing and placed over the flaps to hold them in position.

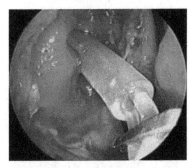

Fig. 8. Intraoperative endoscope view showing right dacrocystorhinostomy with stent in situ an adult patient presenting with unresolving right tearing.

Saline irrigation is started within 3 to 4 hours of surgery. The patient is commenced on broad spectrum antibiotics for 5 days and eye drops are used for 3 weeks. The O'Donoghue tubes are removed in the clinic after 4 weeks. It is rare to see any granulation tissue but if they are present they should be removed. The patient is reviewed for a further 18 months before discharge.

2.5 Laser assisted DCR

For osteotomy, laser was used exclusively in the early part of the series in 1992 and 1993. The preferred site for osteotomy was the thinnest bone located in the infero-posterior parts of the lacrimal fossa, which corresponds to the brightest area in the nasal cavity as demonstrated by the transilluminator. The authors concluded that the success rate of laser-assisted DCR was around 78%, which was much lower than that of conventional DCR. Beginning in 1999 and 2000, osteotomy was performed with either a drill, a punch, or both, which enabled removal of thicker bone. The site of the osteotomy was moved to the level of medial canthus, which was anterior and superior to that of previous surgeries. When the osteotomy was completed, the common internal punctum was visible on endoscopy. With this approach, the success rate improved to 92%(Lee et al, 2004).

In another interesting study in 65 patients with a mean follow-up of 74 months, the authors found the success rate of endoscopic laser assisted DCR has gradually declined over the years to 56%. The authors do not advocate the use of laser in endonasal DCR with epiphora (Umapathy et al, 2006).

3. Endoscopic applications in orbital surgery

3.1 Endoscopic blow out fracture repair

Fractures of the roof of the maxillary sinus with herniation of the orbital content (blow-out fracture), often produce strangulation of the inferior rectus or inferior oblique muscles and thereby impairing movement of eyeball (Fig 9). They can present with periorbital ecchymosis and subconjunctival hemorrhage. Those with fracture of medial wall of orbit without prior surgical intervention can present with enopthalmos.

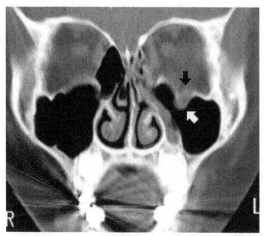

Fig. 9. Coronal CT scan of the paranasal sinuses showing a 'tear drop' sign resulting from a blunt trauma to the left eye in a patient presenting with diplopia

Passage of the endoscope through the intranasal maxillary antrostomy may provide superb visualization of the posterior orbital floor which is the most difficult area to view by transconjunctival or subciliary approach. Anatomically, this area of the orbital floor commonly lies behind the middle half of the globe on axial view. This posterior view may furthermore be obscured because the orbital floor angulates 15 degrees superiorly as one proceeds from the orbital rim toward the orbital apex. Therefore, the endoscope is an extremely useful means of safely and definitely identifying the posterior edge of the defect and ensuring that the posterior edge of the orbital implant do not compromise the optic nerve or other structures at the orbital apex (Hartstein et al, 2004). In many small fractures for which an implant is not required, endoscopic examination and reduction may be sufficient, thus avoiding an external incisional approach.

It is doubtful that endoscopy alone will replace standard CT scanning in the evaluation of orbital fractures. Thus, combining forced duction testing with endoscopic visualization of a fracture may prove to be useful diagnostic tool.

3.1.1 Indications

This include fractures with extension to the middle and posterior portions of the orbital floor, in delayed or secondary fracture repair.

3.1.2 Surgical technique

Orbital fracture repair is normally performed using general anaesthesia. Some author's have reported the use of purely endoscopic approach for the repair of orbital floor fracture (Ikeda et al, 1999). The procedure is commenced by enlarging the maxillary ostium and then introducing an angled endoscope. Bony fragmenst in the fracture site are removed endoscopically until an improvement in forced duction testing is noted. Subsequently, a uretheral balloon catheter is introduced through the ostium into the maxillary sinus. In some patients with trap-door-type fractures, successful fracture repair may be possible with endoscopic approach alone, with removal of the displaced bony fragment and relieve of the entrapment. Saline is used to inflate the balloon which elevates the contents out of the fracture site. The balloon is removed approximately two weeks after surgery.

Tips for successful surgery

Endoscopic visualization of fractures of the posterior aspect of the orbital floor and medial orbit may facilitate safe and secure implant placement and ensures that no residual orbital soft tissue is entrapped within the fracture site or beneath the implant. The endoscopic technique minimizers the uncertainty of implant placement posteriorly in both primary and secondary repairs. It may help to minimize the number of additional incisions required in the medial orbit, maxillary sinus and even the eyelid. The increased accuracy of implant placement may help to reduce the risks of residual exopthalmos postoperatively. This technique is useful in the more complex fractures involving the posterior orbital floor and medial wall.

3.2 Endoscopic orbital decompression of complications of thyroid-related orbitopathy

Graves' disease is an autoimmune disorder affecting the thyroid, orbit and skin. Approximately 50% of patients with this disorder develop orbital manifestation of dysthyroid orbitopathy. Fewer than 5% of such patients have disease that is severe enough to require surgical decompression of the orbit (Metson and Samaha, 2004). The extensive muscle enlargement limits globe movement in extremes of gaze which will cause diplopia. Visual loss in Grave's disease is uncommon, occurring in only 2 to 7% of patients (Kountantakis et al, 2000; Kuppersmith et al, 1997). Exopthalmos in Grave's disease is thought to result from the deposition of immune complexes in the intraocular mucles and fat which in turn leads to edema and fibrosis (Tandon et al, 1994). The resultant increase in intraorbital pressure pushes the globe forward causing proptosis. If this proptosis become severe enough, the eyelids cannot close properly and chemosis with or without exposure keratitis of the cornea may occur. Furthermore, the crowding of the orbital apex by the obviously enlarged extraocular muscles places pressure on the optic nerve. Stretching of the optic nerve by increasing proptosis may result in the development of optic neuropathy and visual loss. If medical treatment fails (high dose steroids with or without low-dose radiotherapy) , surgical decompression of eyelid is indicated(Cook et al, 1996).

Removing one or more of the bony walls can decompress the contents of the orbit. The least amount of decompression would be achieved with medial wall removal , but the most physiologic and least to cause complications like globe displacement and diplopia. Endoscopic orbital decompression affords maximal orbital decompression at the orbital apex, an area that is not fully accessible via the external or transantral routes (Metson et al, 1994). Many techniques have been described for decompressing the orbit but the order of the procedures is that orbital decompression first, then strabismus and lastly the eyelid.

3.2.1 Indications and contraindications

The primary indication for the surgery is exopthalmos, either for cosmetic reasons or when vision is deteriorating and steroids and radiotherapy treatment has failed. The most common indications for such surgery are exposure keratopathy and optic neuropathy that have been refractory to conservative measures. Patients with diplopia from dysthyroid orbitopathy may require decompression before strabismus surgery to reaccess the globe and improve the predictability of muscle adjustments. Some surgeons who consider aesthetically undesirable proptosis to be an indication for orbital decompression have performed such surgery for its cosmetic benefits.

Contraindications to endoscopic orbital decompression include acute sinusitis and anatomic abnormalities of the maxillary bone. Endoscopic decompression may be technically difficult in patients with very small maxillay sinuses or thick orbital walls. These features are easily identified on computed tomography(CT) scan of the orbit and sinuses, which should be obtained on all patients before surgery.

3.2.2 Useful instruments

-   A long-shanked drill with a course diamond burr (Medtronic Xomed, Jacksonville, Florida, USA) and good irrigation system to keep the bone cool.
-   Image guided surgery

3.2.3 Endoscopic technique

The patient is placed in a supine position with head slightly elevated. Packing that has been soaked in a 4% cocaine solution is placed in the nasal cavity to initiate mucosal vasoconstriction. Both eyes are exposed in the surgical field. If general anaesthesia is used, the corneas are covered with protective shells. Under endoscopic visualization, submucosal injections of 1% lidocaine with epinephrine are administered along the lateral nasal wall and middle turbinate. If a septal deviation precludes endoscopic access to the middle meatus region, a septoplasty is performed before orbital decompression.

The bones removed in endoscopic decompression include the medial wall of the orbit and the portion of the floor that is medial to the infraorbital canal. The procedure is initiated with an incision through the uncinate process. This incision is made just posterior to the maxillary line, a bony eminence that extends from the anterior attachment of the middle turbinate to the root of the inferior turbinate(Fig 10). The maxillary sinus ostium is then generously enlarged to provide optimal exposure of the orbital floor to prevent obstruction of the maxillary sinus by the decompressed globe. Bone is removed in the posterior direction to the level of the back wall of the sinus. Anterior removal is terminated at the thick bone of the frontal process of the maxilla, which protects the nasolacrimal duct. The ostium is enlarged superiorly to the level of the orbital floor and inferiorly to the root of the inferior turbinate. A 30-degree endoscope is used to identify the infraorbital nerve along the roof of the sinus (Fig 11).

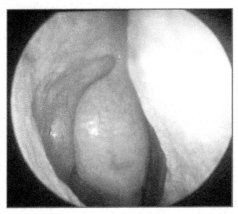

Fig. 10. A zero degree endoscopic view of left lateral nasal wall showing the maxillary line and uncinate process

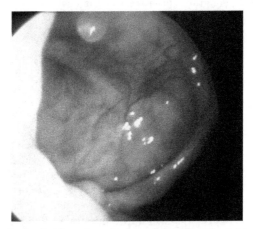

Fig. 11. A 30 degree endoscopic view showing evidence of wide right middle meatal antrostomy with infraorbital indentation in the roof of the maxillary sinus

An endoscopic sphenoethmoidectomy is then completed as described by Stammberger (1991) and Kennedy (1985). The degree of pneumatization of the sphenoid determines whether the optic nerve indents or even dehiscent in its lateral wall. Similarly, if the posterior ethmoid sinuses envelop the optic nerve before it reaches the sphenoid sinus, am Onodi cell may be present (Fig 12).The anterior and posterior ethmoid arteries are identified along the ethmoid roof. The middle turbinate that serves as a landmark during the sphenoethmoidectomy is removed before opening the lamina papyracea to optimize exposure to the medial orbital wall and facilitate postoperative cleaning. The skeletonized lamina papyracea is gently penetrated with a small spoon curette. Bony fragments of lamina papyracea is lifted in a medial direction to avoid perforation of the underlying periorbita. This elevation may also be performed with a periosteal elevator or delicate Blakesley forceps(Stortz, Germany). If surgery is performed using local anaesthesia, additional injections may be necessary to desensitize the medial orbital wall. Anaesthetic agent is injected just deep to the periorbita through the bony opening in the lamina.

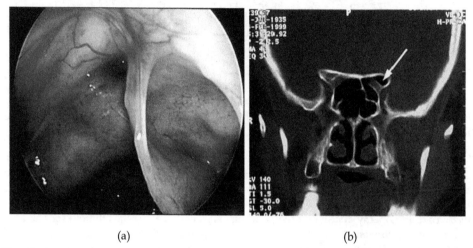

(a)   (b)

Fig. 12. An intra-operative endoscopic view (a) and coronal CT scan view (b) showing an Onodi cell

Bone of the lamina papyracea is removed in a superior direction toward the level of the ethmoid roof. The frontal recess is the most anterior superior portion of the ethmoid sinus, which communicates with the frontal sinus. Removal of the lamina papyracea in this region can cause postoperative obstruction of the frontal sinus by herniated fat. As dissection continous in a posterior direction toward orbital apex, thicker bone and underlying periorbita are generally encounterd within 2 mm of the sphenoid face. This thickening represents the annulus of Zinn, from which the extra ocular muscles(EOMs) originate and through which the optic nerve passes (Fig 13). This landmark represents the posterior limit of dissection and does not need to be removed. In cases of neuropathy, bone removal proceeds more posteriorly and may extend to the lateral wall of the sphenoid sinus.

Fragments of bone are cleared from the anterior end of lamina papyracea where it joins the lacrimal bone. Dissection in this region may be facilitated by use of an angled spoon curette and 30-degree endoscope (Stortz, Germany). The thick white fascia of the lacrimal sac may be uncovered but should not be opened. Firm bone anterior to the maxillary line protects most of the sac, so it should not be removed. Removal of the bone along the medial orbital floor can be most technically challenging aspect of this surgery. A spoon curette is used to fracture the bone in a downward direction. This bone may break apart in several small fragments with a natural cleavage plane along the infraorbital canal. Use of a 30-degree endoscope may facilitate visualization within the maxillary sinus and aid in the identification of the infraorbital nerve which serves as the lateral limit of bone removal.

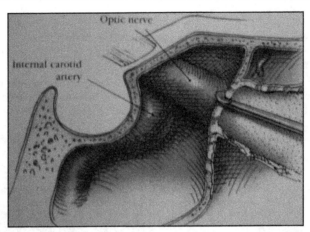

Fig. 13. A diagrammatic sagittal section of left sphenoid and posterior ethmoids showing the thick bone at the annulus of Zinn at the junction of the orbital apex and sphenoid sinus

After the periorbita has been fully exposed and cleared of bony fragments, it is opened with a sickle knife(Stortz, Germany). The incision is usually commenced in front of the sphenoid sinus. Care is taken to keep the tip of the blade superficial to avoid injury of the underlying orbital contents especially the medial rectus muscle, which may be enlarged secondary to dysthyroid orbitopathy. Incision of the periorbita is extended along the ethmoid roof and the orbital floor. A horizontal strip of periorbita overlying the medial rectus muscle is preserved (Fig 14). This fascial sling serves to decrease prolapsed of the muscle and is thought to reduce the incidence of postoperative diplopia (Metson and Samaha, 2002). However, in patients with optic neuropathy, maximal decompression is needed and the fascial sling is sacrificed to allow for wider excision of the periorbita which is removed eventually with angled Blakesley forceps. At the completion of the procedure, the generous prolapsed of the orbital fat into the opened ethmoid and maxillary sinuses should be observed(Fig 15)

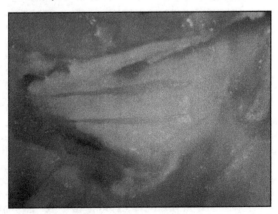

Fig. 14. A 70 degree endoscopic view showing an emergency horizontal orbital decompression incisions of the periorbita extending from the ethmoidal roof to the orbital floor for thyroid related orbitopathy

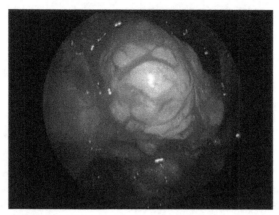

Fig. 15. A 30 degree endoscopic view showing prolapsed of orbital fat into the nasal cavity on balloting the right eye

A lateral orbital decompression may be performed at this time, depending on the extent of patient's disease and the degree of additional decompression desired. Due to the prior medial decompression, the orbital contents are easily retracted in a medial direction to provide excellent exposure of the lateral bony wall, which is removed or contoured. Concurrent excision of excess intraconal fat may also be performed if necessary. Bilateral orbital decompressions may be performed concurrently or as a staged procedure.

Nasal packing is avoided in order to prevent compression of the optic nerve, which is rendered increasingly vulnerable by the decompression. The patient is discharged the morning after surgery with a prescription for oral antibiotics and instructions to begin twice-daily nasal saline irrigations with a bulb syringe. During postoperative visit a week later, residual debri is cleared from the nasal cavity under endoscopic guidance.

In some cases, local anaesthesia may be preferred to general anaesthesia. These situations include patients who have an only-seeing eye, significant medical comorbidity, or a strong preference for local anesthesia.

The use of local anesthetic enables the surgeon to monitor the patient's vision on a continuous basis during the surgery and reduces the likelihood of occult injury to the optic nerve (Metson et al, 1994). Ideal sedation is achieved with intravenous bolus of propofol, 0.4 to 0.8mg/kg, administred before local injection, followed by maintenance infusion of 95 to 75 ug/kg during the procedure. Submucosal infilteration of 1% lidocaine with epinephrine 1:100,000 is performed exactly as described for the procedure utilizing general anaesthesia. Patients may report discomfort during removal of the lamina papyracea, and this may require a small additional infiltration of anaesthetic solution into the periorbita.

3.2.4 Complications

Diplopia is a relatively common sequela of endoscopic orbital decompression reported in 15 to 30 % of postoperative patients. This complication can be the result of change in the vector of pull of the EOMs. Diplopia that is present preoperatively is usually not improved by this surgery. Patients with preexisting or new-onset post-operative diplopia frequently require strabismus surgery. It is essential that all patients be informed of the possibility of postoperative double vision before undergoing orbital decompression.

Techniques to decrease the incidence of new-onset postoperative diplopia, including the preservation of the fascial sling of periorbita to prevent prolapsed of the medial rectus muscle, have been mentioned (Metson and Samaha, 2002). To decrease the incidence of postoperative diplopia, the use of balanced decompression technique is advocated. This technique involves performing external lateral wall decompression at the time of endoscopic medial wall decompression to reduce pressure on the medial rectus muscle while simultaneously increasing the degree of ocular recession.

Postoperative bleeding after endoscopic orbital decompression is managed by direct caurterization of the bleeding site. Nasal packing is avoided in these patients to avoid pressure in the region of the optic nerve. The incidence of sinonasal infection post-surgery is minimized with the routine use of postoperative antistaphylococcal antibiotics.

Postoperative epiphora may occur if the nasolacrimal duct is transected during the maxillary antrostomy. This complication is readily treated with an endoscopic DCR. Blindness and cerebrospinal fluid rhinorrhea are also potentially serious complications of orbital decompression but rare.

Endoscopic orbital decompression should be performed only by surgeons with extensive experience in endoscopic intranasal techniques. A team approach, which uses the skills of both an Otolaryngologist and an Opthalmologist during the performance of this procedure is highly recommended.

Tips for successful surgery

Orbital decompression for thyroid-related orbitopathy is an effective method for reduction of proptosis for cosmetic proptosis, eye complications from exposure of the cornea and visual loss. The amount of regression of proptosis is related to the number of walls removed during surgery. It is believed that three-walled decompression may give a more balanced decompression with less likelihood of postoperative diplopia.

3.3 Endoscopic orbital decompression for acute orbital hemorrhage

The procedure of choice is lateral canthotomy and inferior cantholysis with of course cold dry compresses as tolerable. This is performed for 'orbital compartment syndrome' due to orbital bleeding, emphysema or tumor. For orbital decompression, lateral canthotomy alone is not sufficient and the inferior eyelid should be completely free to allow anterior displacement of the globe. Drainage of any kind is only indicated if this is not helpful. The problem with drainage is that the bleeding is diffuse and not confined to one compartment. Endoscopic drainage is actually performed to remove adjacent orbital wall and open the periosteum to allow decompression of orbital soft tissues. It is important to note that the same can be achieved with the faster canthotomy and inferior cantholysis.

Invariably the anterior ethmoidal artery(AEA) can be located one cell behind the frontal recess(Fig 16 a, b). The size of the so called supra-orbital cell (Bolger & Mann, 2001) varies: it can be small or large. The AEA can often be seen on CT scan, (Fig 10) particularly as it enters the orbit where it produces a fluted defect in the lamina papyracea(LP). The more pneumatized the supra-orbital recess, the more vulnerable it is to damage. Often the ethmoidal bulla (EB) attaches to the skull base and the AEA lies within the roof and is 1-2 mm behind the attachment of the anterior wall of the EB to skull base. If the frontal recess (FR) does require opening, it is best approached anteriorly, away from AEA if the landmarks are poor owing to previous surgery or bleeding. As the AEA is sometimes dehiscent, it is advisable not to grasp polyps in this area if one is unable to identify the anatomy clearly. Often the FR can be found by following the intact anterior wall of the ethmoidal bulla superiorly.

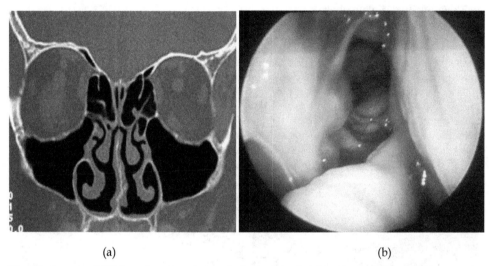

(a)   (b)

Fig. 16. A coronal CT imaging showing an indentation of right anterior ethmoidal artery at the region of frontal recess (a) and a 70 degree endoscopic view showing indentation of the artery in the same patient(b).

The AEA is dehiscent at some point in the majority of patients (Lang, 1989). It is essential to avoid tearing it for it can cause marked bleeding. If it is transected and retracts into the orbit, a marked increase in pressure in the posterior compartment of the eye can occur and place the retinal artery and its supply to the retina at risk. If it is torn, gentle bipolar diathermy will arrest the bleeding but this should be performed with great care to avoid transecting the remaining segment of the artery.

3.3.1 Bleeding

If there is obvious bleeding into the posterior compartment of the eye, the eye will prop out, the orbit will become very firm and within a few minutes the swinging flash light test will reveal an afferent defect. An awake patient will complaint of discomfort and loss of vision. An orbital tourniquet should be tried on immediate recognition. This involves placing a cotton wool over the closed eyelid and applying an orbital tourniquet over the cotton wool and around the head and then inflating it to systolic pressure. This is performed for one minute and then it should be removed and the pupil reflexes and/or the vision checked. If the vision or pupil reflex has improved, the orbital tourniquet should be reapplied and the process repeated every minute for up to 5 minutes. If this is performed soon after injury, it may be sufficient to stop bleeding into the orbit and it can arrest the process.

It is advisable to monitor vision for 6 hours postsurgery to ensure that no further bleeding occurs into the posterior compartment. If this maneuver fails then the orbit must be decompressed. A lateral canthotomy and inferior cantholysis is quick and efficient technique for up to one hour and it is best to decompress the orbit as early as possible (Jones, 1997). Moreover, one should not wait for an opthalmological colleague to arrive unless they do so within an hour. Assessing the vascular supply of the retinal vessels with an opthalmoscope is inadequate.

3.3.2 Lateral canthotomy and inferior cantholysis

Local anesthetic is placed around the lateral canthus of eye and it is divided using small straight scissors down to the bone of the orbital rim and to the depth of the lateral sulcus of the conjunctiva. A corneal abrasion or conjuctival damage can be avoided by protecting the globe. The lower lid is then retracted downward for good expose. The scissors is angled at 45 degree to the horizontal axis and the lateral ligament and septum is divided and the globe and contents of the orbit will then prolapse forward (Fig 17). The pupil reflexes, the pressure of the orbit and vision should all be checked. The orbit will retract to its normal position over the next 2-3 days. Suturing is usually performed a week or so after the procedure.

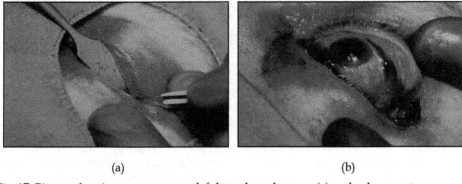

(a)   (b)

Fig. 17. Picture showing an emergency left lateral canthotomy (a) and subsequent cantholysis (b) being performed in the same patient for iatrogenic orbital hemorrhage

This procedure is normally sufficient to decompress the posterior compartment of the eye. If inadequate a surgical decompression should be undertaken. It can be done either endoscopically by removing the LP widely and incising the orbital periosteum or externally via a Lynch-Howarth incision. Preserving vision takes priority over producing an external scar. If the orbit is decompressed by an external approach, the AEA will not be found as it will have retracted into substance of the orbit.

3.3.3 Medial rectus damage

Medial rectus damage occurs when there is disinsertion of the muscle, damage to the muscle nerve or intramuscular bleeding. In damage encountered during enscopic sinus surgery, a vigilant assistant should look out for movement of the globe which occurs unintentionally. As a precautionary measure, the assistant should repeatedly ballot the eye when the surgeon is operating on the lateral nasal wall. Anatomically the medial rectus muscle is located closer to LP posteriorly then anteriorly (Fig 18). The suction port of the powered shaver should preferably be directed medially away from the LP to minimize the risk of damaging the structures in the lateral nasal wall. Damage to medial rectus occurs through deeper penetration into the orbit. Unfortunately, it is very difficult to prevent the scarring and diplopia that are likely to occur if recognized then. Moreover, expert strabismus surgeons have difficulty in correcting the problems caused by damage to the medial rectus. It is a medical negligence and should preferably be settled out of court.

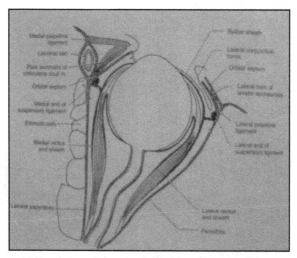

Fig. 18. Axial section of the relationship of right medial rectus and optic nerve to the lamina papyracea

3.3.4 Optic nerve damage

The optic nerve can be damaged by penetration of the orbit through the lamina papyracea. Therefore, it is important for the assistant to look for eye movements when the surgeon is operating on the lateral nasal wall. Moreover, the optic nerve can be damaged if it is exposed in a sphenoethmoid air cell(Onodi cell)(Fig 19). An Onodi cell should be identified on routine pre-operative imaging and care taken in removing polyps lateral to the sagittal plane of the medial wall of the maxillary sinus. It is advisable to identify the sphenoid sinus ostia medially and then work forward. The optic nerve indentation can be prominent in 20% of patients in the upper half of lateral wall of sphenoid sinus but is rarely dehiscent (Fig 20). The carotid artery lies in the lateral and inferior aspect of the sphenoid sinus. Therefore, it is advisable to avoid the lateral wall of sphenoid sinus by directing the suction port of the powered shaver medially away from the lateral wall of sphenoid sinus to minimize the risk of damaging the structures present there.

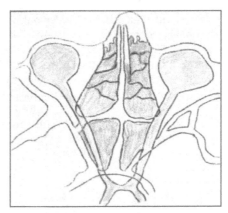

Fig. 19. A diagrammatic axial view of the paranasal sinuses showing a rare bilateral Onodi cell

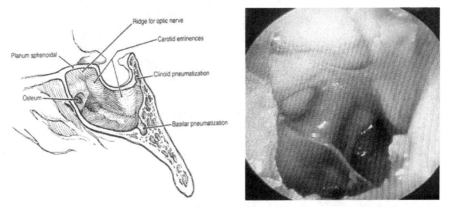

Fig. 20. Diagrammatic sagittal section and endoscopic view of the sphenoid sinus showing indentations of the lateral wall by internal carotid artery inferiorly and optic nerve superiorly

3.3.5 Post-operative complications

3.3.5.1 Bleeding

Sitting the patient 30% head up at end of procedure is often adequate for minor general ooze. Coughing during extubation will result in temporarily more bleeding due to increase in venous pressure. A nasal pack soaked in 1:10,000 epinephrine is helpful for more than minor ooze and removed in the recovery or left in position for 12 hours if oozing continues. Prophylactic antibiotics are advocated for nasal packs left in position for more than 24 hours. Rarely, torrential reactionary bleeding can occur in the first 12 hours due to these vessels initially going into spasm intra-operatively when the platelet plug and clotting factors block them but with due time either due to relaxation of artery or fibrinolysis reverses this process and bleeding commences. Usually it is impossible to locate the bleeding site. If a local nasal pack with vasoconstrictor and local anesthetic is not helpful to control the bleeding, then bipolar caurtery of the offending vessel may be helpful. If this too fails, then reinserting a nasal pack and/or balloon may be necessary to tamponade the bleeding until the spheno-palatine artery(SPA) can be ligated under general anesthesia. If a large sphenoidotomy has been performed, the bleeding could be due to the damaged septal branch as it crosses the anterior wall of the sphenoid (Fig 21).

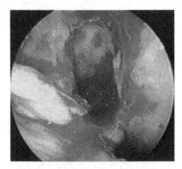

Fig. 21. Intraoperative Endoscopic view showing a right low sphenoidotomy with evidence of sphenopalatine bleed

3.3.5.2 Adhesions

Mucosal damage to adjacent surfaces can result in adhesions (Fig 22). Adhesions can be minimized by topical and local corticosteroids application. If adhesions are present pre-operatively, they need removal with a through-cutting punch followed by douching and debridement at one week.

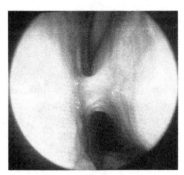

Fig. 22. Endoscopic view showing adhesions between left septum and inferior turbinate after nasal surgery

3.3.5.3 Epiphora

The lacrimal sac or naso-lacriminal duct can be damaged if the middle meatal antrostomy(MMA) is extended too far anteriorly. If middle meatus needs to be enlarged anteriorly to allow improved access or drainage, then the uncinate process (UP) is removed retrograde with Stammberger Rhinoforce antrum punch (Stortz, Germany). If patient complaints of watery eyes post surgery, it is best not to intervene as it will often resolve on its own. If the epiphora is persistent, an endo-nasal DCR will be helpful.

3.3.5.4 Periorbital emphysema

Peri-orbital emphysema or air in the soft tissues around the eye is due to intra-operative breach of the LP and the patient unknowingly blown their nose(Fig 23).The anesthetist should be advice to take care on extubating the patient and not to use too much force if patient needs to be ventilated with face mask. The emphysema will resolve in due time provided the patient does not blow any more air into the area. Prophylactic antibiotics are administered for active sinusitis or history of sinusitis.

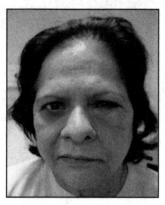

Fig. 23. Left periorbital emphysema post powered endoscopic sinus surgery which resolved spontaneously

3.3.5.5 Anosmia

Smell is a precious sense and every effort should be made to preserve or improve it. The olfactory mucosa extends from the cribriform plate to cover almost all the medial side of middle turbinate and the same area on the septum with a little inferior extension.

Pre-operative oral steroids are helpful in preventing damage to the mucosa, especially if polyps are medial to the middle turbinate (MT) when assessed as an outpatient. If the polyps remain medial to middle turbinate at surgery, perform an ethmoidectomy and then gently lateralize the MT to open the olfactory cleft which allows better access to topical steroid spray. If the patient has hyposmia or anosmia post-surgery and the MT is adherent to the septum, it is worth resecting and lateralizing the MT as an elective procedure when mucosal edema has settled down.

3.3.5.6 Frontal recess stenosis

The frontal sinus is often opaque on CT scan in nasal polyposis and it is normally due to retained secretions. It is rare to find polyps within the frontal sinus. Often opening the middle meatus and de-bulking polyps in region below the frontal recess with a shaver or through-cutting forceps (Stortz, Germany) followed by washing and topical nasal steroids may be adequate to allow the patients disease to be controlled.

It is essential not to denude the frontal recess of its mucosa since this may predispose to stenosis. If there is purulent disease within the frontal sinus causing symptoms, then it is advisable to open the recess, preserving as much mucosa as possible. This is ideally performed by dissecting the mucosa off the agger nasi cells with a ball probe and pulling it down on the shell of the cell and removing the fragments of bone and carefully preserving the mucosa. Any loose fragments of mucosa are best left alone. Large fragments of redundant mucosa around the frontal recess can be trimmed using a shaver or through-cutting forceps (Stortz, Germany). If there is a bony partition between the supra-orbital cell and frontal recess or a high frontal cell, the partition between them should be removed sub-mucosally.

3.3.5.7 Crusting

Crust results from mucosal damage. If there is full thickness mucosal damage, the mucus produced stagnates because there is no functioning cilia to clear it and it may take up to a year for the cilia to start to function synchronously again. Therefore, mucosal damage should be minimized and a full thickness defect should be avoided at all cost.

3.3.5.8 Infection

Superficial infection of stagnant mucus is common and usually resolves with douching. Sometimes, staphylococci multiply in a sump of mucus that collects in the maxillary sinus and may be slow to clear with douching alone. Topical nasal mupirocin ointment sniffed liberally after douching 6 times a day for 3 weeks can be very helpful.

3.3.5.9 Osteitis

Local osteitis due to exposure of bone is a rare complication resulting in severe pain. It produces a very dull, severe crippling nagging ache that causes tears to the patient. This condition is very distressing to the patient and worrying for the surgeon. Major analgesics are required and local treatment appears to provide little relief. Patients undergoing surgery for inverted papilloma where mucosal preservation is not practiced are at risk.

Tips for successful surgery

Intraobital hemorrhage should be managed with lateral canthotomy and cantholysis followed by orbital decompression with removal of the medial orbital wall. Orbital decompression can be performed without canthotomy and cantholysis if the complication is notice intraoperatively

3.4 Endoscopic orbital decompression for orbital sub-periosteal abscess

Rhinosinusitis in children is not a surgical disease, and therefore the treatment is medical with systemic antibiotics such as clavulinic acid and ampicillin(Augmentin). The priority should be safety in any treatment as the problem usually resolves with time without intervention. Growth and maturation of the immunological response to pathogens play a major role in resolution of the disease (Jones, 1999; Howe & Jones, 2004).

Patients presenting with orbital complications of sinusitis commonly have a degree of cellulitis and edema (chemosis) around the eye with associated proptosis (Fig 24). This may be associated with some restriction of eye movement. Patients typically present with history of nasal obstruction, purulent rhinorrhea and facial pressure or pain. Nasal endoscopy reveals an inflamed and oedematous nasal mucosa with usually presence of pus in the middle meatus.

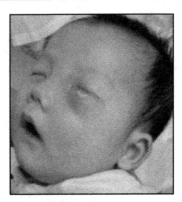

Fig. 24. Picture of a child with a left orbital cellulitis

If a subperiostal abcess is suspected, a CT scan of the parananasal sinuses with contrast will present a mass located on the lamina papyracea or in relation to the frontal sinus. The rim of the mass will enhance with the contrast. Moreover, the proptosis will be visible on the axial scans.

The external approach is quick and easy and the abscesss can usually be rapid and safely drained. If the surgeon is a skilled and experienced endoscopic sinus surgeon, endoscopic drainage of the subperiosteal abscess can be performed. The problem with this procedure is the significant vascularity that is associated with acute sinusitis. If the mucosal surface is touched with an instrument or endoscope, it will usually bleed and an inexperienced surgeon may lose orientation and complications may occur as a result of poor visibility during the surgery. Frequent packing with decongested soaked neuropatties throughout the procedure helps to minimize the bleeding but will not control it entirely. In a patient with acute sinusitis, the anaesthetist needs to optimize the patient's hemodynamics parameters to create an optimal surgical field.

The surgical approach is to perform an uncinectomy and enlarge the maxillary ostium to a moderate degree. Uncinectomy alone without antrostomy carries the risk of postoperative closure of the maxillary sinus because the inflammation and edema predisposes to scarring and adhesion formation. Clearance of the frontal sinus depends on whether the frontal sinus is thought to be the origin of the subperiosteal abscess. If the abscess is located adjacent to the ethmoidal sinuses, clearance of the bulla ethmoidalis and posterior ethmoids is performed with identification of the lamina papyracea. The lamina papyracea over the subperiosteal abscess is widely exposed and removed. If the abscess is related to the floor of the frontal sinus, it can still be drained endoscopically. A minitrephine is usually placed in the frontal sinus before dissection of the frontal recess. This aids in identification of the frontal outflow tract. The frontal recess is cleared and the frontal ostium identified. The lamina papyracea directly behind the the lacrimal sac is removed and using a curette, the orbital periostium is kept intact and gently pushed laterally while the curette advances into the subperiosteal abscess and the abscess drained (Wormald PJ, 2005).

A malleable suction (Medtronic Xomed, Jacksonville, Florida, USA) is introduced into the cavity and any fibrin within the cavity is removed. A corrugated Pendrose drain is slid into the abscess cavity and left in place, draining the abscess cavity into the ethmoid sinuses for 1 to 2 days before being endoscopically removed. Endoscopic removal of the subperiosteal abscess remains highly effective but it must be emphasized that the surgeon should be very experienced.

Although endoscopic drainage of subperiosteal and other orbital abcesses is becoming more common, the efficiency of narrow surgical drainage via an endoscopic approach has not been thoroughly been evaluated (Page and Wiatrak, 1996). Similarly, although endoscopic treatment of frontal sinus is less invasive than open frontal surgery, it also has a lower reported success rate (Metson and Gliklich, 1998).

Indications for CT scan

- Unable to accurately assess vision, gross proptosis, opthalmoplegia, deteriorating visual acuity or colour vision, bilateral edema, no improvement or deterioration at 24 hours or a swinging pyrexia that does not resolve within 36 hours

Tips for successful surgery

Endoscopic decompression of a subperiosteal abscess should only be performed by very experienced endoscopic sinus surgeons because the surgical field can be very bloody, which can significantly increase the degree of difficulty and the likelihood of complications. If the surgeon is not experienced, then the abscess should be drained via an external incision.

3.5 Endoscopic optic canal decompression

The most common indication for endoscopic optic canal decompression is traumatic optic nerve neuropathy(TON). Currently it is thought that 5% of severe head injuries will have concomitant injury to the optic nerve, optic tract or optic cortex (Tandon et al, 1994; Kountantakis et al, 2000; Kuppersmith et al, 1997). Since major brain injury takes precedence over traumatic optic neuropathy, it may result in the optic nerve injury being diagnosed somewhat later then the brain injury. Some authors feel that early diagnosis and treatment of traumatic optic neuropathy may be of greater benefit to the patient(Lubben et al, 2001, Sofferman, 1995) and advocate diagnosis of optic nerve deficit by the presence of an absolute or relative afferent pupillary defect supported by disc edema and congestion of the vessel walls. These findings in addition to CT scan and possibly MRI scan and visual evoked potentials are sufficient to undertake optic canal decompression. Currently there is no properly conducted randomized controlled trials comparing high-dose steroid therapy, surgical decompression and observation (Steinsapir et al, 2002).

Traumatic optic neuropathy is believed to result from two distinct injuries to the nerve. The primary injury is the result of either a direct contusive force on the optic canal and nerve or elastic deformation of the sphenoid, with transfer of the force on the intra-canalicular optic nerve disrupting the axons and blood vessels (Steinsapir & Goldberg, 1994). This primary injury may result in compression of the nerve by bony fragments or in hemorrhage into the nerve sheath. A secondary injury may occur if the primary injury is not treated in due time. Compression of the blood vessels occur if there is bleeding into the dura resulting in ischaemia and continued axon loss (Sofferman, 1995; Steinsapir & Goldberg, 1994).

We have adopted a conservative approach to traumatic neuropathy with all patients undergoing high-dose steroid treatment before being offered surgical intervention. The exception is when bony fragments are found to impinge on the optic nerve.

A randomized clinical trial demonstrated no benefit of either high-dose corticosteroids nor optic nerve decompression. Both are still employed because the alternative may be irreversible blindness. However, at the initial presentation, the visual performance of visual fields is correlated to the final outcome.

3.5.1 Medical therapy for traumatic optic neuropathy

Presently megadose intravenous methylprednisolone is helpful. Methylprednisolone 30mg/kg IV loading dose is given followed by 5.4 mg/kg/hr thereafter (Cook et al, 1996). The patient's visual acuity is monitored hourly and surgical intervention is considered if the patient shows or fails any of the criteria below:

- A dilated optic nerve on CT scan
- Fracture of optic canal on CT scan with vision less than 6/60
- Fracture of optic canal with vision more than 6/60 but the patient's vision deteriorates on steroids
- Vision is less than 6/60 after 48 hours of steroids with likely canal injury (indicated by the presence of fluid levels in the posterior ethmoids and sphenoids and/or the presence of fractures of the ethmoids, orbital apex and sphenoid).

3.5.2 Surgical therapy for traumatic optic neuropathy

Optic nerve decompression (OND) is an extension of orbital decompression when the optic nerve in the lateral wall of the sphenoid is decompressed.

3.5.3 Indications

Optic nerve injury is usually and should be recognized immediately by the existence of relative afferent papillary defect (RAPD) or inverse RAPD. It always appears in optic nerve injury even if visual acuity is relatively preserved initially. If it occurs in traumatic setting, the visual acuity will always deteriorate to no light perception. One should suspect this injury whether the ocular media are clear or opaque. It may be inappropriate for the patient to undergo surgery if they have a Glasgow coma scale of less than eight (Jones et al, 1997). Several studies suggest that with retro-orbital hemorrhage, decompression of the orbit needs to be done in less than one hour (Mason et al, 1998). However, where there is no hemorrhage, it is less understood under what circumstances it is beneficial to decompress the nerve pathway. If there is an anatomical constriction on CT scans affecting the course of the optic nerve and the patient is fit for anesthesia, then it seems reasonable to remove bone pressing on the nerve.

3.5.4 Useful instruments

- A long-shank drill with a course diamond burr and good irrigation system (Medtronic Xomed) to keep the bone cool.
- Image guided surgery

3.5.5 Surgical technique

The standard preparation of the nose is performed with decongestants and infilteration. An uncinectomy with exposure of the maxillary ostium is performed (Fig 25). An axillary flap is performed and the agger nasi cell removed for acess to skull base. The fovea ethmoidalis is exposed in the region above the bulla ethmoidalis. If there is disruption of the cells of the frontal recess, then this will be cleared. In some patients with severe sinus fracture, the entire skull base may be mobile.

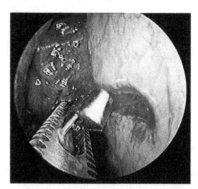

Fig. 25. A zero degree endoscopic view showing a left uncinectomy being performed

In majority of patients, the posterior ethmoid cells will be full of blood and when combined with mobility of lamina papyracea, the skull base surgeon can become disorientated. Thus, this surgery should be undertaken only by highly experienced endoscopic sinus surgeons. A posterior ethmoidectomy and sphenoidotomy should be performed. In the posterior ethmoids, the posterior lamina papyracea and fovea ethmoidalis should be identified. If significant disruption of the posterior ethmoids and lamina papyracea has occurred, then a large middle meatus antrostomy provides an extra reference point and lessens the likelihood of the surgeon becoming disorientated. The natural ostium of the sphenoid sinus should be identified and anterior face of the sphenoid widely opened.

The anterior face of the sphenoid needs to be taken as high as possible so that the roof of the sphenoid and the posterior ethmoids is continuous (Kuppersmith et al, 1997; Luxenberger et al, 1998; Chow and Stankiewicz, 1997). The sphenoid should be inspected and the optic nerve, carotid artery and pituitary fossa identified (Luxenberger et al, 1998; Chow and Stankiewicz, 1997). If there is significant disruption of the orbital apex or the lateral wall of the sphenoid, the identification of these basic structures can be difficult and image guidance may be helpful here.

The thick bone overlying the junction of the orbital apex and sphenoid sinus is known as the optic tubercle. This bone is normally too thick to flake off and an irrigated 15 degree angled diamond burr(Medtronic Xomed, Jacksonville, Florida, USA) is used to thin this bone down until it is almost transparent (Luxenberger et al, 1998; Chow and Stankiewicz, 1997). A blunt Free's elevator is pushed through the lamina papyracea 1.5 cm anterior to the junction of the posterior ethmoids air cell(s) and the sphenoid. While performing, care should be taken to keep the orbital periosteum intact, otherwise prolapsed of the orbital fat can severely obstruct the dissection of the optic nerve. The bone of the posterior orbital apex is flaxed off the underlying orbital periosteum (Luxenberger et al, 1998; Chow and Stankiewicz, 1997).

The bone over the optic canal is approached once the bone over the orbital apex is removed. This bone is usually quite thin and in majority of the cases can simply be flaked off the underlying nerve (Fig 26). Sometimes, the bone over the nerve can be too thick and will need to be thinned with diamond burr prior to removal. When the bone is thin enough to be flaked off the underlying nerve, suitable instruments like the Beale's elevator and the House curette, both from the ear tray should be used.

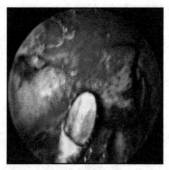

Fig. 26. A 45 degree endoscopic view showing bone being cleared off the optic canal with underlying optic nerve sheath clearly visible in a patient with traumatic optic neuropathy

When all the bone has been cleared off the optic canal and underlying optic nerve sheath is clearly visible, the sheath should be incised (Luxenberger et al, 1998; Chow and Stankiewicz, 1997). The location of the ophthalmic artery should be noted for it usually runs in the posteriorinferior quadrant of the nerve. Occassionally, this artery can migrate around the lower edge of the nerve and potentially into the surgical field (Steinsapir et al, 2002). However, if the nerve is incised in the upper medial quadrant, the risk to this artery should be minimal(Luxenberger et al, 1998; Chow et al, 1995). A sharp sickle knife is used to incise the sheath of the optic nerve. Usually the swollen nerve is under pressure and the sheath splits as it is incised and nerve will protrude through the incision.. The incision is continued onto the orbital periosteum of the posterior orbital apex with resultant protrusion of orbital fat. The orbital fat covering this area of the medial rectus muscle is thin and care should be taken to avoid injuring this muscle (Fig 27). No packs are placed on the nerve or in the sinuses.

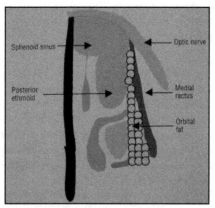

Fig. 27. A diagrammatic axial section of the paranasal sinuses and the orbit showing the anatomical relationship of the medial rectus muscle to fat and periorbita

It is vital to monitor the vision post-operatively quarter-hourly for one hour and then hourly for 4 hours. The immediate or early results of decompression are frequently extremely gratifying. The patient should be instructed not to blow their nose or sniffle sneezes for 4 days to avoid surgical emphysema.

Tips for successful surgery

Optic nerve decompression is a highly complex procedure and should be undertaken by endoscopic sinus surgeon with significant experience and skill. Potential injury to the skull base with a resultant CSF leak may occur and in addition an associated injury to the internal carotid artery may be present. Injudicious manipulation of bony fragments may have catastrophic consequences for the patient. A trial of medical therapy should be advocated before surgery is contemplated unless there is an obvious bony fragment impinging on the optic nerve. Literature review suggests that patients should be operated upon if medical therapy fails to improve the vision within 24 to 48 hours. Significant delays would seem to lessen the potential for success of the surgery. Great care should be considered in exposing the optic nerve especially when flaking the bone from the nerve. Injudicious use of inappropriate instruments has the potential to worsen the vision. In the hands of an experienced endoscopic sinus surgeon, this procedure is relatively safe with low morbidity and has the potential to improve and in some cases restore lost vision, especially after blunt trauma.

4. Endoscopic applications to the pterygopalatine and infratemporal fossa for resection of benign pathological lesions

The most common benign tumor involving the pterygo-palatine and infra-temporal fossa is the juvenile angiofibroma(Fig 28). These tumors originate in the region of spheno-palatine foramen and expand into pterygo-palatine fossa. Large tumors may extend into infra-temporal fossa and usually have a large intranasal component that may extend into nearby sinuses especially the sphenoid sinus. Other benign tumors in this region are inverting papilloma extending from the nasal cavity or rare tumors arising from the nerve sheath (schwannomas)(Fig 29), cartilage or muscle. Meningoceles extending into this area from the middle cranial fossa are rare.

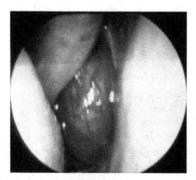

Fig. 28. Endoscopic view of a right juvenile angiofibroma in a teenage male presenting with recurrent epistaxis.

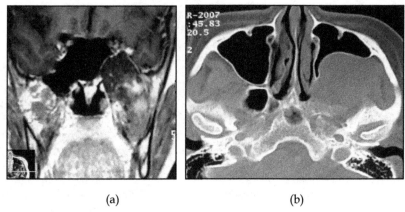

(a)   (b)

Fig. 29. A coronal(a) and axial(b) MRI view of the paranasal sinuses showing a left maxillary nerve schwanomma

4.1 Surgical technique for endoscopic modified medial maxillectomy

The nasal cavity is prepared by placing cocaine and adrenaline-soaked neuropatties in the nasal cavity. The lateral nasal wall and septum are infiltrated with 2% lidocaine and 1:80,000 adrenaline. Using 2 ml of lidocaine and adrenaline, a pterygo-palatine fossa block is placed via the greater palatine canal which greatly helps to reduce vascularity during dissection of medial wall of the maxilla and pterygo-palatine fossa.

The initial step in endoscopic modified medial maxillectomy is to remove the uncinate process and perform a large middle meatal antrostomy. Moreover, the maxillary antrum is enlarged posteriorly up to posterior wall of maxillary sinus. This provides visualization of the medial orbital wall and aids in removal of residual medial maxilla without endangering the orbit. Majority of tumors of maxillary sinus and pterygo-palatine fossa will involve the posterior ethmoids and sphenoid. The bulla ethmoidalis is removed and a posterior ethmoidectomy and sphenoidotomy are performed. The inferior turbinate is medialized and its posterior two-thirds removed. A right angled phako-knife is used to make mucosal incisions from just below the orbit, through the anterior one third of the inferior turbinate onto the floor of the nasal cavity. The incision is continued along the floor of the nose to the posterior region of the inferior turbinate and on to the maxillary sinus. A sharp chisel is used to cut the bone under the mucosal incisions

If the bone forming the medial maxillary wall is mobilized, the naso-lacrimal duct will tether the bone anteriorly and the duct will be visualized which can be transected with a scalpel (Fig 30). Subsequently, a DCR spear knife (Metronic Xomed) is used to open the lower half of the sac, creating an anterior and posterior flaps and rolling these out (Wormald et al, 2003; Wormald & van Hasselt, 2003; Vrabac, 1994). This prevents stenosis of the sac postoperatively (Wormald et al, 2003; Wormald & van Hasselt, 2003). The edges of the resected maxilla are cleaned with micro-debrider (Metronic Xomed). Using a 70 degree endoscope the entire maxillary sinus can be visualized including the anterior wall and floor. The tumor can now be removed from the maxillary sinus under direct vision. A canine fossa puncture can be performed, if additional access is required which can be useful to access areas within the sinus that may otherwise be difficult to access. Malleable suction dissector's are useful because these instruments can be bent to the required angle for dissection in difficult areas like the anterior wall or antero-lateral region of the lateral wall of maxillary sinus.

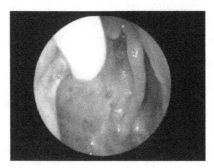

Fig. 30. A 30- degree endoscopic view showing evidence of right modified medial maxillectomy performed for an inverted papilloma.

4.2 Exposure of the pterygo-palatine fossa

Exposure of the pterygo-palatine fossa via a wide medial maxillary antrostomy is necessary for tumors the occupy the ptergo-palatine fossa and extending into the infra-temporal fossa. The mucosa from the posterior wall of the maxillary sinus is elevated and preserved and the exposed bone removed to access the pterygo-palatine fossa. A 45 degree through-bitting Blakesley forceps is used to remove the bone anterior to the spheno-palatine artery and continued to the posterior wall of the maxillary sinus exposing the contents of the pterygo-palatine fossa. Traction is vital for tumors that extend into the infra-temporal fossa because it allows the surgeon to identify the areas of attachment of the tumor to the surrounding tissues and to dissect these free with suction dissector. Thus the entire tumor can be mobilized and its pedicle identified.

Tumors that extend into the infra-temporal fossa will usually be closely associated with the maxillary nerve in the pterygo-palatine fossa. This nerve should be identified both distally and proximally early in the dissection and preserved. Suction dissection instruments are used to separate the nerve from the tumor. Fibrous tissue is easily divided with endoscopic soft tissue scissors.

Feeding blood vessels can either be cauterized with suction bipolar diathermy forceps or clipped and cut. Once the tumor is removed, the tumor bed can be closely inspected to ensure no tumor remnant remains. Once hemostasis is achieved with suction bipolar forceps, the preserved mucosa from the posterior wall of the maxillary sinus is replaced. Surgicel can be placed in the cavity if required. Finally, ensure that the lacrimal sac is adequately exposed to prevent postoperative stenosis and epiphora. The incidence of postoperative epiphora has been described as high as 30% (Bolger et al, 1992).

Endoscopic two-surgeon technique for tumors of the pterygo-palatine and infra-temporal fossa

The key to successful endoscopic removal of large tumors in this region is having two surgeons operating at the same time. This can be achieved by providing access to the tumor bed for the second surgeon through the septum from the opposite nasal cavity. A hemi-transfixation(Freer's) incision is made on the opposite site of tumor. Using standard septoplasty techniques, the mucosa is elevated off the cartilage of the septum which is preserved but most of posterior bony septum is resected. A horizontal incision is made in the opposite septal mucosa to allow instruments placed through the opposite nostril and into the Freer's incision to cross the septum and access the tumor on the contra-lateral side of the nose.

During tumor removal, the second surgeon can provide significant traction on the tumor and when the feeding vessel from the maxillary artery is cut, large volume suction in the field can allow the suction bipolar cautery to be used to identify and cauterize the large bleeding vessel.

4.3 Juvenile angiofibroma with pterygo-palatine and infra-temporal fossa extension

Angiofibromas that significantly extend into pterygopa-latine fossa can be removed after endonasal endoscopic medial maxillectomy (Kennedy et al, 1990) and embolization within the preceding 24 hours. This reduces the vascularity of the tumor and allows dissection around the tumor without major hemorrhage. The second surgeon can keep the surgical field clear using a large suction in the area of dissection while the other surgeon holds the telescope and suction dissection instrument.

4.4 Schwannoma involving the pterygo-palatine and infra-temporal fossa

Endoscoopic medial maxillectomy also provides access to other tumors that may involve the pterygo-palatine and infra-temporal fossa. Schwannoma of the maxillary nerve involves the entire ptrygo-palatine fossa and extends significantly into the infra-temporal fossa. Endoscopic medial maxillectomy allows access to the entire posterior wall of the maxillary sinus and after its removal, to the tumor.

4.5 Post-operative care

Douching of the nose with saline is started immediately postoperatively. Local and systemic antibiotics and corticosteroids are usually helpful. Crusting will usually continue for a few weeks until the cavity epithelializers but has not proved to be problematic in the long run. Benign tumors do not usually need any adjuvant treatment but malignant tumors may require postoperative radiotherapy.

5. Endoscopic resection of benign pathological lesions of paranasal sinuses

5.1 Mucoceles

Mucocele is a chronic, expansile, benign cystic lesion limited by the mucosa of the paranasal sinus, with thick, translucent mucous secretions (Fig 31). The most common are the frontoethmoidal mucoceles which presents with headaches and orbital symptoms. The expansile character of the mucocele promotes slow erosion of the adjacent bone via compression and consequent bone absorption. This disease is usually secondary to obstruction to sinus drainage, leading to stagnation of the secretion within the cavity. The predisposing factors can be fractures, mucosal edema, polyps, tumors, surgical trauma and chronic sinusitis. Mucoceles are classified according to the sinus of origin. The frontal sinus being the most common site, followed by the ethmoid, maxillary and sphenoid sinuses.

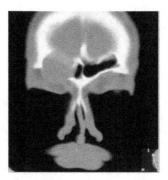

Fig. 31. Coronal CT imaging of the right frontal sinus with evidence of a right mucocele showing expansile erosion of right orbital floor with lateral extension

Fronto-ethmoidal sphenoidal and the rare maxillary sinus mucoceles are ideal cases for endoscopic approach provided wide marsupilization can be achieved (Hehar & Jones, 1997). Mucoceles accessible with the endoscope should be opened as widely as possible using through-cutting forceps in order to minimize the amount of scar tissue that forms around the edges and which might lead to recurrence. Coronal CT scan is helpful to show whether the lesion can be approached via the nasal cavity and whether it is unilocular or multilocular. In the frontal sinus, a small mucocele may be drained via the endoscopic approach (Fig 32) but mucoceles with lateral extension may be difficult to access via the nose. Therefore, an external and endoscopic approach can be usefully combined, preserving lateral support of the frontal recess and avoiding a stent.

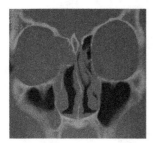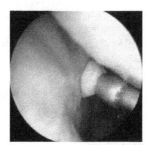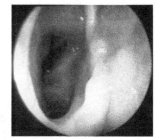

Fig. 32. Coronal CT imaging showing a right iatrogenic frontoethmoid mucocele and intraoperative endoscopic drainage and follow up a 3 months post surgery showing a patent frontal sinustomy in an adult presenting with frequent right headaches and heavy eyes

Preoperative evaluation of patients with frontal mucoceles should include careful evaluation of the lesion relative to the skull base. Endoscopic decompression is probably the best initial therapy for these lesions. It is particularly true of mucoceles that have eroded the posterior table of the frontal sinus and become adherent to the dura.An uncinectomy is performed with an axillary flap as advocated by Wormald PJ(2005). Often in surgery of these lesions, the skull base is identified within the posterior ethmoids and then followed anteriorly until the bone of the lesion is identified. The mucosal covered mass at the frontal recess area is opened with Blackesley's straight forceps (Stortz, Germany). As the lesion is approached or entered, mucoid or mucopurulent material is sucked out. The frontal sinustomy is enlarged upto about 2cm and the edges of exposed mucosa marsupilized. It is essential to remove all osteitic intersinus septa if recurrence of disease is to be avoided. If the bony margins are not flushed with the surrounding wall, narrowing of the opening, due to scarring and closure may occur (Kennedy et al, 1989). Once a frontal and/or ethmoid mucocele has been marsupilized, the expanded "shell" of bone that remains can be pushed manually to correct any bony swelling that may cause a cosmetic defect or displacement of the orbit intraoperatively. Sometimes a posteriorly placed mucocele may leave the orbit displaced even after marsupilization and then the orbit may need to be decompressed by removing its lateral wall (Conboy & Jones, 2003).

The majority of mucocels can be marsupilized endoscopically with minimal morbidity and long-term results as compared to other techniques. The wider the mococele is marsupilized, the better the result. Majority of mucoceles can be marsupilized well with the endoscope except those lying in the lateral aspect of the frontal sinus, those that are secondary to malignancy(require an en-bloc and a craniofacial resection) and those secondary to pathology like Paget disease of fibrous dysplasia (Kennedy et al, 1989; Beasley & Jones, 1995).

In the postoperative period, the mucosal lining the mucocele cavity may undergo significant hypertrophy and secretions may accumulate, necessitating suction from time to time. However, mucociliary clearance becomes reestablished, typically in a few weeks and the mucosal hypertrophy resolves over time (Kennedy et al, 1989). Hospitalization usually is less than 24 hours. As with other endoscopic sinus surgery, meticulous postoperative care is essential.

Relative contraindications for endoscopic marsupilization

- Abnormally thick bone (Paget's disease (Fig 33), fibrous dysplasia (Fig 34)).
- Revision surgery where an external fronto-ethmoidectomy was performed and if the recurrence is located lateral to area accessible via a median drainage procedure
- A laterally placed frontal mucocele
- Malignancy associated with a mucocele

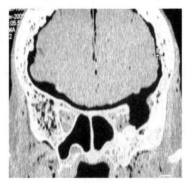

Fig. 33. A coronal CT scan view of paranasal sinuses and skull showing evidence of Pagets disease

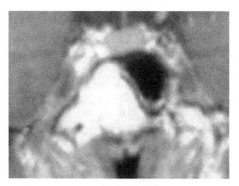

Fig. 34. A coronal CT scan of the paranasal sinuses showing evidence of fibrous dysplasia involving the sphenoid sinus

6. Endoscopic applications to the sellar, parasellar and clival for resection of benign pathological lesions

6.1 Endoscopic pituitary micro-adenoma and macro-adenoma surgery

6.1.1 The various approaches to the pituitary include

- Trans-septal, trans-sphenoidal
- Trans-nasal
- Transcolumellar approach(Fig 35)
- Via an external ethmoidectomy approach
- Through the upper buccal sulcus of the mouth and then trans-septal, trans-sphenoidal
- Via a craniotomy eg an anterolateral or a frontal approach

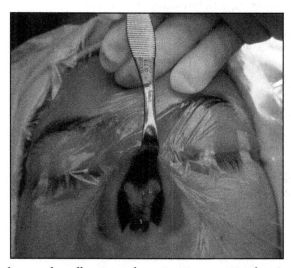

Fig. 35. A picture of transcolumella approach as an access route to the pituitary

6.1.2 Indications

Pituitary tumors occur in 9 in 10,000 pupulation and comprise 10% of intracranial tumors. The commonest pituitary tumors in patients under 35 years secrete prolactin and adrenocorticotropin whereas after 35 to 50 years they generally secrete growth hormone. In the latter, non-secreting tumors are more common. Symptoms can be caused by pressure on the anterior pituitary and hypo-pituitarism or by extra-sellar growth that can produce headaches, pressure on the optic chiasma or brain (Fig 36). Surgery is usually the treatment of choice. Surgery is the first-line treatment in acromegaly, where up to 90% of micro-adenomas are cured but the outcome is not as good as in large tumors.

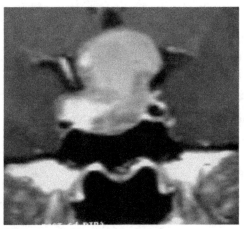

Fig. 36. A coronal MRI of the paranasal sinuses showing a suprasellar extension of a pituitary adenoma presenting with headaches and visual symptoms

Surgery for pituitary disease must be based on an assessment of the patient by a multidisciplinary team (Gendeh, 2006). The medical management of many pituitary tumors has reduced the frequency of the need for surgery in many patients. Medical management is rarely indicated in tumors that extend into the supra-sellar region and extending above the diaphragma sellae.

The endoscope gives excellent visibility within the sphenoid sinus and with a 45 degree endoscope it is possible to see more detail within the pituitary fossa than with the microscope. The advantages of the trans-nasal, trans-septal or lower buccal approach is that it avoids an external scar and by removing the posterior part of the septum, vomer and anterior wall of sphenoid, this approach allows wide access. In the endoscopic trans-nasal technique, mucosal preservation is an added advantage and allows the surgeon to work bimanually if necessary. The advantage of the two nostril technique is when there is moderate or severe bleeding, it can be controlled more readily. An external ethmoidectomy approach produces a scar and has the potential to cause stenosis of the frontal recess. Pituitary surgery has been routinely been performed with endoscopic endonasal approach at our referral center since 1990. (Gendeh, 2010)

6.1.3 Surgical anatomy

The vomer consistently joins the sphenoid in the mid-line and this is a very reliable landmark. The sphenoid inter-sinus septum is often asymmetric(more than 75%) and its essential to review the CT scans pre-operatively. The degree of pneumatization of the sphenoid sinus also varies greatly (Lang, 1989). A chonchal sinus is small and confined to the anterior aspect of the sphenoid in 5% of cases. A pre-sellar sinus extends to the coronal plane level with the anterior wall of the sphenoid in 28% of cases. In 67% of cases it is sellar type(Fig 37). Agenesis of the sphenoid sinus occurs in 0.7% of patients. The carotid artery bulges into its lateral wall and it can be dehiscent in up to 30% of patients. Axillary imaging cuts complement coronal sections and sagittal reconstruction helps. The natural sphenoid sinus is relatively high in the posterior wall of the sphenoid and is often placed at the level of the superior turbinate which may be readily visible after gentle lateralization of the middle turbinate. The bony anterior wall of the sphenoid sinus is often thin or deficient 1 to 1.5 cm above the posterior choana. The lateral wall of the sphenoid sinus has indentations from various structures (Fig 38):

- The optic nerve can indent its surface in the upper third
- The maxillary nerve can form an almost horizontal semicircular intrusion that may be mistaken for optic nerve in its medial third
- The degree of pneumatization of the sinus varies and influences how prominent structures are in its lateral wall. Pneumatization can extend to the clivus, the lesser wing and the root of the pterygoid process).
- The vidian nerve can bulge into its floor

1. Choncal (5%)
     - Common in children below 12 years
     - Area below sella is complete block of bone
2. Presellar (28%)
     - Posterior limit of air cavity is perpendicular to sella
3. Sellar (67%)
     - Commonest,
     - Air cavity extended into body of sphenoid below sella and may extend as posterior as clivus

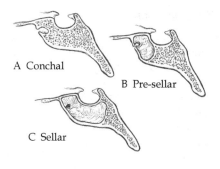

A Conchal

B Pre-sellar

C Sellar

Fig. 37. Types of sphenoid sinus pneumatization

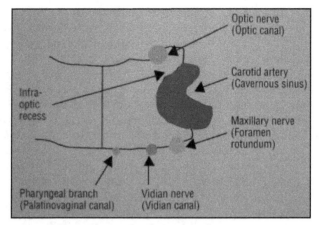

Fig. 38. A diagrammatic coronal section of the sphenoid sinus showing the anatomical indentaions of vital structures in its roof, lateral wall and floor.

6.1.4 Useful instruments

- Hajek-Koffler punch (Stortz, Germany) to remove thick bone. The rotating sleeve allows its jaws to be pointed in any direction and for the handle to be in a comfortable position for the operator
- A Kerrison punch (Stortz, Germany) allows fine controlled removal of small segments of bone and the slight reversed angle of its jaws help to remove the back of the vomer
- A long-shanked drill with a coarse diamond (Metronic Xomed) to remove any bone in the roof of the sphenoid bone in a controlled way
- A computer guided systems

6.1.5 Surgical technique

The trans-nasal endoscopic approach commences by making a sphenoidotomy on the side of the tumor or when it is in the midline opening, the side where the sinus is larger. The sphenoidotomy is opened up to the level of the skull base using a sphenoid punch. Suction diathermy will be needed to stop the bleeding from the posterior branch of spheno-palatine artery when opening the sphenoidotomy inferiorly. Any vomerine spur should be removed. After careful CT examination and endoscopically inspecting the sphenoid sinus to check on the proximity of the lateral structures, the lateral aspect of the anterior wall can be removed if necessary. A Kerrison antrum punch (Stortz, Germany) is useful for performing this as its small diameter means that the bone can be removed in small pieces with good visibility. If more space is required across the midline, the vomer can be fractured across or it can be incised 1cm in front of the sphenoid and removed. The vomer can be very thick where it joins the sphenoid but it rarely needs drilling (Fig 39). The pituitary often bulges into the roof of the sphenoid and the bone may be very thin (Fig 40). If the bone is thick, a course diamond burr (Metronic Xomed) should be used to thin it. A diathermy point is useful to open the dura by making a cross-shaped incision through it. A 45 degree endoscope gives excellent visibility and helps to avoid going through the diaphragm sellae. A Hajek punch (Stortz, Germany) helps to remove the bone over the pituitary. The tumor is often grey in colour, but occasional it can be vascular and ooze moderately. The pituitary fossa can be closed at the end of the procedure with raised naso-septal flap placed onto the bony defect. If there is a CSF leak, in addition an underlay duragen(collagen matrix graft) is placed before a naso-septal flap is placed as overlay flap and secured in position by Tisseel and gel-foam over it.

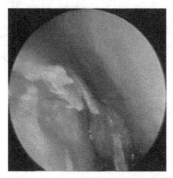

Fig. 39. Intraoperative endoscopic view showing a transseptal transsphenoidal approach to pituitary adenoma exposing the sphenoid rostrum

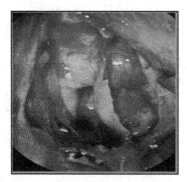

Fig. 40. A 45 degree endoscopic view of exposed sphenoid sinus showing a intersinus septum and an enlarged sella

It is possible to approach the pituitary via a limited sphenoidotomy, although it reduces access and visibility. It may be useful to trim the middle turbinate on one side for better access and visibility utilizing a four hand technique.

7. Endoscopic repair of skull base CSF fistula

CSF leak results from a breach in the dura, which may be spontaneous, secondary to a fracture, related to a surgical trauma or associated with pathology of the skull base and/or secondary to a high-pressure system (Fig 41).

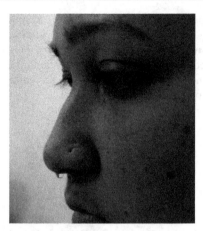

Fig. 41. Picture of an adult obese female presenting with unilateral clear watery spontaneous CSF rhinorrhoea on exertion

7.1 Indications

The main indications for repairing a CSF leak is its association with a 10% risk per year of developing meningitis (Gendeh et al, 1998). Those who have a leak from a fracture of the anterior skull base repaired still have a slightly increased risk of developing meningitis in the future but this is less than those whose leak stops spontaneously. Therefore, active leaks should probably be repaired at any stage.

7.2 Surgical anatomy

The skull base is made up anteriorly of the posterior wall of the frontal sinus, which is a thick frontal bone that extends posteriorly to form roof of ethmoid sinuses(fovea ethmoidalis) on either side of the cribriform plate. The cribriform plate joins the fovea through the lateral lamella and can be almost non-existent when the cribriform plate and fovea ethmoidalis are on the same plane or it can form the thin vertical bone connecting them, depending on how far the cribriform plate dips into the nose (Fig 42). Posteriorly, the sphenoid sinus and posterior ethmoidal air cells form the inferior relationship of the skull base.

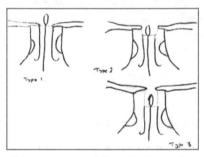

Fig. 42. Keros classification of the anatomy of the cribriform plate which may lie at different level in relation to the anterior skull base

The commonest site of a spontaneous CSF leak is the area of the cribriform plate where dura around the olfactory nerves appears to have extended through the cribriform plate and ruptured (Fig 43). The next most commonest leak is from a very well-pneumatized sphenoid sinus (Fig 44). A high-pressure system may be a contributing factor in these cases and a shunt or venrticulostomy may be required.

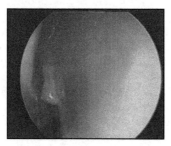

Fig. 43. Intraoperative endoscopic view showing arachnoid granulations arising from the left cribriform area in an obese female presenting with spontaneous cerebro-spina fluid rhinorrhea

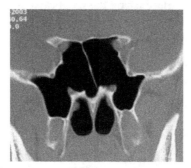

Fig. 44. A coronal CT scan showing a well pneumatized sphenoid sinus

Iatrogenic CSF leaks are often found around the lamina lateralis (the vertical thin bone joining the cribriform plate to the fovea ethmoidalis) near the anterior ethmoidal artery. Post neurosurgical procedure leaks most commonly follow pituitary surgery, come from the posterior wall of frontal sinus when it has not been cranialized and more likely if a peri-cranial flap has not been used to repair any dural defect.

7.3 Diagnosis

- It is vital to localize the site of a leak (Marshall et al, 2001)
- Fluid collected should be tested for immune-fixation of beta-2-transferrin
- Rule out any high- pressure system leak
- Successful closure depends on localizing the exact site of the fistula

It is essential to confirm the diagnosis with immune-fixation of beta-2-transferrin which is extremely specific and sensitive test (Eljamel, 1993). Unilateral autonomic rhinitis is unusual but can mimic CSF rhinorrhea.

Site of any defect should be defined using high-resolution coronal CT (Lloyd et al, 1994). If CT fails to define the site of the defect, T2-weighted MRI may help which has superseded CT cisternography (Stafford et al, 1996). In a few post-trauma patients the site of leak is uncertain or it could be that there is more than one leak. In dural defects less than 15mm, the 'bath plug' technique is encouraged which consists of introducing a fat plug with vicryl suture into the intra-dural space (Wormald & McDonough, 1997) It is believed that this technique would prevent high pressure from pushing the graft away from the defect (Gendeh et al, 2002). The fat pug can be harvested from the ear lobule. A 4 0 vicryl suture is knotted through one end of the fat plug and the suture is passed down the length of the fat plug. A free mucosal graft about 3 x 3 cm is harvested anterior to the middle turbinate from the contralateral lateral nasal wall. The fat plug is placed below the defect and the malleable frontal sinus probe (Metronic Xomed, Jacksonville, Florida, USA) is used gently to introduce the fat plug through the defect (Wormald and McDonough, 1997). Once the fat plug has been safely introduced through the defect, the plug is stabilized with the probe and the vicryl suture is gently pulled. The seal is tested by placing the patient head down and asking the anaesthetist to perform a forced-inspiration maneuver. No Fluorescein-stained CSF should be seen. The patient is placed head-up (15 degrees) and the free mucosal graft is slid up the vicryl suture until it covers the defect (Fig 45). Ensure that the graft is correctly orientated with the mucosal surface facing the nasal cavity. Fibrin glue is applied and the vicryl suture cut. Gelfoam is placed over the free mucosal graft and fibrin glue is reapplied. No other nasal packing is used.

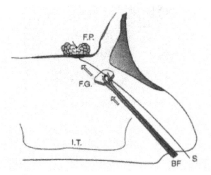

Fig. 45. A diagrammatic sagittal section of the nose showing the a free mucosal graft being slid up the vicry suture to cover the protruding fat plug and skull base defect. Adapted with permission from Wormald and McDonough. Americal J Rhinol 2003; 17:299-305

A diagnostic or pre-operative sodium fluorescein lumbar puncture will help define the source of leak(Fig 46 a). It is vital to ensure that there is a free flow of CSF before proceeding to inject any sodium fluorescein. The patient was skin tested with 2% sodium flourescein eye drops one day before surgery. A lumbar drain was inserted on the day of surgery and intrathecal sodium fluorescein 10%(0.1% of sodium flourescein is diluted with 10ml of withdrawn CSF) was given in a slow bolus over 10 minutes to identify site of fistula (Gendeh et al, 2005). The ideal time for the sodium fluorescein to be injected is one hour beforehand. It is a great help to place the patient in a 10 degree head-down position. The fluid will appear bright yellow, unless a blue filter is used when it appears fluorescent green (Fig 46 b). The systemic clearance of fluorescein is essentially complete by 48 to 72 hours from the patient's body.

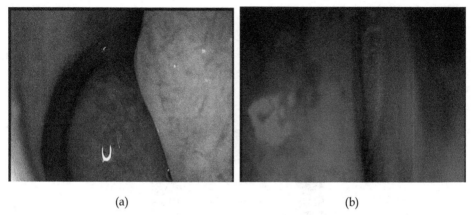

(a)   (b)

Fig. 46. A 30 degrees endoscopic view showing a spontaneous CSF leak from the anterior cribriform plate using intrathecal sodium fluorescein(a) and highlighted using blue blue filter(b) in the same patient

The adverse reactions of intrathecal fluorescein administration are nausea, vomiting, gastrointestinal distress, headache, syncome and hypotention. Cardiac arrest, basilar artery ischaemia, severe shock, convultions, thrombophlebitis at the injection site and rare cases of death have been reported.

7.4 Surgical technique

Initially the repair of CSF fistula involved the use of multi-layered barrier comprised of free tissue grafts harvested from the nasal perichondrium or temporalis fascia. On top of the on lay graft, an abdominal fat graft was used as a bolster and a biological dressing. A fibrin sealant was applied to help fixate the fat graft. Sponge packing (Merocel tampons) were placed intra-nasally to support the fat graft and provide some compression.

We adopted the use of collagen matrix graft (duragen, Intra Life Sciences, USA), which was easy to maneuver, is soft and pliable, thus decreasing the risk of injuring any critical structures as we tuck the graft to overlap the surrounding dural edges of the defect. Duragen is an absorbable and sutureless collagen onlay indicated as dura substitute for the repair of dura mater. We eliminated the routine use of lumbar drains and reserved them for high-risk situations or secondary repairs.

The latest intervention to decrease CSF leaks employs vascularized mucosal flaps which hastens the healing process, especially in patients with prior radiation therapy and make patients more suitable for early postoperative radiation therapy. Hadad and Bassagasteguy from Argentina developed the nasoseptal flap, supplied by the posterior nasoseptal arteries which are branches of the posterior nasal artery. A mucoperichondrial/mucoperiosteal flap pedicle on the posterior nasal arteries provides a long flap that has a wide arc of rotation and a potential for area of coverage that is superior to any other flap previously described(Fig 47). The flap may be harvested to cover the entire anterior skull base from the frontal sinus to the sella or cover a clival defect from the sella to second cervical vertebra (C2). Use of this flap has to be anticipated in advance, since a posterior septectomy and a wide large slphenoidotomy removes the vascular pedicle. This flap is very reliable and is typically positioned over a fascial graft or fat graft and held in place with fibrin glue and a balloon catheter. We have not observed any significant donor site morbidity with the use of this flap and the septum becomes remucosalized within several months of surgery

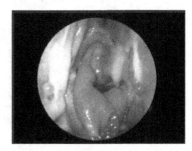

Fig. 47. Endoscopic view of a healed nasoseptal flap repair at 3 months post surgery for a pituitary macroadenoma with evidence of CSF fistula

8. Recent advances in technology and its application to anterior and ventral skull base lesions

There is an ongoing revolution in multiple surgical specialties with the introduction of minimally invasive techniques. A natural extension of ESS has been the application of endoscopic techniques for the surgical treatment of pathologic conditions of the cranial base. This has been driven by the ongoing development of endoscopic technology increasing consumer demand. Furthermore, as the limits of ESS is tested, the possibilities for cranial base surgery are expanded. Truly, it is a maximally invasive endoscopic surgery than minimally invasive surgery.

The Expanded Endo-nasal Approach(EEA) to the ventral skull base provides endoscopic access from the frontal sinus to C2 in the sagittal plane and from the midline to the jugular foramen, internal acoustic canal(IAC) and lateral mass of C2 in the coronal plane (Fig 48). Potential advantages of the EEA not only include improved cosmesis but more importantly, the potential for much less neurovascular manipulation in well selected cases. In pediatric patients, preservation of facial skeleton avoids disruption of growth centers and development of facial asymmetry with further growth. In contrast to an intracranial approach, an endo-nasal approach avoids the need for any brain retraction and may result in less damage to brain tissue. Improved visualization and better access to difficult sites may result in improved oncological outcomes.

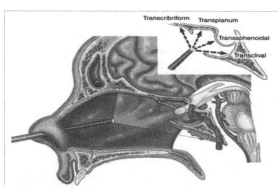

Slide Courtesy of the Pittsburgh Otolaryngologists & Neurosurgical team

Fig. 48. Expanded endonasal approaches to base of skull

Advances in cranial base surgery over the last two decades have only been possible with the collaboration of multiple surgical specialities (Kassam et al, 2007). This is more obvious with endoscopic skull base surgery. Rather than working sequentially as is often done with open approaches, surgeons from different speciality work together simultaneously as a team: one person maintaining a view with the endoscope and the other working bimanually to dissect the tissues. The benefits of the two team surgery include improved visualization, increased efficiency and the ability to deal with a crisis such as vascular injury. There is added value of having a 'co-pilot' for problem solving, avoiding complications and modulating enthusiasm.

The primary advantage of the endoscope compared to other methods is improved visualization which accounts for an increased access to difficult to reach areas and may facilitate complete tumor resection and avoidance of complications due to poor visualization. Other potential benefits of endoscopic surgery include improved cosmesis and decreased morbidity from tissue trauma and manipulation of vessels and nerves. The consequences of decreased morbidity are a faster recovery, shortened hospitalization and decreased cost of medical care (Gendeh, 2009).

Familiarity with endoscopic anatomy, proper instrumentation, an experienced surgical team and adherence to endoscopic surgical principles are essential ingredients for avoiding severe complications. The basic principle of endoscopic cranial base surgery is internal debulking of tumor to allow extra-capsular dissection of tumor margin with early identification of neural and vascular structures. This principle is the same for open neurosurgical procedures and sharp dissection of tumor margins is performed without pulling on tumor. Adherence to these fundamental principles minimizes the risk of neural or vascular injury.

In the late 1970s and early 1980s, the combined effort between the Otolaryngologist and neurosurgeons worldwide, made significant strides in the surgical removal of tumors at the base of the skull and brain. These procedures were however disfiguring and painful for the patient. Furthermore, patients encountered long recovery periods and significant risk of complications because the procedures involved large incisions in the face and scalp and removal of parts of the skull to reach the abnormality at the cranial base.

In 1998, a group of Otolaryngologist and neurosurgeons at UPMC in Pittsburgh, USA initiated the first systemic approach to using the nose as a minimally invasive passageway to the brain. They began the extensive process of mapping anatomy and in collaboration with the medical device manufacturers, designed new instruments to make this idea a reality.

By 2000, the Pittsburgh team of doctors had developed the necessary tools and techniques to access tumors located inside the skull by the way of the nose known as EEA. In EEA, the surgeons use endoscopes with light source as well as other instruments especially designed, to treat various types of brain and spinal abnormality. Hence, today surgeons can take out baseball-sized growths without pulling on the brain or touching the normal tissue. This continued refinement of EEA now allows access to an expanded region of the brain, skull base and spine. The classification of endoscopic approaches to cranial base are listed in Table 3.

SAGGITAL PLANE

- Transfrontal
- Transcribriform
- Transplanum (Suprasellar/Subchiasmatic
- Transsphenoidal (Sellar/Medial transcavernous)
- Transclival
  - o Posterior clinoid
  - o Mid-clivus
  - o Foramen magnum
- Transodontoid

CORONAL PLANE

- Transorbital
- Petrous apex (Medial transpetrous)
- Lateral transcavernous
- Transpterygoid
- Transpetrous
  - o Superior
  - o Inferior
- Transcondylar
- Parapharyngeal space

Snyderman CH.2007. Acquisation of surgical skills for endonasal skull base surgery: a training program. Laryngoscope 117(4): 699-705

Table 3. Classification of endoscopic approaches to cranial base

The collaborative effort has put the Otolaryngologist and the neurosurgeon to work closely via the nose using the two-nostril and four hand technique was first advocated by Prof. Dr Heinz Stammberger from Graz, Austria for endoscopic cranial base surgery.

Standardization of training and the adoption of modular, incremental training program are expected to facilitate the gradual training of endo-nasal surgeons in Otolaryngology and Neurosurgical disciplines. Stages of training are established for both surgical speciality based on level of technical difficulty, potential risk of vascular and neural injury and unfamiliar endoscopic anatomy. Mastery of each level is recommended before attempting procedures at higher level. Adherence to such a program during the growth phase of endoscopic skull base surgery may decrease the risk of complications as the surgeon's knowledge and surgical expertise develop (Snyderman et al, 2007).

Complications of EEA are the same as open approaches: neural and vascular injury, infection and CSF leak. Literature report of neural and vascular injury are fortunately rare accounting for 1% incidence. These can be avoided with attention to anatomical landmarks and proper dissection techniques. An experienced team can effectively control venous bleeding from the cavernous sinus or basilar plexus. Peri-operative antibiotic prophylaxis, multilayered repair of dural defects and aggressive management of postoperative CSF leaks are contributing factors. One of the biggest remaining challenges is repair of large dural defects and prevention of post-operative leaks. With the advent of the septal mucosal flap, the Pittsburgh group suggest an incidence of 6% of CSF leak. Developments that have decreased the incidence of postoperative CSF leaks include a multilayered closure, direct suturing of grafts to dural edges, use of biological glues, coverage with vascularized septal mucosal flap and supporting the reconstruction with an intranasal balloon catheter.

9. Acknowledgements

I wish to acknowledge with gratitude the co-operation of the Departments of Otorhinolaryngology - Head and Neck Surgery, Neurosurgery, Endocrinology and Ophthalmology of the National University Malaysia Medical Faculty (UKMMC).

10. References

Beasley N and Jones NS. 1995. The role of endoscopy in the management of mucoceles. *American Journal of Rhinology* 9(5): 251-256

Bolger WE, Parsons DS, Mair EA, Kuhn FA. 1992. Lacrimal drainage system injury in functional endoscopic sinus surgery: Incidence, analysis and preventions. *Archives of Otolaryngol Head Neck Surg* 118(11): 1179-1184

Bolger WE and Mann CB. 2001. Analysis of the suprabullar and retrobullar recesses for endoscopic sinus surgery. *Annals of Otology, Rhinology and Laryngology* Supplement 186 110(5 part 2): 3-14

Chow PI,Sadun A, Lee H. 1995. Vascular and morpheometry of the optic canal and intracanalicular optic nerve. *J Neuroopthalmol* 15: 186-190

Chow J and Stankiewicz. 1997. Powered instrumentation in orbital and optic nerve decompression. *Otolaryngol Clin North Am* 30: 467-478

Conboy PJ and Jones. 2003. The place of endoscopic sinus surgery in the treatment of paranasal sinus mucoceles. *Clin Otolaryngol* 28: 207-210

Cook M, Levin L, Joseph M, Pinczower E. 1996. Traumatic optic neuropathy: a meta-analysis. *Arch Otolaryngol Head Neck Surg* 122: 389-392

Eljamel MSM. 1993. The role of surgery and beta-2-transferrin in the management of cerebrospinal fluid fistula. *MD thesis*. University of Liverpool.

Gendeh, B.S, Selladurai B.M, Selvapragasam T, Khalid B.A.K, Said H. 1998. The transseptal approaches to pituitary tumours: Technique, rhinologic functions and complications *Asian J Surgery* 21(4): 259-265

Gendeh BS, Wormald PJ, Forer M, Goh BS, Misiran K. 2002. Endoscopic repair of spontaneous cerebro-spinal fluid rhinorrhoea: a report of 3 cases. *Med J Malaysia* 57(4): 503-508

Gendeh BS, Mazita A, Selladurai BM, Jegan T, Jeevanan J, Misiran K. 2005. Endoscopic repair of Anterior Skull Base Fistula: The Kuala Lumpur Experience. *J Laryngol Otol* 119: 866-874

Gendeh BS. 2006. Minimally invasive surgical approaches to the sphenoid sinus, sell, parasellar and clival region. Current and future perspectives. *Med J Malaysia* 61(3); 274-277

Gendeh BS, Salina H, Selladurai B, Jagan T. 2007. Endoscopic assisted craniofacial resection: A case series and post-operative outcome. *Med J Malaysia*   62(3); 234-237

Gendeh BS. 2010. Extended applications of endoscopic sinus surgery and its reference to cranial base and pituiatary fossa. *Indian J Otolaryngol Head Neck Surg* 62: S 68-S 80.

Gendeh BS, 2009. Advances in technology and its application to rhinology. In Gendeh BS Ed. Clinical atlas of nasal endoscopy. *UKM Publication*. Pg 114-117

Hartstein ME, Kokoska M. Woog JJ. 2004. Endoscopic techniques in orbital fracture repair. In Woog JJ, ed *Manual of endoscopic lacrimal and orbital surgery*. Butterworth Heinemann, pp 175-182.

Hehar SS and Jones NS. 1997. Fronto-ethmoidal osteoma: the place of surgery. *J Laryngol Otol* 111: 372-375

Howe L and JonesNS. 2004. Guidelines for the management of periorbital cellulitis/abcess. *Clin Otolaryngol* 29: 725-728

Ikeda K, Suzuki H, Oshima T, Tomonori T. 1999. Endoscopic endonasal repair of orbital floor fracture. *Arch Otolaryngology Head Neck Surg* 125; 59-63

Jones NS. 1997. Visual evoked potentials in endoscopic and anterior skull base surgery. *Journal of Laryngol and Otology* 111: 513-516(OMIT)

Jones NS, Bullock P, Hewitt s et al. 1997. Head injuries and the principles of craniofacial repair. In Jones NS, ed. *Craniofacial Trauma: An interdisciplinary approach.* Oxford: Oxford University Press, pp. 18-60

Jones NS. 1998. Microendoscopy in rhinology. *Minimally Invasive Therapy and Allied Technologies* 7: 149-154

Jones NS. 1999. Current concepts in the management of paediatric rhinosinusitis. *Journal of Laryngology and Otology* 113: 1-9

Kassam A, Snyderman, CH and Carrau RL et el. 2007.Introduction, Conclusion. In *The Expanded Endonasal Approach to the Ventral Skull Base: Sagittal Plane*, edited by Snyderman CH. Tuttlingen: Endo-Press

Kennedy DW. 1985. Functional endoscopic sinus surgery technique. *Arch Otolaryngol Head Neck Surgery* 111:643-649

Kennedy DW, Josephson JS, Zinreich SJ, Mattox DE, Goldsmith MM. 1989. Endoscopic sinus surgery for mucoceles: a variable alternative. *Laryngoscope* 99:885-889

Kennedy D.W, Goodstein M.L, Miller N.R, Zinreich. S.J. 1990. Endoscopic transnasal orbit decompression. *Archives of Otolaryngology Head and Neck Surgery*. 116: 275-282

Khairullah A, Gendeh BS. 2011. Tube extrusion and cheese wiring 5 years post dacryocytorhinostomy: case report. *Phillipine Intn J of Otolaryngol* 26(2): 34-36

Kountantakis S, Maillard A, El-Harazi S, Longhini L, Urso R. 2000. Endoscopic optic nerve decompression for traumatic blidness. *Otolaryngology Head Neck Surg* 123: 34-37

Kuppersmith R, Alford E, Patrinely J, Lee A, Parke R, Holds J. 1997. Combined transconjunctival/intranasal endoscopic approach to the optic canal in traumatic optic neuropathy. *Laryngoscope* 107: 311-315

Lang J. 1989. *Clinical anatomy of the nose, nasal cavity and paranasal sinuses*. Stuttgart: Georg Thieme Verlag

Lee TS, Shin JC, Woog JJ. 2004. Endoscopic dacryocystorhinostomy: An eastern perspective. In Woog JJ, ed *Manual of endoscopic lacrimal and orbital surgery*. Butterworth Heinemann, pp 123-133.

Lubben B, Stoll W, Grenzebach U. 2001. Optic nerve decompression in the comatose and conscious patients after trauma. *Laryngoscope* 111: 320-328

Luxenberger W, Stammberger H, Jebeles J, Walch C. 1998. Endoscopic optic nerve decompression: The graz experience. *Larygoscope* 108: 873-882

Marshall A, Jones NS, Robertson IJA. 2001. CSF rhinorrhoea: a multidisciplinary approach to minimise patient morbidity. *British Journal of Neurosurgery* 15(1): 8-13

Mason JDT, Haynes RJ, Jones NS. 1998. Interpretation of the dilated pupil during endoscopic sinus surgery *J of Laryngol and Otology* 112: 622-627

Metson R, Dallow R, Shore J. 1994. Endoscopic orbital decompression. *Laryngoscope* 104: 950-957.

Metson R, Gliklich RE. 1998. Clinical outcomes of endoscopic surgery for frontal sinusitis. *Otolaryngol Head Neck Surg* 124(10): 1090-1096

Metson R, Samaha M. 2002. Reduction of diplopia following endoscopic orbital decompression: The orbital sling technique. *Laryngoscope* 112: 1753-1757

Metson R, Samaha M. 2004. Endoscopic orbital decompression. In *Manual of endoscopic lacrimal and orbital surgery*. Editor Woog JJ. Butterworth Heinemann, Elsevier, pg 167-173

Page EL,Wiatrak BJ. 1996. Endoscopic versus external drainage of orbital subperiosteal abscess. *Arch Otolaryngol Head Neck Surg* 122(7): 737-740

Setliff R.C. 1994. The "Hummer": New instrumentation for functional endoscopic sinus surgery. *Am J Rhinol*. 8: 275-278.

Sofferman B. 1995. The recovery potential of the optic nerve. *Laryngoscope* 105: 1-38

Stafford JDB, Brenan P, Toland J, O'Dwyer AJ. 1996. Magnetic resonance imaging in the evaluation of cerebrospinal fluid fistula. *Clinical Radiology* 51:837-841

Stammberger H. 1991. *Functional endoscopic sinus surgery*: The Messerklinger Technique. Philadelphia: Brian C Decker

Steinsapir K, Goldberg R. 1994. Traumatic optic neuropathy. *Surv Opthalmol* 38: 487-518

Steinsapir K, Seiff S, Goldberg R. 2002. Traumatic optic neuropathy: where do we stand? *Ophthal Plast Reconstr Surg* 18: 232-234

Snyderman CH, Kassam A and Carrau RL et al. 2007. Acquisition of Surgical Skills for Endonasal Skull Base Surgery: A Training Program. *Laryngoscope* 117: 699-705

Tandon DA,Thakar A, Mahapatra AK, Ghosh P. 1994. Transethmoid optic nerve decompression. *Clin Otolaryngol* 19: 98-104

Umapathy N, Kalra S, Skinner DW, Dapling RB. 2006. Long-term results of endonasal laser dacrocystorhinostomy. *Otolaryngol Head Neck Surgery* 135(1): 81-84

Vrabac DP. 1994. The inverted Schneiderian papilloma: a 25 year study. *Laryngoscope* 104: 582-605

Woog JJ. 2004.Endoscopic dacryocystorhinostomy and conjunctivodacryostorhinostomy. In Woog JJ, ed *Manual of endoscopic lacrimal and orbital surgery*. Butterworth Heinemann, pg 105-121.

Wormald P, McDonough M. 1997. Bath plug technique for the endoscopic management of cerebrospinal fluid leaks. *J Laryngol Otol* 111: 1042-1046

Wormald P.J. 2002. Powered endoscopic dacryocystorhinostomy. *Laryngoscope.* 112(1): 69-72.

Wormald PJ and van Hasselt CA. 2003. Endoscopic removal of juvenile angiofibroma. *Otolaryngol Head Neck Surgery* 129: 684-691

Wormald PJ, Ooi E, van Hasselt CA, Nair S. 2003. Endoscopic removal of sinonasal inverted papilloma including endoscopic medial maxillectomy. *Laryngoscope* 113: 867-873

Wormald PJ. 2005. Endoscopic orbital decompression for exopthalmos, acute orbital hemorrhage and orbital subperiosteal abscess. In Wormald PJ, ed. *Endoscopic sinus surgery: Anatomy, three-dimentional reconstruction and surgical technique*. Thieme Medicl Publishes, Inc, New York. Stuttgart, pg135-140

Permissions

The contributors of this book come from diverse backgrounds, making this book a truly international effort. This book will bring forth new frontiers with its revolutionizing research information and detailed analysis of the nascent developments around the world.

We would like to thank Shimon Rumelt, MD, MPA, for lending his expertise to make the book truly unique. He has played a crucial role in the development of this book. Without his invaluable contribution this book wouldn't have been possible. He has made vital efforts to compile up to date information on the varied aspects of this subject to make this book a valuable addition to the collection of many professionals and students.

This book was conceptualized with the vision of imparting up-to-date information and advanced data in this field. To ensure the same, a matchless editorial board was set up. Every individual on the board went through rigorous rounds of assessment to prove their worth. After which they invested a large part of their time researching and compiling the most relevant data for our readers. Conferences and sessions were held from time to time between the editorial board and the contributing authors to present the data in the most comprehensible form. The editorial team has worked tirelessly to provide valuable and valid information to help people across the globe.

Every chapter published in this book has been scrutinized by our experts. Their significance has been extensively debated. The topics covered herein carry significant findings which will fuel the growth of the discipline. They may even be implemented as practical applications or may be referred to as a beginning point for another development. Chapters in this book were first published by InTech; hereby published with permission under the Creative Commons Attribution License or equivalent.

The editorial board has been involved in producing this book since its inception. They have spent rigorous hours researching and exploring the diverse topics which have resulted in the successful publishing of this book. They have passed on their knowledge of decades through this book. To expedite this challenging task, the publisher supported the team at every step. A small team of assistant editors was also appointed to further simplify the editing procedure and attain best results for the readers.

Our editorial team has been hand-picked from every corner of the world. Their multi-ethnicity adds dynamic inputs to the discussions which result in innovative outcomes. These outcomes are then further discussed with the researchers and contributors who give their valuable feedback and opinion regarding the same. The feedback is then collaborated with the researches and they are edited in a comprehensive manner to aid the understanding of the subject.

Apart from the editorial board, the designing team has also invested a significant amount of their time in understanding the subject and creating the most relevant covers. They scrutinized every image to scout for the most suitable representation of the subject and create an appropriate cover for the book.

The publishing team has been involved in this book since its early stages. They were actively engaged in every process, be it collecting the data, connecting with the contributors or procuring relevant information. The team has been an ardent support to the editorial, designing and production team. Their endless efforts to recruit the best for this project, has resulted in the accomplishment of this book. They are a veteran in the field of academics and their pool of knowledge is as vast as their experience in printing. Their expertise and guidance has proved useful at every step. Their uncompromising quality standards have made this book an exceptional effort. Their encouragement from time to time has been an inspiration for everyone.

The publisher and the editorial board hope that this book will prove to be a valuable piece of knowledge for researchers, students, practitioners and scholars across the globe.

List of Contributors

Irina Gout, Faye Mellington, Vikas Tah
Mahmoud Sarhan, Sofia Rokerya, Michael Goldacre and Ahmed El-Amir, Oxford University, England

Xiao-Xu Zhou and Jian-Guo Wu
Tianjin Medical University Eye Center, Tianjin, People's Republic of China

Yan-Ping Song, Yu-Xing Zhao and Jian-Guo Wu
Department of Ophthalmology of PLA Wuhan General Hospital, Wuhan, People's Republic of China

Mario Bradvica, Tvrtka Benašić and Maja Vinković
University of Josip Juraj Strossmayer, Medical School Osijek, University Hospital Osijek, Croatia

Irina Golovleva and Marie Burstedt
University Hospital of Umeå, Umeå, Sweden

Qianying Gao
State Key Laboratory of Ophthalmology, Zhongshan Ophthalmic Center, Sun Yat-sen University, Guangzhou, China

Phillip S. Coburn and Michelle C. Callegan
University of Oklahoma Health Sciences Center, Dean McGee Eye Institute, Oklahoma City, Oklahoma, USA

Venugopal Gunda and Yakkanti A. Sudhakar
Cell Signaling, Retinal and Tumor Angiogenesis Laboratory, Department of Genetics, Boys Town National Research Hospital, Omaha, NE, USA

Yakkanti A. Sudhakar
Department of Biochemistry and Molecular Biology, University of Nebraska Medical Center, Omaha, NE, USA

Yan Chen, Zhenyang Zhao, Paul Sternberg and Jiyang Cai
Vanderbilt Eye Institute, Vanderbilt University Medical Center, Nashville, TN, USA

Anne Kasus-Jacobi, Lea D. Marchette, Catherine Xu, Feng Li and Huaiwen Wang
Oklahoma University Health Sciences Center, USA

Mark Babizhayev
Innovative Vision Products, Inc., USA

Ayub Hakim
Department of Ophthalmology, Western Galilee - Nahariya Medical Center, Nahariya, Israel

Balwant Singh Gendeh
Department of Otorhinolaryngology – Head and Neck Surgery, UKM Medical Center, Jalan Yaacob Latif, Bandar Tun Razak, Kuala Lumpur, Malaysia